Practical Cardiac Diagnosis

Medical Care of the
Cardiac Surgical Patient

General Series Editor

Stephen C. Vlay, M.D., F.A.C.P., F.A.C.C.
  Associate Professor of Medicine
Director, The Stony Brook Arrhythmia Study
  and Sudden Death Prevention Center
Director, The Coronary Care Unit
  University Hospital
Division of Cardiology, Department of Medicine
  State University of New York at Stony Brook

Other titles in the series:

Practical Cardiac Diagnosis

Medical Care of the Cardiac Surgical Patient

edited by

Stephen C. Vlay, M.D., F.A.C.P., F.A.C.C.

Associate Professor of Medicine
Director, The Stony Brook Arrhythmia Study and
Sudden Death Prevention Center
Director, The Coronary Care Unit, University Hospital
Division of Cardiology, Department of Medicine
State University of New York at Stony Brook

Boston
Blackwell Scientific Publications
Oxford   London   Edinburgh   Melbourne
Paris   Berlin   Vienna

Blackwell Scientific Publications

Editorial offices:
Three Cambridge Center, Cambridge, Massachusetts 02142, USA
Osney Mead, Oxford OX2 0EL, England
25 John Street, London, WC1N 2BL, England
23 Ainslie Place, Edinburgh, EH3 6AJ, Scotland
54 University Street, Carlton, Victoria 3053, Australia

Other editorial offices:
Arnette SA, 2 rue Casimir-Delavigne, 75006 Paris, France
Blackwell-Wissenschaft, Meinekestrasse 4, D-1000 Berlin 15,
    Germany
Blackwell MZV, Feldgasse 13, A-1238 Wien, Austria

Distributors:
USA and Canada
Blackwell Scientific Publications
Three Cambridge Center
Cambridge, Massachusetts 02142
(Orders: Telephone: 800-759-6102)

Australia
Blackwell Scientific Publications (Australia) Pty Ltd
54 University Street
Carlton, Victoria 3053
(Orders: Telephone: 03-347-0300)

Outside North America and Australia
Blackwell Scientific Publications, Ltd.
c/o Marston Book Services, Ltd.
P.O. Box 87
Oxford OX2 0DT
England
(Orders: Telephone: 011-44-865-791155)

Typeset by Huron Valley Graphics
Printed and bound by BookCrafters
Designed by Joyce C. Weston

© 1992 by Blackwell Scientific Publications
Printed in the United States of America
91 92 93 94 5 4 3 2 1

Library of Congress Cataloging in Publication Data
Medical Care of the Cardiac Surgical Patient / edited by Stephen C. Vlay.
        p.   cm.—(Practical cardiac diagnosis)
    Includes bibliographical references and index.
    ISBN 0-86542-143-9
    1. Heart—Surgery—Risk factors.   2. Coronary artery bypass—Risk
factors.   3. Surgical indications.   I. Vlay, Stephen C.
II. Series.
    [DNLM: 1. Heart Surgery.   2. Risk Factors.   WG 169 E92]
RD598.E83   1991
617.4′12059—dc20
DNLM/DLC
for Library of Congress   91-12440
                                                              CIP

Contents

Contents

Contributors

Constantine E. Anagnostopoulos, M.D., Sc.D., F.A.C.S., F.A.C.C.
Professor of Surgery
Chief, Cardiothoracic Surgery
State University of New York at Stony Brook
Stony Brook, New York

Richard L. Barnett, M.D.
Assistant Professor of Medicine
State University of New York at Stony Brook
Northport Veterans Administration Medical Center
Stony Brook, New York

Thomas V. Bilfinger, M.D.
Assistant Professor of Surgery
Division of Cardiothoracic Surgery
State University of New York at Stony Brook
Stony Brook, New York

Thomas R. Eide, M.D.
Director of Clinical Services
Associate Professor of Anesthesiology
State University of New York at Stony Brook
Stony Brook, New York

Mark J. Greco, M.D.
Assistant Professor of Clinical Medicine
School of Medicine
State University of New York at Stony Brook
Stony Brook, New York

Andrew J. Green, M.D.
Assistant Professor of Clinical Medicine
Division of Endocrinology
State University of New York at Stony Brook
Stony Brook, New York

Alan R. Hartman, M.D., F.A.C.S., F.A.C.C., F.C.C.P.
Clinical Associate Professor of Surgery
Division of Cardiothoracic Surgery
University Hospital at Stony Brook
Stony Brook, New York

Adam N. Hurewitz, M.D.
Director of Fellowship Program
Associate Professor of Clinical Medicine
State University of New York at Stony Brook
Stony Brook, New York

William E. Lawson, M.D.,
F.A.C.C., F.C.C.P.
Associate Professor of Medicine
Interventional Cardiology
State University of New York at
Stony Brook
Stony Brook, New York

Robert Mason, M.D., F.A.C.S.
Associate Professor of Surgery
State University of New York at
Stony Brook
Stony Brook, New York

Frank C. Seifert, M.D.,
F.A.C.S., F.A.C.C.
Associate Professor of Surgery
State University of New York at
Stony Brook
Stony Brook, New York

Stephen C. Vlay, M.D.,
F.A.C.P., F.A.C.C.
Associate Professor of Medicine
Director, The Stony Brook
Arrhythmia Study and Sudden
Death Prevention Center
Director, The Coronary Care
Unit, University Hospital
State University of New York at
Stony Brook
Stony Brook, New York.

Foreword

The number of patients undergoing cardiac surgery in the United States remains substantial despite the inroads made by percutaneous transluminal coronary angioplasty and to a much lesser extent, other "medical" procedures such as balloon valvuloplasty. Indeed, the number of cardiac surgical procedures in the United States remains in excess of 250,000 per year. Appropriate selection of patients who are to undergo cardiac surgery involves not only the clinical indications per se but also evaluation of *any* factors that might reduce the chances of a good surgical result. These factors include pulmonary and renal status and complicating peripheral vascular disease, or diabetes mellitus. In his current monograph, Dr. Vlay has assembled a series of experts to review specific areas of concern for patients referred for cardiac surgery. These experts include medical specialists, cardiac and vascular surgeons, and anesthesiologists. Their well-written and to-the-point chapters make this text extremely helpful in formulating strategies for referring and evaluating patients for cardiac surgery, and in managing them before, during and after the actual surgical procedure.

Peter F. Cohn, M.D.
Professor of Medicine
Chief of Cardiology
SUNY Stony Brook

Preface

The concept of this text was formulated by considering the multiple factors involved when a patient undergoes cardiac surgery. First, one must determine whether cardiac surgery is appropriate or would benefit the patient. Many potential candidates for cardiac surgical procedures have other serious medical problems that not only require attention but also affect the surgical risk. Management of the patient before surgery centers on optimizing the medical condition and minimizing the risk.

In this volume, we have attempted to focus on the most critical factors involved with the adult patient scheduled for coronary artery bypass graft surgery, valvular surgery, and some other common referrals to the cardiac surgeon.

The indications for cardiac surgery are discussed in detail. A brief overview of cardiac diagnostic techniques presents the vital facts that the physician should be aware of when ordering the test and describes the salient critical findings that will assist in the decision-making process. Next, hemodynamic evaluation is presented in detail, because these measurements are important before, during, and after cardiac surgery.

The most frequent complicating medical problems in patients with severe cardiac disease requiring surgery are pulmonary, renal, metabolic, or vascular in origin. Consequently, we have asked these consultants to review the way they evaluate the risks from each subspeciality viewpoint and provide advice on methods to minimize the probability of an adverse event.

The anesthesiologist is critical to the successful outcome of the procedure and assists not only by administering anesthesia but also by constantly monitoring the rhythm and hemodynamics together with the cardiac surgeon. Our consultation informs us how risk is evaluated and minimized from the anesthesiology viewpoint. The cardiac surgeon evaluates surgical risk from another perspective. The referring physician should not expect the surgeon to take a patient to cardiac surgery if the risk is unacceptable. Furthermore, the referring physician should realize that sometimes the expectations must be limited.

Our cardiac surgeons then describe the important aspects of cardiac surgery including myocardial preservation techniques, the salient points of aortocoronary bypass, valvular repair or replacement, and immediate postoperative care. The potential new directions and problems facing cardiac surgery are reviewed.

This text has been written for the clinician by the clinicians. Every author is on the frontlines every day, dealing with complex patient care problems. The practical information contained reflects actual hands-on clinical experience and reflects state-of-the-art medical and surgical care in the 1990s. I thank all my collaborators who have helped put this volume together. It was no easy task for any of us to write a chapter in addition to our busy schedule caring for critically ill patients. I thank James Krosschell of Blackwell Scientific Publications for encouraging us to compile this volume, Victoria Reeders, M.D. and Patricia Tyler of Blackwell for their assistance in its production.

Stephen C. Vlay, M.D.

Notice

The indications and dosages of all drugs in this book have been recommended in the medical literature and conform to the practices of the general medical community. The medications described do not necessarily have specific approval by the Food and Drug Administration for use in the diseases and dosages for which they are recommended. The package insert for each drug should be consulted for use and dosage as approved by the FDA. Because standards for usage change, it is advisable to keep abreast of revised recommendations, particularly those concerning new drugs.

Medical Care of the Cardiac Surgical Patient

Candidates for Cardiac Surgery

Stephen C. Vlay, M.D.

1

Managing the patient with cardiac problems requires an understanding of the pathophysiology of the condition as well as the various therapeutic options available. In this chapter the critical issues involved with the most common referrals to the cardiac surgeon are discussed. The emphasis is on the indications for surgery and the type of procedures to consider. Ischemic heart disease, valvular disease and a variety of other common problems are considered. The chapter concludes with a general approach to the patient before considering specific diagnostic techniques in chapter 2.

ISCHEMIC HEART DISEASE

Atherosclerotic coronary artery disease, one of the major causes of cardiovascular morbidity and mortality, was once treated by little more than bed rest, sedation, and analgesics. At one time, the only available anti-ischemic medication was nitroglycerin, and that was prohibited during the acute phase of myocardial infarction (MI). Therapies once "contraindicated" now appear in the forefront of therapy for acute MI. These include intravenous nitroglycerin, intravenous β-blockers, thrombolytic agents, aspirin, all in addition to oxygen, morphine, and bed rest. In certain selected situations, mechanical revascularization with percutaneous transluminal coronary angioplasty (PTCA) or cardiac surgery is considered. Thus, the advances and innovations achieved during the past 30 years have been astonishing and will continue to evolve.

Coronary artery bypass graft (CABG) surgery is performed primarily for chronic and acute myocardial ischemia, with surgery for acute MI a very small percentage. In 1988, more than 200,000 patients underwent CABG. Adjunct procedures include resection or plication of a ventricular aneurysm, surgery for arrhythmias, and valve repair/replacement. Acquired valvular heart disease represents the other major referral to the cardiac surgeon. Congenital heart disease ranks third. Pacemaker implantation, surgery for aortic dissection, and cardiac transplantation comprise most of the remaining indications.

As these procedures have become common, it is appropriate that we review the indications so that the proper referrals can be made after the appropriate medical evaluation. In this chapter, indications for CABG surgery and valve repair/replacement, the two major referrals of the adult cardiac patient, will be discussed. It is not our purpose to present a comprehensive historical review of cardiac surgery, but rather to highlight the accepted indications, the necessary diagnostic evaluation, and the possible alternatives. In the subsequent chapters, we ask the medical and surgical subspecialists for their perspectives.

Coronary artery bypass graft surgery

Since its introduction by Favolaro in the late 1960s, CABG surgery has undergone major improvement. Advances in myocardial preservation along with technical developments have reduced mortality and morbidity. Current practice will be described in later chapters by my surgical colleagues. The present discussion will review the major trials in CABG surgery, to enable the reader to understand how the current indications were determined.

The three major studies are the Coronary Artery Surgery Study (CASS) and its subgroup analyses, the Veterans Administration Cooperative Study (VA), and the European Cooperative Study (ECS). These studies are not exactly comparable because each included patients with different entry criteria. Table 1-1 lists the Canadian classification of angina. The VA study had the most symptomatic patients (class III-IV) with more than 50% severely symptomatic. The ECS looked at Canadian class III (40% severely symptomatic), whereas CASS included mildly symptomatic stable angina patients (class I-II).

Table 1-1   Canadian Classification of Effort Angina

I. No angina with ordinary activity (angina occurs with strenuous activity)

II. Slight limitation of ordinary activity (walking >2 level blocks, climbing >1 flight of stairs, walking rapidly causes angina)

III. Marked limitation of ordinary physical activity (walking 1–2 level blocks, climbing 1 flight of stairs causes angina)

IV. Inability to carry on any physical activity without discomfort—angina may be present at rest

Modified from Campeau L. Grading of angina pectoris. *Circulation.* 1975;54:522.

One must also remember that these studies were performed years before our current armamentarium of anti-ischemic drugs (including β-blockers and calcium antagonists) were available or widely used. Similarly, angioplasty was not routinely performed except during some of the later trial years. Thus, with these caveats in mind, we will review the results of these studies.

The VA study was completed first and also reported the highest morbidity and mortality in some centers. One must consider the early time of this study, especially in terms of myocardial preservation, the fact that the most symptomatic patients were included, and realize that in 1972 we were on the learning curve in terms of cardiac surgery. In the VA study, the patients who had a superior result with cardiac surgery included those with triple vessel disease, impaired left ventricular function, hypertension, prior MI, and resting ischemia on electrocardiography (ECG). These results were observed at 11 years. Patients experienced less angina, required fewer medications, and described an improved quality of life. In addition, left ventricular dysfunction improved as did functional class and exercise capacity.

The ECS demonstrated better survival in patients with triple vessel or left main coronary artery disease. Demonstration of ischemia on the ECG was better treated with surgery. If the left anterior descending artery was involved with two or three vessel disease, bypass surgery improved survival. It is important to note that this study involved patients with relatively preserved left ventricular function (ejection fraction

[EF] > 50%) as the CASS study conclusions indicated better survival with surgery for those with left ventricular dysfunction. (Again remember CASS dealt with only mildly symptomatic patients, the European study dealt with very symptomatic patients.)

CASS excluded severely symptomatic patients and found no overall difference between surgery (92% survival) and medical (90% survival) therapy. In the subgroup analysis, those with triple vessel disease and left ventricular EF between 35% and 50% fared better with CABG surgery (P < .01). A trend was seen with single or double vessel disease and moderate left ventricular dysfunction (EF < 50%) in favor of bypass. The CASS study has been criticized because it considered only mildly symptomatic patients and entered less than 5% of those screened. Furthermore, analysis was done on the "intention to treat" basis and did not consider crossover from medical to surgical therapy (25%) nor did it consider those who died prior to surgery.

Certainly criticisms can be made about all of these studies as well as clinical research in general. There will always be deficiencies and what some consider better ways to analyze the problem. Nevertheless, if one is careful about drawing conclusions, each study provides important data with which to develop a set of indications for surgery. Although the CASS did not consider severely symptomatic individuals, it provided vital information about the beneficial nature of medical therapy. Some patients eventually required CABG on clinical grounds, in fact crossing over to the other therapy. Taking a more global perspective, one can argue that they moved out of the CASS entry criteria and into the VA trial or ECS entry criteria. They then would be expected to fare better with surgery. Current practice today is to provide maximal medical therapy for those mildly symptomatic patients and consider surgery (or angioplasty when appropriate) when ischemia becomes unmanageable. Anatomy (e.g., left main disease) becomes important in making a recommendation for surgery.

Surgery today is more difficult because the patient referred to the surgeon is older and sicker. Since operation is not performed until ischemia is medically refractory, the extent and severity of coronary artery disease is worse and the left ventricular function poorer. Our surgeons favor different procedures today with the internal mammary artery (IMA) considered the optimal graft. Unfortunately, the time needed for dissection often prohibits its performance in emergency revascularization. IMA grafts were infrequently used in the three cited studies. In CASS, patients who received IMA grafts experienced better survival than those with traditional saphenous vein grafts.

Disease of the *left main coronary artery* is unquestionably better treated with a surgical approach. Medically treated patients in both the VA study and ECS trial exhibited a poorer survival rate (65% to 67%) as compared to the 4–5-year survival rates of those treated with bypass (93% and 89%, respectively). Today we also are aware that angioplasty is contraindicated in left main disease, with coronary bypass the treatment of choice.

CASS also noted a less favorable outcome in medical therapy of *unstable angina.* CABG surgery was associated with better survival regardless of left ventricular EF and was most noticeable in patients with two or three vessel disease.

Another CASS analysis described a less favorable result after CABG in women. Although this finding is not completely understood, women tend to have small coronary arteries, a technically limiting factor in achieving favorable coronary blood flow rates.

The morbidity and mortality of cardiac surgery depends on a number of variables (Tables 1-2 and 1-3). *Advanced age* is certainly a factor, but also certainly *not* a contraindication. Elderly people are more likely to have multisystem disease (or certainly diminished function of organ systems such as the kidney), have more extensive cardiac disease, are more likely

---

Table 1-2   High Risk Candidates for Coronary Artery Bypass Grafting

Advanced age
Reoperation (prior CABG)
Diffuse severe coronary artery disease
Unstable angina or unstable hemodynamics
Accompanying severe systemic disease
   Chronic obstructive pulmonary disease
   Peripheral vascular disease
   Prior cerebrovascular accident
   Diabetes mellitus
Obesity and other technical difficulties such as inadequate vein

---

Table 1-3   Variables Associated with Increased Operative Mortality

Advanced Age
Left main stenosis ($\geq 90\%$)
Female gender
Left ventricular dysfunction as measured by both regional contraction
    abnormalities and elevated left ventricular end-diastolic pressure
Pulmonary vascular congestion (rales) and congestive heart failure
Unstable angina
Extensive severe coronary artery disease
Small size of vessels

Table 1-4   Risks for Prolonged Hospitalization

Advanced age
Emergency procedure
Unstable angina or ongoing MI
Congestive heart failure
Female gender

to have vascular complications, and are slower to heal (higher incidence of wound infections) and recover from their surgery. Some of these same factors predict a risk of prolonged hospitalization (Table 1-4). An elderly patient with severe ischemic heart disease and left ventricular dysfunction is less likely to fare well from surgery than the same age patient with pure valvular disease (e.g., severe aortic stenosis with normal coronary arteries and normal left ventricular function). Whether it is desirable or even advantageous for an octogenarian to undergo bypass becomes an individual decision depending on the individual patient. It is my personal bias to be extremely conservative when the patient nears or exceeds the age of 80.

Other variables that indicate high risk include severe diffuse coronary disease, severe left ventricular dysfunction, chronic lung disease, diabetes mellitus, prior stroke, and previous CABG or chest surgery. Dissection after prior bypass is a lengthy procedure and occasionally may compromise remaining viable grafts. Finally, the more unstable the patient, the greater the risk for perioperative MI. In the three studies cited, perioperative MI occurred in 6.4%, less than 8%, and 10% (CASS, European, VA studies, respectively) (Table 1-5). Note

Table 1-5   Perioperative Myocardial Infarction

VA Coop study	10%
ECS	<8%
CASS	6.4%

Table 1-6   General Risks of Mortality

CABG—Optimal patient   1%
         Overall mortality 3%
         Neurologic event 3%
         Perioperative MI 5%

Table 1-7   Risk Factors for Early Death after Bypass Surgery

Older age
Left ventricular dysfunction
Hemodynamic instability at operation
Recent MI
Severity of coronary artery disease
Associated mitral regurgitation
Ventricular aneurysm
Ventricular tachycardia
Longer aortic cross clamp time
Nonuse of IMA for graft

Modified from Kirklin JW, Naftel DC, Blackstone EH, et al.: Comment: Summary of a consensus concerning death and ischemic events after coronary artery bypass grafting. *Circulation.* 1989; 79 (suppl. I): I-81-I-91.

that myocardial protection techniques today have improved, with the risk of perioperative MI approximately 5%.

In general, the risks of mortality for the optimal patient should be under 1%. Considering the vast majority of low to moderate risk patients referred to the surgeon, the mortality should range from 1% to 3% (Table 1-6). Neurologic events may be seen in up to 2% to 3%. Risk factors for early death after CABG have also been identified (Table 1-7).

The morbidity and mortality rates are much higher when CABG is performed during the acute phase of MI and may reach 25% to 30%. Certainly the more emergent the surgery, the greater the chance of further infarction, compromised left ventricular function, and death. Outcome depends on the amount of reversibly and irreversibly damaged myocardium. The experience from the Spokane group indicates that bypass surgery can be performed in this time period with complication rates not very much higher than with elective procedures. In a 13-year follow-up, surgically treated patients fared better than medically treated patients within the first 6 hours of MI. The advantage was greater with anterior wall MI, reflecting the amount of jeopardized myocardium. However, before one can become enthusiastic about this approach, one must recall that this study was done at a time when we did not have the medical therapeutic options and angioplasty widely available today. Furthermore, the study was neither controlled nor randomized. What the study does tell us is that carefully selected patients who undergo CABG in the first few hours of acute MI can survive the procedure and experience a beneficial long-term result. Perhaps the ideal patient would be one with left main disease and anterior wall MI who starts to decompensate hemodynamically despite medical therapy and for whom angioplasty of the culprit lesion is contraindicated by its anatomic location. Operative mortality in surgery for acute MI varies with severity with 2% to 3% for one vessel disease, 4% to 5% for two vessel disease and 8% to 10% for three vessel disease.

The other situation in which CABG is performed emergently is when angioplasty results in abrupt closure of the vessel resulting in impending MI. Fortunately, this complication is infrequent, 1% to 2% in most series. Damage may be held to a minimum by placement of a perfusion catheter until the patient is taken to the operating room. Other rare referrals from the angioplasty suite to the cardiac surgeon result from the inability to remove all or part of an angioplasty catheter or guidewire. Statistics from the National PTCA Registry indicate a 7% mortality and 38% infarction rate for emergent CABG after failed angioplasty.

Cardiac surgery may be performed urgently after acute MI when the MI is complicated by rupture of the interventricular septum causing a ventricular septal defect (VSD), rupture of a papillary muscle causing acute mitral regurgitation, and pseudoaneurysm. Pseudoaneurysm is a type of myocardial rupture where the overlying pericardium forms an adhesive seal over the ruptured segment. Obviously this weak link must be repaired. Acute rupture of the ventricular free wall results in acute pericardial tamponade. The patient usually dies before the diagnosis is made or the patient can be taken to the operating room. Obviously, acute surgical repair is the only way to save the patient.

At one time, operation for acute VSD or acute mitral regurgitation related to MI was delayed in the hopes that the tissue would become more scarred and allow an easier repair. Suturing into acutely necrotic tissue is extremely difficult due to its friability. Unfortunately, delay in operation resulted in a worse outcome. Often these patients had remaining ischemic myocardium in another distribution and the pressure-volume overload worsened the ischemia. Congestive heart failure is another possibility. Today the patient is stabilized with an intra-aortic balloon pump (IABP) and medical therapy consisting of vasopressors and vasodilators. Surgery is accomplished within the next 2–3 days. Septal defects are closed, sometimes with a Dacron patch reinforced with felt pledgets. Mitral valve replacement is simpler because the valve is placed on the mitral annulus, which does not involve suturing the papillary muscle.

The benefits of CABG correlate with patency of the bypass grafts. In the three cited studies, patency ranged from 69% (VA) to 89% (ECS) to 90% (CASS) (Table 1-8). As previously stated, most of these were saphenous vein grafts. Today we know that these grafts have at best a 55% patency rate at 10 years and at worst 45%. In comparison, the IMA graft has a greater than 90% early patency rate and 80% (free IMA) to 85% to 90% (in situ IMA) patency rate at 10 years (Table 1-9). Nevertheless, the saphenous vein graft has done yeoman's work in restoring blood flow and will continue to be used as an adjunct procedure. The surgeon is limited with the availability of only two mammary arteries and many more obstructed coronary arteries requiring bypass. Thus the saphenous vein graft will be utilized to complete the revascularization. The advantage of complete revascularization is well recognized. Handling of the saphenous vein is critical, because poor technique in harvesting or handling may condemn the graft to

Table 1-8 Early Graft Patency	
VA Coop Study	69%
ECS	89%
CASS	90%

Table 1-9   Graft Patency

Saphenous vein grafts
Occlusion Rate 12–20% 1 y
    2–4%/y for next 4–5 y
    4–8%/y for next 4–5 y
At 10 y 50% occluded
IMA grafts
Patency >90% at 7 y
Can be used for up to 70% of all distal anastomoses
    and in 95% of patients
Patency rates at 10 y

Saphenous vein	45–55%
In situ IMA	85–90%
Free IMA	80%

failure as much as suboptimal anastomotic technique. Injury to the vein results in endothelial damage and predisposes to platelet deposition. As platelets start to adhere in layers and mural thrombus forms, both may contribute to intimal smooth muscle proliferation and connective tissue synthesis. Eventually these events accelerate the atherosclerotic process and may lead to occlusion. Disproportion between vein size and artery size may also be a factor in limiting success.

The medical physician must emphasize the need to stop smoking and lower the serum cholesterol level after surgery because these factors are associated with less favorable long-term benefit. Recently, the administration of fish oils has been advocated to maintain graft patency but has not been substantiated in large studies. One intervention with demonstrated benefit is the administration of aspirin and dipyridamole, both antiplatelet agents. In fact, many surgeons start dipyridamole in doses up to 100 mg four times daily, 1–2 days before surgery and start aspirin 6–24 hours (325 mg daily) after surgery. Dipyridamole is continued chronically in doses of 25–75 mg orally, three to four times daily (Table 1-10).

Obviously, the care of the patient requires a team effort, using the expertise of the referring physician, cardiologist, and cardiac surgeon to achieve the most optimal long-term benefit. The correct diagnosis must be made and the severity of the coronary artery disease and left ventricular dysfunction assessed. Based on the response to medical therapy and anatomic

Table 1-10   Current Recommendations for Antiplatelet Therapy

1. No ASA prior to surgery
   Start ASA 325 mg od 6–7 h after surgery
2. Dipyridamole 75–100 mg po tid-qid starting 1–2 days prior
   to CABG

Table 1-11   Advantages of Coronary Artery Bypass Graft Surgery for Exercise-Induced Myocardial Ischemia

Improve survival
Left main disease (VA Study)
3 vessel—Normal left ventricle (ECS)
3 vessel—Abnormal left ventricle (VA, CASS)
Proximal left anterior descending as part of two or three vessel
   disease (ECS)
Positive exercise test (ECS)
Improve symptoms
Less angina
Fewer medications
Improved functional class
Improved exercise capacity
Better quality of life
Less left ventricular dysfunction

factors (such as left main disease indicating CABG), a decision will be made to continue medical therapy, recommend angioplasty, or advise CABG surgery. The responsibility does not end there as postoperative management regarding risk facors, diet, exercise, and medical therapy including antiplatelet drugs is just as critical.

Surgery is better than medical therapy for improving survival in left main or triple vessel disease, double vessel disease involving the left anterior descending artery; for relieving exercise-induced ischemia, or chronic ischemia leading to left ventricular dysfunction, and for improving the quality of life (Table 1-11). Surgery does not always prevent MI (a common misconception). Medical therapy is recommended when ischemia is prevented by anti-ischemic drugs that are well tolerated. With one or two vessel disease not involving the left anterior descending artery, medical therapy (or angioplasty) is recommended first with CABG reserved for refractory ischemia. If left ventricular dysfunction is not related to coronary artery disease but instead to a nonischemic cardiomyopathy, CABG to borderline significant narrowings would not be expected to improve the function.

With limited coronary artery disease refractory to medical therapy, angioplasty should be considered before recommending surgery unless there is a compelling reason such as left main disease. If angioplasty is high risk (see below), or the lesions are technically unsuitable, CABG is the correct way to proceed. Success with angioplasty depends on the skill of the physician performing the procedure. Some very experienced operators may be able to successfully dilate multiple lesions in multiple arteries, even at one procedure. Unquestionably the referring physician must know the track record of the center and physician performing the procedure. This same caveat holds true for the cardiac surgeon and surgical center.

Left ventricular aneurysm

Surgery for left ventricular aneurysm may be performed to improve the overall efficiency of the heart, which is obviously impaired after MI. Part of the cardiac output is directed into the aneurysm, which does not contract effectively. Left ventricular aneurysm often contains thrombus, which is a risk to the patient during life and certainly at the time of the procedure. Resection or plication of the aneurysm is not always desirable and quite often not feasible. If the MI was extensive, the aneurysm may be diffuse and impossible to resect or plicate because insufficient ventricle might be left and fill with blood and pump. Some procedures have involved reconstruction of the ventricle with prosthetic material interposed between remaining viable myocardium. Preserving the geometry may benefit the function and preserve cardiac output.

The ideal candidate for resection or plication has a discrete aneurysm, usually with a well-defined neck. Aneurysms may involve any segment of ventricular myocardium. Locations on the anterior wall or apex are obviously the easiest to deal with. Operation is usually inadvisable if the patient already has severe end-stage heart failure.

Refractory ventricular arrhythmias

When a patient suffers from recurrent life-threatening ventricular arrhythmias such as ventricular tachycardia or ventricular fibrillation, every effort is made to define the anatomy (cardiac catheterization) and the electrical substrate (electrophysiology study). If the patient is refractory to medical therapy, two further options are available. One is implantation of the automatic internal cardioverter defibrillator (AICD). This device is lifesaving and reduces the mortality associated with recurrent ventricular tachycardia fibrillation from 25–40% to 2%. The procedure does not involve opening the ventricle and may be performed alone or in conjunction with other cardiac surgical procedures.

In a patient with a well-defined aneurysm in whom plication or resection is anticipated, every effort should be made to eradicate the irritable focus at the same time. This involves mapping of the ventricular tachycardia in the electrophysiology laboratory before surgery and intraoperatively at the time of surgery. Rapid hypotensive ventricular tachycardias or ventricular fibrillation usually cannot be mapped. It is important to perform the mapping in those who can tolerate the procedure in the electrophysiology laboratory, because the arrhythmia may not always be inducible in the operating room after general anesthesia. Map-guided resection is superior to blind resection in preventing recurrence. Resection may be accomplished by surgical subendocardial scraping with a scalpel, with cryoablation, and with laser. Often the procedure is combined with placement of an AICD or at least the patch electrode(s) should the primary procedure fail to control the arrhythmia. With the excellent results of the AICD alone, entry into the left ventricular cavity is not usually undertaken unless there is a specific indication for left ventricular aneurysm resection, because the additional procedure increases the operative and perioperative morbidity and mortality.

Surgery directed at ventricular arrhythmias may be combined with other necessary procedures such as CABG or valve repair/replacement. The number of procedures increases the risk of surgery, but one cannot treat the arrhythmia alone without treating the underlying heart disease.

Recommendations

Current indications for CABG are summarized in Table 1-12.

Addendum: As this text goes to press, the American College of Cardiology and the American Heart Association published a special report on guidelines for coronary artery bypass

Table 1-12   Indications for Coronary Artery Bypass Graft Surgery

Elective

1. Symptomatic angina pectoris due to documented myocardial ischemia refractory to appropriate medical therapy
2. Significant left main coronary artery narrowing (>50%); (many would consider the need for CABG urgent if the degree of stenosis is >75%).
3. Severe triple vessel disease associated with impaired left ventricular function. (If left ventricular function is normal, medical therapy is indicated with surgery a consideration if ischemia persists.)
4. Severe two vessel disease involving the proximal left anterior descending artery that is not amenable to angioplasty

Urgent

1. Unstable angina pectoris despite appropriate medical therapy
2. Rare patients in the early phase of acute MI who have not suffered extensive irreversible myocardial damage

---

graft surgery which summarizes many of the important issues addressed in this chapter. This article is recommended for reference.

Kirklin JW, Akins CW, Blackstone EH, et al.: ACC/AHA Guidelines and Indications for Coronary Artery Bypass Graft Surgery. *Circulation* 1991 83:1125–1173.

Percutaneous transluminal coronary angioplasty

Another procedure for coronary revascularization is angioplasty, a procedure in which a stenotic coronary artery obstruction is reduced by balloon inflation. In 1988, 235,000 procedures were performed. If successful, the risks, complications, discomfort, and longer hospitalization with surgery may be avoided. The appropriate referral should be made by the physician because there are specific situations in which one procedure is not only preferable but superior to the other.

Indications for angioplasty have changed with a result of greater operator experience and new technology. Today multiple lesions in a single vessel and multiple vessels are dilated as are stenoses in saphenous vein and IMA grafts. In some cases, angioplasty may delay the need for cardiac surgery, a particularly desirable aspect because saphenous vein and even IMA grafts may have a finite time of patency.

The interventional cardiologist and cardiac surgeon will often make a joint decision regarding the best approach for an individual patient. There is certainly no reason to consider the two approaches, PTCA versus CABG, adversarial since they are complementary. In certain cases, both procedures may be performed because all lesions may not be suitable for surgical anastomosis.

Early graft closure may be rescued by angioplasty if the vessel is not yet completely occluded. Late graft stenosis is also amenable to angioplasty although the success rate depends on the extent of narrowing and intimal hyperplasia. In some patients with left main disease requiring further revascularization after initial surgery, angioplasty may even be possible on the left main lesion if there is a patent graft to the left anterior descending artery. Angioplasty is always performed in a facility with cardiac surgical backup.

Angioplasty is not without risk, cost, or potential complications. Success varies with both the severity of lesions and operator experience. Restenosis may occur in 20% to 30% of cases. Cost must take into account catheterizations before and after PTCA, the cost of surgical and anesthetic backup, the repeated noninvasive tests (such as exercise testing) to assess efficacy, and the need for repeat PTCA if restenosis occurs.

Guidelines for PTCA were published by the ACC/AHA Task Force on Assessment of Diagnostic and Therapeutic Cardiovascular Procedures (Subcommittee Percutaneous Transluminal Coronary Angioplasty), a worthwhile reference to include in one's library.*

Table 1-13 summarizes current indications for PTCA. One must have confidence in the operator, the center, and the surgical backup. One must correctly assess the suitability of the patient and the lesion for PTCA. The question must be asked, "Is surgery a better alternative?" If abrupt closure occurs during PTCA and necessitates emergent cardiac surgery, bypass is limited to saphenous vein grafting since the time necessary for IMA dissection cannot be expended. Consequently, when the lesion predicts a low chance of success with PTCA, e.g., a type C lesion (high risk of abrupt closure), surgery may be a better consideration if IMA grafts would be advantageous. Nevertheless, suitable lesions may have a 95% to 99% success

*Circulation. 1988;78:486–502.1

Table 1-13   Indications for Percutaneous Transluminal Coronary Angioplasty*

Symptomatic ischemia despite medical therapy
1. Single vessel disease with significant narrowing or *recent* total occlusion
2. Multiple vessel disease with suitable narrowings amenable to angioplasty
3. Multiple narrowings in a single coronary vessel or a major epicardial and a branch vessel
4. Narrowing in a bypass graft either saphenous vein or IMA graft, if approachable
5. Restenosis in a previously angioplastied vessel

Acute MI (acute phase)
1. For appropriate patients who fail to respond to (or have contraindications to) standard therapy (including β-blockers, thrombolysis, aspirin) and develop hemodynamic deterioration

Adjunctive procedures
1. To complete revascularization in patients undergoing CABG surgery in whom certain coronary lesions are not amenable to surgery but may not benefit from PTCA

---

* In patients with with anatomically suitable coronary stenoses

---

Table 1-14   The Ideal Lesions for Percutaneous Transluminal Coronary Angioplasty

Single
Short
Smooth (concentric, not eccentric)
Not calcified
No side branch(es)
Good collateral flow

---

rate and be associated with a beneficial long-term result. Table 1-14 lists the ideal lesions for PTCA.

Neither surgery nor angioplasty should be considered unless the patient has accepted indications for intervention because both procedures have associated potential morbidity and mortality. In general, indications include continued myocardial ischemia despite adequate medical therapy, poor prognosis in the absence of intervention, and occasionally as a rescue procedure in suitable patients with cardiogenic shock in the acute phase of MI.

Table 1-15 Contraindications to Percutaneous Transluminal Coronary Angioplasty

1. Left main disease in the absence of a patent bypass graft to the left anterior descending or left circumflex artery
2. Severe diffuse triple vessel disease better approached by CABG
3. High-grade stenosis with remaining viable myocardium in a patient with coronary occlusion and prior MI in another vascular distribution in whom a complication of PTCA would pose an unacceptable risk
4. Ostial right coronary artery disease
5. Long-standing complete occlusion
6. Absence of cardiac surgical program within the institution
7. Coagulopathy
8. No evidence for myocardial ischemia
9. Vasospastic angina with narrowing <60%
10. Low anticipated rate of success
    Chronic total occlusion (older than 3 months)
    Subtotal narrowing longer than 20 mm
11. Noninfarct-related artery in patient having procedure during acute MI

Table 1-16 Risks of Percutaneous Transluminal Coronary Angioplasty

Mortality	1% (in-hospital)
Nonfatal MI	4%
Need for emergency CABG★	3.5%
Usual risks of cardiac catheterization	

★This procedure is associated with a 25% to 40% incidence of nonfatal new Q wave MI

Table 1-15 describes the contraindications to angioplasty. It may be briefly summarized by stating that placing large amounts of viable myocardium in jeopardy when the procedure has a low chance of success and a high risk of abrupt closure with hemodynamic deterioration is not advisable. In addition, specific types of lesions such as left main, ostial right coronary artery, and chronic occlusions are contraindications. Looking at the risk of angioplasty (Table 1-16), one can see that the mortality (1%) and morbidity (nonfatal MI 4%) are comparable to the risks of surgery in most low–risk candidates. Not surprisingly, catastrophic results in the angioplasty laboratory are associated

Table 1-17 Potential Success/Risk Rate for Percutaneous Transluminal Coronary Angioplasty

TYPE A	*High Success Rate ($\geq$85%)* **Low risk of abrupt closure**
Discrete Concentric Easily accessible Nonangulated Smooth Noncalcified Residual lumen Nonostial location Absence of branch disease Absence of thrombus	
TYPE B	*Moderate Success Rate (60% to 85%)* **Moderate risk of abrupt closure**
Tubular ostial location Eccentric Moderately tortuous accessibility Angulated (>45° <90°) Irregular Moderate to severe calcification Thrombus Bifurcation lesion requiring two guidewires Total occlusion <3 months old	
TYPE C	*Low Chance of Success (<60%)* **High risk of abrupt closure**

Long narrowing (>2 cm)
Excessive tortuous of proximal
    segments
Angulated segment (>90°)
Total occlusion >3 months old
Inability to protect major side
    branches
Degeneration of older grafts with
    friable lesions	

Modified from Ryan TJ, Faxon DP, Gunnar RM, et al.: Guidelines for PTCA. *Circulation.* 1988; 78:486–502.

with higher operative mortality and morbidity. Thus, the success rate/risk rate (Table 1-17) must be weighed before deciding on the type of procedure recommended to the patient.

Both angioplasty and surgery are options for revascularization. It is up to the clinician to make the appropriate referral.

VALVULAR HEART DISEASE

In patients with coronary artery disease, the decision to recommend surgery is based on the extent, location, and severity of arterial narrowings, the extent of left ventricular dysfunction, as well as refractoriness to medical therapy. In valvular heart disease, the pressure gradient, the valve area, the resistance (particularly the pulmonary vascular resistance), and the involvement of multiple valves are critical to the decision to operate. In addition, patients' symptoms are important, such as syncope, congestive heart failure, or chest pain in patients with aortic stenosis, or dyspnea in mitral stenosis (also for mitral or aortic regurgitation). When the symptoms do not correlate with the severity of disease, other causes should be excluded to avoid unnecessary surgery.

The most common aortic valvular abnormality is congenital, a bicuspid aortic valve. With aging, the leaflets become calcified and stenotic, requiring aortic valve replacement. For selected patients too ill or debilitated to undergo surgery, aortic valvuloplasty in the catheterization laboratory has been palliative, at least for a short period of time. Acquired valvular disease may be a result of calcification, rheumatic processes, ischemic heart disease, just to mention the three most common varieties. Rheumatic heart disease was in decline but nevertheless remained prevalent in certain areas, particularly those with less access to modern medical care. Recently, certain areas have reported a resurgence of rheumatic fever. Not only the valves (usually more than one involved) but also the myocardium can be involved with this disorder.

The purpose of this book is not to review in depth the pathophysiology of valvular disease, but rather to mention the salient features as they apply and present the indications for operation. The surgeon will describe factors pertinent to the operative procedure because they vary with each indication. Often the choice of procedure depends on the severity, extent of associated disease, as well as the age and general state of health of the patient.

Aortic stenosis

As mentioned above, aortic stenosis in the adult may be related to calcification of a bicuspid valve, scarring or calcification of a rheumatic valve, or to calcification of a porcine aortic prosthesis. Once a patient with aortic stenosis develops symptoms of syncope, left ventricular dysfunction, or chest pain related to the valvular obstruction, it is time to intervene because 50% will die within 3–4 years.

Cardiac catheterization will provide the valve gradient, the cardiac output, and the calculation of the aortic valve area. It is important to note that a small gradient with a low cardiac output may still reflect a significant stenosis since the valve area calculation is a function of both the pressure difference and the flow across the valve.

If a patient has critical aortic stenosis with an aortic valve area less than 0.75 cm², operation is recommended, particularly in the presence of syncope or congestive heart failure. If the patient has NYHA class IV heart failure, severe left ventricular dysfunction, severe associated coronary artery disease, and is elderly, the surgical procedure may have unacceptable risks. In this situation, aortic valvuloplasty may provide palliation, either as a single procedure or in anticipation of later surgery if the patient's condition improves and surgery can be performed with lower risk.

Even if patients with critical aortic stenosis are asymptomatic, operation can be justified, especially if left ventricular dysfunction or progressive cardiomyopathy is present. Some physicians and surgeons have suggested additional criteria to help make a decision for surgery. These include:

1. Aortic stenosis, peak gradient >50 mm Hg with normal cardiac output
2. Aortic stenosis, peak gradient >50 mm Hg with pulmonary hypertension or left ventricular hypertrophy
3. Aortic stenosis, peak gradient >75 mm Hg, even if asymptomatic
4. Aortic stenosis, peak gradient <50 mm Hg, valve area ≤0.8 cm² in the presence of calcification and left ventricular hypertrophy

If severe coronary artery disease has brought the patient to the attention of the cardiologist and moderately severe aortic stenosis is also discovered, medical therapy may be risky. Many of the drugs used for ischemia may lower the blood pressure, heart rate, and cardiac output and are contraindicated in the presence of aortic stenosis. If the patient is not a candidate for angioplasty of the coronary artery, it may be prudent to recommend both CABG surgery and aortic valve replacement.

In general, few patients with aortic stenosis are considered inoperable because of age, but only because of associated heart failure or extensive coronary artery or other multisystem disease. In fact, the elderly patient who has preserved left ventricular function, minimal coronary artery disease, who is otherwise in good medical condition, may fare better with aortic valve replacement (even if age 90) than a younger patient with severe diffuse coronary disease and severe left ventricular dysfunction undergoing CABG surgery and aneurysmectomy.

Aortic regurgitation

Aortic regurgitation may be valvular in origin or may be related to disease of the aorta. Valvular causes include rheumatic disease, or endocarditis resulting in a flail leaflet. Aortic diseases include all that result in dilatation of the ascending aorta and aortic root. At one time, syphilis was a common cause of aortitis. Due to dilatation of the entire aortic root (often an aneurysm) the murmur of aortic regurgitation was heard to the right of the sternum. Today other causes are more commonly seen, including collagen vascular disorders such as Marfan syndrome, ankylosing spondylitis, or disease of the aorta such as cystic medial necrosis. Severe hypertensive disease leading to aortic dissection may involve the aortic root and cause acute aortic regurgitation, a surgical emergency.

Aortic valve replacement is performed for symptomatic (usually severe dyspnea on minimal exertion) severe aortic regurgitation. The goal is to operate before serious and irreversible left ventricular dysfunction occurs. If patients with chronic severe aortic regurgitation are asymptomatic, have good exercise tolerance, and normal left ventricular function, medical follow-up may continue until the noninvasive cardiac tests indicate a change. Note that chronic aortic regurgitation can be well tolerated for a long period of time while irreversible damage occurs. Consequently, careful and periodic follow-up is a *must*.

When aortic regurgitation is only mild to moderate, the

10-year survival rate is 85% to 90%. When it is severe, the survival rate drops to 70% at 10 years and 50% within 20 years. After left ventricular failure develops, half the patients will die in the following 2 years. Severely symptomatic patients (NYHA class III–IV) have even worse survival (4% at 10 years). After successful surgery the chances for survival improve to 84% at 1 year and 50% at 10 years. The vast majority improve symptomatically. Thus, the timing of aortic valve replacement is critical. It may be better to operate a little too soon than a little too late.

Noninvasive procedures such as echocardiography and radionuclide angiography provide guidance for the timing of surgery in the asymptomatic patient. Previously the end-systolic dimension was considered the best index. If surgery was postponed until the dimension was larger than 55 mm, half the patients died or developed heart failure. Thus, one should consider operation when the measurement approaches 55 mm. An end-diastolic dimension greater than 75 mm is also a poor omen. Fractional shortening on the echocardiogram may be the most useful measurement, with 5-year survival 100% if greater than 35% and 30% if the value is less than 30%. The EF represents another cutpoint, with 3-year survival 91% if the left ventricular EF is greater than 50% and only 64% if the EF is less than 50%. Note that with regurgitant lesions, a higher than normal EF is expected because the heart must pump the blood forward but a significant proportion also flows backward. Thus, when the EF in aortic regurgitation starts to fall into the "normal" range, it is a sign of progressive deterioration. The gated blood pool scan (MUGA) may be performed both at rest and with exercise. Normally with exercise, the EF should rise. If it decreases or remains the same, it is an indication of an impaired cardiovascular reserve. In symptomatic patients, the exercise EF will fall in 95%; in asymptomatic patients 67% will have a reduced stress EF. The chest x-ray may also be helpful, with increasing cardiomegaly an indication of deterioration. If the cardiothoracic ratio is less than 0.57, the 5-year survival rate is 84%. If greater than 0.61, the 5-year survival rate is 46%.

These general guidelines should provide the practitioner with the information necessary to know when to refer the patient for surgery. Remember, asymptomatic does not mean that left ventricular function is not deteriorating. Unfortunately, we sometimes encounter patients who have waited too long before seeking medical attention or those who have previously refused surgery. Although impaired left ventricular function is usually not a contraindication to aortic valve replacement, left ventricular function may not be expected to improve significantly. If improvement occurs, it is usually noted early after operation.

To summarize, operate on patients with aortic regurgitation if they are severely symptomatic (NYHA class III–IV), when the left ventricular end-systolic dimension on echo is greater than 55 mm, or if the other noninvasive indices provide evidence of progressive left ventricular dilatation and dysfunction.

Mitral stenosis

Mitral stenosis is most often the result of rheumatic disease; congenital mitral stenosis is rare. Sometimes patients have mixed mitral disease with combination of obstruction to inflow into the left ventricle along with abnormal closure resulting in regurgitation. The major symptom reported in mitral stenosis is dyspnea, followed by fatigue, and poor exercise tolerance. Although it may be an oversimplification, the obstruction to flow across the mitral valve results in an increased pressure in and size of the left atrium. The increased size may predispose to atrial arrhythmias, particularly atrial fibrillation. Furthermore, these events may predispose to the development of thrombus and emboli. The increased pressure eventually backs up through the entire system including the pulmonary veins, lungs, pulmonary artery, and eventually the right ventricle and atrium. Pulmonary hypertension is a late sign and a fixed pulmonary vascular resistance an ominous and pessimistic finding. Severe pulmonary hypertension and right ventricular pressure-volume overload may eventually lead to tricuspid regurgitation. Thus, it is little wonder that the primary complaint is dyspnea. End-stage mitral stenosis with severe pulmonary hypertension is devastating both for the patient and family. The patient may get to the point where it is impossible to take a step without losing breath. It is a horrible way to spend one's last days. Consequently, it is important to make the diagnosis of mitral stenosis, follow the patient until it is appropriate to operate, and then make a decision about commissurotomy (cracking the valve leaflets) or valve replacement. Today, mitral valvuloplasty is also a possibility, but again is reserved for those patients who are not operative candidates.

The diagnosis of mitral stenosis can be made by classic features on physical examination including increased intensity of S_1, a diastolic rumble, and occasionally an opening snap (depends on pliability of valve and absence of calcification). The echocardiogram reveals classic features. Cardiac catheterization is performed when it is thought that symptoms indicate surgery. The purpose of the catheterization is to measure the cardiac output, the pressures, determine the gradient, calculate the valve area and resistances as well as to exclude other valvular involvement or coronary artery disease.

Reasons to operate in mitral stenosis include increasing symptoms of dyspnea and evidence of moderate to severe mitral stenosis as measured by a valve area of less than 1.0 cm^2/m^2 body surface area. Other compelling reasons include prior episodes of pulmonary edema, a significantly increased pulmonary vascular resistance, or multiple arterial embolic events. Thromboemboli are readily apparent if the terminal place of lodgment is the cerebral artery (stroke), coronary artery (MI), or arterial supply to extremity (loss of pulse), but multiple small emboli to kidney, spleen, or other internal organs may go unrecognized.

Mitral commissurotomy may still be performed today if the patient is younger, still in sinus rhythm with a left atrium that is not severely enlarged or containing thrombi. As previously noted, the presence of an opening snap suggests that the valve is still pliable. Confirmation is obtained by the demonstration of good excursion of the leaflets. Certain patients may not get a good result from commissurotomy. They include those with heavy calcification and those with subvalvular disease. Remember that it is not only the valve leaflets that play a role—one must also consider the chordae and the papillary muscle. For these and other patients in whom commissurotomy would be unwise, mitral valve replacement is indicated. The choice of valve, bioprosthetic or mechanical, depends on a number of factors, which will be evaluated by the cardiac surgeon in a later chapter.

As noted above, the presence of advanced mitral disease may result in tricuspid regurgitation. Often the surgeon will also perform tricuspid annuloplasty to restore competence. Tricuspid stenosis on a rheumatic basis is rare but may occur in combination with mitral stenosis and also requires attention at the time of surgery.

Thus, for mitral stenosis, symptoms of dyspnea in addition to evidence for significant valvular obstruction determine the time of surgery.

Mitral regurgitation

Mitral regurgitation has many more causes than mitral stenosis. In addition to rheumatic heart disease, ischemic heart disease is important as an etiology and is perhaps one of the most prominent. It is also one of the most difficult to deal with since the patient is likely to also have left ventricular dysfunction ranging from mild to moderate to severe. Myxomatous degeneration is fairly common but only a few patients progress to valve replacement. When it does occur, the patient frequently presents with acute pulmonary edema due to rupture of part of the valvular apparatus. Endocarditis may also result in acute pulmonary edema due to an infectious process eating away part of the valvular structure or substructures. The latter two causes are reasons for urgent surgery as is acute mitral regurgitation related to acute MI. Each has a different prognosis. The patient with a myxomatous valve and normal left ventricular function will fare the best. The prognosis for the patient with endocarditis will depend on the ability to eradicate the infection. The prognosis for the patient with MI will depend on the state of the left ventricle and extent of coronary artery disease. The above three cases of acute mitral regurgitation are different, in terms of timing of surgery and outcome, than patients with chronic mitral regurgitation who require other considerations.

Chronic mitral regurgitation is a valvular disorder that can be well tolerated for a long period of time. With afterload reduction by medications, the regurgitant fraction can be decreased and the patient made relatively asymptomatic or minimally symptomatic. Nevertheless a time will come when left ventricular dysfunction will become irreversible. As with aortic regurgitation, it is important to operate before this occurs, although objective parameters are not as clear. Today some physicians are leaning toward earlier surgery.

It is easy to recommend surgery when the patient is in NYHA class III or IV and is severely symptomatic. If the patient is only minimally symptomatic, medical therapy should be continued unless the left ventricle starts to dilate. Certain echocardiographic guidelines were once proposed to aid in this decision and include a left ventricular end-diastolic dimension greater than 80 mm and an end-systolic dimension greater than 50 mm. Impairment of left ventricular contractility with an EF of less than 55% and fractional shortening less than 30% support the recommendations for surgery. Just as with aortic regurgitation, the ventricle in mitral regurgitation must work harder to maintain cardiac output since half the blood is being ejected back into the left atrium. Thus, one would expect a higher than normal EF before left ventricular dysfunction occurs. One other calculation has been proposed—the ratio of end-systolic wall stress: end-systolic volume index, to assist in the decision for surgery.

Depending on the state of the ventricle, the condition of the mitral leaflets, and the experience of the surgeon, a decision can be made to proceed with valve replacement with a bioprosthetic or mechanical valve or to attempt valve repair. The latter avoids many of the complications of the prosthetic valves and may obviate the need for chronic anticoagulation. Due to time constraints, valve repair is usually not a consideration when one is dealing with an ischemic ventricle with a need for multiple CABGs as well as a procedure for mitral regurgitation.

Of all the valvular problems discussed, ischemic mitral regurgitation perhaps has the worst prognosis, even if the patient survives the surgery. Often the patient also has ventricular arrhythmias sometimes necessitating antiarrhythmic drugs or possibly arrhythmia surgery or an AICD in addition to valve replacement. This type of patient is at high risk for anesthesia, for the surgery, and during the postoperative course.

Thus, the indications for surgery in mitral regurgitation and the prognosis thereafter vary with the acuity, the underlying etiology, and the general state of the patient's health. One must intervene quickly in acute mitral regurgitation and one would endeavor to intervene before left ventricular dysfunction occurs in chronic mitral regurgitation.

Tricuspid valve stenosis and regurgitation

Isolated tricuspid valve disease is uncommon. Rather, it is most likely to occur in combination with mitral or aortic valve disease (or both). Involvement of the valve may result in tricuspid stenosis or regurgitation or both.

Tricuspid regurgitation may be rheumatic in origin or result from mitral valve disease with pressure-volume overload.

More often than not, severe tricuspid regurgitation may be treated by valvular repair, often with insertion of a Carpentier ring. The necessity for tricuspid valve surgery is determined after the mitral valve surgery is completed.

The rare patient with isolated tricuspid stenosis or regurgitation is taken to surgery only when the patient's functional class deteriorates to NYHA class III or IV. At this point the tricuspid regurgitation is usually severe and the patient with tricuspid stenosis has a mean diastolic gradient exceeding 5 mm Hg and a valve area of less than 2.0 cm^2.

Pulmonic valve disorders

The majority of pulmonic valve disorders are related to congenital heart disease (e.g., tetralogy of Fallot) and are not considered in this text. Pulmonic valve regurgitation is usually a result of left-sided pressure-volume overload and is not treated surgically.

Combined valvular disease

Frequently, patients with valvular heart disease have multiple valves involved. Hemodynamically, the severity of the distal lesion may be masked by a proximal one. Aortic regurgitation and mitral regurgitation are relatively frequent. More than half the patients with mitral stenosis have aortic regurgitation of varying severity. Mitral stenosis and aortic stenosis may occur together. Aortic stenosis combined with mitral regurgitation is a bad combination because forward cardiac output is severely compromised. Tricuspid valve disease usually occurs with or as a result of mitral valve disease.

It is important to identify all valvular lesions before surgery using techniques including echocardiography and cardiac catheterization. The surgeon will make a final determination at the time of surgery. Surgery is usually scheduled once the patient's functional class reaches NYHA class III and before irreversible damage occurs. If more than one valve needs replacement, the surgeon will usually use both mechanical or both bioprosthetic valves depending on the patient's age and need for or contraindication to anticoagulation.

Balloon valvuloplasty

After the development of balloon angioplasty for coronary artery disease, it became reasonable to consider adaptation of this technique for stenotic cardiac valves, with the hopes of achieving relief of obstruction to outflow without the need for cardiac surgery. "A consummation devoutly to be wished!" While the initial enthusiasm has dampened somewhat, balloon valvuloplasty still can provide palliation and short-term symptomatic relief. We shall consider aortic and mitral valvuloplasty separately.

Valvuloplasty for aortic stenosis

Valvuloplasty achieves its success by causing fractures of the calcific plates and nodules holding the aortic valve leaflets together. The valve structure itself changes little after the procedure. After inflation of the balloon and successful valvuloplasty, the gradient may decrease by half and the valve area may increase by 0.2–0.4 cm^2. Most patients, however, continue to have severe although no longer critical aortic stenosis. Many of these patients still describe symptomatic improvement.

Restenosis develops in 50% to 75% of patients after a 6-month period and is one of the major limiting factors when considering valvuloplasty versus aortic valve replacement. Aortic regurgitation may result in a small percentage of cases. Other complications include stroke and perforation of the left ventricle. Tears of the aorta or aortic annulus may occur but are rare.

In some patients, aortic valvuloplasty may be performed to improve hemodynamics to the point where aortic valve surgery may be performed more safely. Patients in cardiogenic shock due to critical aortic stenosis may otherwise not even tolerate anesthesia induction. In general, if a patient can tolerate aortic valve replacement for severe or critical aortic stenosis, that procedure is the treatment of choice. For the severely symptomatic patient, usually the elderly, for whom surgery presents too high a risk, balloon valvuloplasty may provide short-term symptomatic improvement albeit with some risk of complication.

Valvuloplasty for mitral stenosis

For patients with mitral stenosis, the outlook may be somewhat more optimistic, provided that the valve is not too immobile or heavily scarred. A rule of thumb may be that patients who are candidates for mitral commissurotomy rather than replacement may be the ideal candidates for valvuloplasty. In these patients the leaflets are mobile and not thickened, and there is little subvalvular disease or calcification. They may be expected to have good short- and long-term results. The opposite is true for those with heavily calcified thickened valves and substructure with little leaflet mobility.

Successful valvuloplasty may result in a 6–15 mm Hg reduction in transvalvular gradient and an increase in mitral valve area from an initial value of 0.9 to 2.0 cm^2. These results may be comparable to those achieved by surgery.

Complications are possible, the worst being death in 1% to 3% of procedures. Obviously, a patient with left atrial thrombus is a poor candidate due to the chance of systemic embolization. Since the procedure is performed by crossing the atrial septum, an atrial septal defect (ASD) may remain. Some patients may be left with mitral regurgitation. Finally, the long-term follow-up is not yet available.

Consequently, the place of mitral valvuloplasty remains to be clearly defined. Selected patients may have an excellent result, but it is in these same patients that surgery can be performed with minimal risk. Thus, the physician must evaluate each patient individually before recommending a specific therapy.

OTHER REFERRALS TO THE CARDIAC SURGEON

Atrial septal defect

Most ASDs are recognized in childhood and undergo surgical repair. The goal is to avoid long-term complications, particularly pulmonary vascular disease. Occasionally some ASDs escape medical attention and are noticed later in adulthood, often presenting with atrial arrhythmias. Unless the defect is trivial, surgery is still indicated, because the potential for complications remains.

Small ASDs, particularly the secundum variety, are most likely to be noted later. The defect involves the fossa ovalis. The ECG will often demonstrate a conduction defect, incomplete or complete right bundle branch block (RBBB) and a rightward axis. The physical examination is remarkable for a systolic ejection murmur in the second left intercostal space, due to increased flow across the pulmonic valve. Splitting of the S_2 is wide and fixed.

Primum defects are often associated with endocardial cushion defects (common atrioventricular [AV] canal) and usually come to medical attention early. Mitral regurgitation may be present. In addition, other problems may be present. In primum ASD, the ECG will demonstrate RBBB and a leftward axis.

High ASDs of the sinus venosus variety may be associated with anomalous venous return. The echocardiogram aids in the diagnosis but cardiac catheterization is necessary to assess the degree of shunting, regardless of location of the defect. Initially shunts are left to right. The serious problems begin if the shunt reverses.

Operation is indicated for significant left-to-right shunts in which the ratio of pulmonary:systemic blood flow is greater than 1.5:1.0. If the defect is small and the flow is less, surgery is not necessary.

It is too late to perform surgery if the patient has severe pulmonary vascular disease. If the ratio of the pulmonary: systemic vascular resistance is greater than 0.7:1.0 and there is no significant left-to-right shunt, surgery will not be beneficial.

Surgery can be performed with minimal risk, usually with a mortality rate of less than 1%. The patient usually makes an uncomplicated recovery. Endocarditis prophylaxis is not necessary for patients with repaired ASDs unless other associated turbulent lesions are present.

Ventricular septal defect

Most VSDs are noted in childhood and either close spontaneously or require surgical closure. Repair is indicated for hemodynamically significant left to right shunts. If the ratio of pulmonary:systemic flow is less than 1.5–2.0:1 and the pulmonary artery pressure is not elevated, surgery is usually not necessary.

The majority of adult patients requiring closure of a VSD have ischemic heart disease, MI, and acute rupture. More often than not, these patients are in cardiogenic shock and must be stabilized with an IABP. The diagnosis is made by demonstration of an oxygen saturation step-up in the right ventricle. The ventriculogram will show the defect angiographically. VSD may occur with either anterior or inferior wall MI. The larger the defect, the more extensive the remaining ischemic myocardium, the worse the prognosis.

Constrictive pericarditis

An uncommon referral to the cardiac surgeon is for the surgical treatment of constrictive pericarditis, a process in which ventricular filling and cardiac output are limited by a dense adhesive process involving the pericardium. Actually, in most cases, the cause of the process is never determined. In past years when tuberculosis was more rampant, tuberculous pericarditis leading to a dense scar was more prevalent, but not today. Right-sided heart failure with hepatic congestion, hepatosplenomegaly, and even ascites may be the presenting symptom. The patient may be short of breath and complain of a lack of exercise capacity. Due to the inability to fill the ventricles, the cardiac output cannot increase the significantly.

The diagnosis can be suspected from the presenting symptoms, the physical examination of the jugular venous pulse (rapid x or y descent), the echocardiogram, and the chest x-ray. Hemodynamic tracings confirm the finding with diastolic equilibration of the intracardiac pressures as well as a "dip and plateau" pattern on the ventricular diastolic tracings (blood volume expansion is quickly restricted). The y descent is prominent and deeper than the x descent.

Therapy is surgical with removal of the pericardium, which can be a time-consuming and delicate procedure.

Pericardial tamponade

Pericardial tamponade may be treated initially by a cardiologist or a cardiac surgeon, because the first step is emergency pericardiocentesis. The reason for the tamponade determines the ultimate prognosis. Most cases the author has seen in a university medical center result from a malignant pericarditis (i.e., metastatic disease) and have a very poor outcome. Nevertheless, the patients often require a surgical approach once the initial pressure is relieved since the fluid usually continues to accumulate.

Tamponade occurs as the result of the rapid accumulation of fluid in the pericardial space, resulting in the inability of the heart to fill with blood and maintain the cardiac output. Frequent causes of pericardial tamponade include rupture of the free wall of the ventricle 2–5 days after MI, dissection of the aorta, or trauma (perforation of the ventricle with a scalpel or catheter; violent due to a knife or bullet). Some patients with postcardiotomy syndrome, heart failure, collagen vascular disease, infectious pericarditis, uremia, or myxedema develop pericardial effusion, but only rarely develop tamponade.

The deterioration of the patient may be rapid or slow,

depending on the mechanism. Symptoms often start with dyspnea, fatigue, and dizziness (related to a poor cardiac output). One looks for a pulsus paradoxus (inspiratory fall in systolic blood pressure greater than 15 mm Hg) although this finding may also be seen in constrictive pericarditis, right ventricular infarction, obstructive lung disease, cor pulmonale, or hypovolemic shock. The pulse rises, the patient becomes hypotensive, and the renal perfusion and urine output fall. The diagnosis is confirmed by evaluation of the pressures during pulmonary artery catheterization.

Echocardiography may be helpful with the diagnosis, but the problem may require more urgent intervention before the study can be accomplished. In addition to revealing both anterior and posterior pericardial fluid, early diastolic collapse of the right ventricle and the right atrium (due to the intrapericardial pressure) are suspicious for tamponade. If the diagnosis is in doubt, a pulmonary artery catheter may be inserted. Diastolic equilibration of intracardiac pressures is observed.

Once the diagnosis is confirmed, relief is obtained with needle aspiration of the pericardial fluid, often leaving a pigtail catheter in for drainage. If the cause is rupture of the free wall, only immediate surgery is lifesaving. In other situations, continued accumulation of pericardial fluid necessitates a surgical approach. Diagnostic evaluation of the pericardial fluid will provide information about other needed therapy.

The surgeon makes a decision about the extent of the procedure based on the underlying cause as well as other anatomic features.

Endocarditis

The treatment of bacterial endocarditis of a native heart valve is medical, involving appropriate antibiotics for a period of time, usually 6 weeks. Occasionally surgery will be necessary, particularly if the bacterial infection results in destruction of the valve (most often resulting in regurgitation) or if persistent infection results in abscess formation. The timing of surgery depends on the degree of hemodynamic embarrassment caused by the valvular lesion as well as the virulence of the organism. Consultation is usually obtained with the cardiologist, cardiac surgeon, and infectious diseases specialist and a joint decision made.

Prosthetic valve endocarditis is another serious condition.

It may be related to the initial surgical procedure or result from bacteremia. It is imperative that patients with prosthetic valves observe guidelines for endocarditis prophylaxis whenever undergoing dental work or genitourinary or other procedures likely to cause bacteremia. Prosthetic valve endocarditis is associated with a high mortality rate and requires intense antibiotic therapy. Development of regurgitation indicates tissue destruction and dehiscence of the valve, a serious complication requiring surgery. Inability to eradicate the infection with antibiotics makes abscess formation likely. Reoperation is associated with increased risk.

Surgery for aortic dissection

Aortic dissection is a catastrophic disorder that may be amenable to surgical correction if the patient can be first stabilized medically. Most aortic dissections today are related to atherosclerosis in patients who have histories of hypertension and hyperlipidemia. Cystic medial necrosis is seen in the aortic arch. Previously, syphilis was an important cause of aneursym of the ascending aorta but has declined in frequency. Other reasons for aneurysm surgery include disorders of connective tissue such as Marfan syndrome.

Certainly aneurysm can exist for a number of years before dissection, and the location and size often determine the timing of surgery. The vascular surgeon is often involved with fusiform aneurysms involving the celiac, superior mesenteric, or renal arteries or those just below and extending to the illiac arteries. These types of aneurysms may also involve the femoral or popliteal arteries. When the aneursym involves the ascending or descending aorta, a number of factors including the underlying etiology and the presence of hypertension determine how far the dissection will extend.

Depending on the location of the dissection, blood to various end organs can be compromised. Ischemia and infarction may occur in the heart, the brain, kidneys, visceral organs, extremities, or even in the spinal cord. DeBakey has classified dissecting aneurysms according to location. Type I affects the ascending aorta, the arch, the descending aorta, and occasionally the abdominal aorta. Type II is confined to the ascending aorta and does not involve the innominate artery. Type III occurs after the takeoff of the left subclavian artery. If confined to the thoracic aorta above the diaphragm, it is considered IIIa; if the dissection extends to the abdominal aorta, it is classified IIIb.

The presenting symptom is most often chest or back pain, which the patient almost accurately describes as a "tearing" sensation. Death can occur almost immediately if the dissection proceeds proximally and results in pericardial tamponade. As described above, specific vascular beds that are compromised will lead to end-organ damage and the complications.

Once the patient has sought medical attention, the diagnosis must be made quickly. Often the regional pulses and blood pressures give clues (e.g., palpable pulse and blood pressure in right arm, absent in left arm and legs). The critical point is to preserve circulation to the heart, brain, kidneys, and visceral organs. To prevent further dissection, lowering the blood pressure and reducing the contractile force of the heart may be beneficial. β-Blockers and intravenous vasodilators are the pharmacologic agents of choice. Performing arteriography to define the extent of the dissection is the next logical step, although in some cases a computed tomographic (CT) scan will provide vital information. Compromise to critical organs in an acute dissection makes surgery an emergent lifesaving but highly hazardous operation; however, there may be no choice. If the patient stabilizes, surgery becomes elective and somewhat less riskly, although spinal cord injury and injury to internal organs are always concerns. In certain patients, medical treatment is recommended, particularly if the vital organs are not jeopardized and the risk of surgery is too high. Individual decisions must be made.

Ventricular aneurysm and congestive heart failure

The title of this section is a broad topic with many factors that the physician must consider individually before referring a patient to the cardiac surgeon. First, if the patient has heart failure related to myocardial ischemia or valvular dysfunction, revascularization or valve repair may be the answer. However, if the heart muscle is extensively and irreversibly damaged, surgery may be of little benefit. Furthermore, even if a surgeon can be convinced to take a high-risk patient to surgery, the benefits may be limited if cardiac function cannot be improved and the complication rate will be high.

In dealing with patients who have ventricular aneurysm, the main question will revolve about the extent of aneurysm.

An attempt at excision or plication of a diffuse aneurysm will most likely be unsuccessful because the amount of remaining viable myocardium may be too small to permit adequate volume for filling. In addition, the attempts at aneurysmectomy in diffuse aneurysm of the left ventricle may result in inability to be weaned from cardiopulmonary bypass, resulting in intraoperative death.

Surgery is much more likely to be successful for a discrete aneurysm. Location is important in determining risk. A discrete anterior or apical aneurysm will be much easier to deal with from the technical standpoint than one involving the inferoposterior wall. One must then ask, why consider surgery for this discrete aneurysm? Is the patient experiencing congestive heart failure related to the aneurysm, recurrent arterial emboli due to thrombus in the aneurysm, or intractable ventricular arrhythmias that would be amenable to electrophysiologically guided resection? All of these may be reasonable indications. Most often ventricular aneurysm resection or plication will be combined with another surgical procedure including revascularization or implantation of an AICD.

Pseudoaneurysm of the left ventricle is an indication for surgical repair. It occurs after MI and involves full-thickness destruction of myocardium with only adherent pericardium preventing pericardial tamponade. The surgeon must reapproximate sections of myocardium.

Cardiac transplantation

Cardiac transplatation has become highly successful for the treatment of end-stage heart disease. Limiting factors remain and include the necessity for lifelong immunosuppressive therapy as well as the relative lack of availability of donor organs. The restrictions to acceptance of a patient into a transplant program have been relaxed, particularly in regard to age. Usually patients older than 55–60 years are not considered. Nevertheless, the presence of multisystem disease, active infection, fixed pulmonary vascular resistance, or severe psychosocial problems remain exclusion criteria. Insulin-dependent diabetics are at increased risk of infection and are usually not accepted.

Although the surgical technique of transplantation is relatively straightforward, the follow-up and prevention of rejection require great care and meticulous attention. Periodic myocardial biopsies must be performed and immunosuppressive therapy regulated. Coronary arteriography is also recommended at varying intervals to assess the possibility of development of coronary atherosclerosis.

Physicians should consider transplantation in suitable candidates while maximizing medical therapy. Once it is clear that medical therapy or surgical procedures such as revascularization have little to offer, the physician should discuss the possibility of transplantation with the patient and make a referral to the regional transplant center.

Indications for permanent pacing

A fairly common referral to the cardiologist or cardiac surgeon is the patient requiring a permanent pacemaker. Depending on the institution, either of these subspecialists may perform the procedure. Because the implantation procedure is relatively uncomplicated, only the indications will be discussed. The variety of pacemakers available is increasing and now include not only single chamber but also dual chamber and physiologic devices. The more features included, the higher the cost and consequently, the need for careful selection of the appropriate device. The government already regulates reimbursement for pacemakers implanted in Medicare patients. Utilization review organizations decide whether procedures were appropriate.

Bradyarrhythmias

Sick sinus syndrome: Many of these patients have a fast component as well (tachy-brady syndrome). They require negative chronotropic or dromotropic drugs for tachycardias and a pacemaker for the bradyarrhythmias. Sick sinus syndrome may occur in the absence of underlying heart disease and may be seen at both young and older ages in both genders. Since bradycardia is not always present, many of these patients may be treated by single chamber ventricular pacemakers to pace when necessary. Many of these patients also have distal conduction disease.

Symptomatic sinus bradycardia: When patients are truly symptomatic and do not have an escape rhythm, a pacemaker is indicated. Single chamber atrial pacing is rarely used since many of these patients may also be at risk for distal conduction disease. They may be treated with single chamber ventricular or dual chamber (if atrial kick is desirable) pacing.

Sinus arrest or sinoatrial block: Some might consider this entity as a variant of sick sinus syndrome without the tachy component or distal conduction disease. The indications and considerations for pacemaker implantation are the same.

Atrial fibrillation with a very slow ventricular response: If symptomatic (hemodynamically compromised) from a slow ventricular response, single chamber ventricular pacing is indicated. The choice of device depends on whether a fixed pacing rate is desired or one that can be regulated by physiologic need, such as muscle activity.

High degree atrioventricular block (Möbitz II or complete heart block): Some individuals with complete heart block have a relatively fast ventricular escape rate (e.g., 50 bpm), maintain their blood pressure, remain asymptomatic, and are capable of physical activity. They do not need pacemakers. The majority of the remaining individuals will be symptomatic in terms of dizziness, syncope, or fatigue and will benefit from a pacemaker. Often high degree AV block is transient and causes symptoms difficult to correlate to an underlying rhythm disturbance. If ambulatory ECG recording is unable to document the block, electrophysiologic testing can be used to demonstrate block below the His bundle.

Once a decision has been made to recommend a pacemaker, a decision must be made regarding single versus dual chamber pacing. The need for the atrial contribution to the cardiac output will determine whether the patient should receive a dual chamber or a single chamber pacemaker. Obviously if the supraventricular rhythm is atrial fibrillation, only a VVI pacemaker is considered. If one wishes to allow tracking of the atrial (i.e., sinus) rate, then a dual chamber device is chosen. Rate responsive pacemakers are now available which increase the ability to respond to physiologic requirements.

High degree atrioventricular block during anterior wall myocardial infarction: When high degree AV block (Möbitz II or complete heart block) occurs transiently or permanently during anterior wall MI, permanent pacing should be considered before discharge. Even if transient, high degree block may recur. Unfortunately, these patients are at high risk due to extensive loss of myocardium and are likely to have heart failure and occasionally life-threatening ventricular arrhythmias. These latter issues must be individually addressed.

Other more controversial indications: There is not universal agreement on all indications for permanent pacemakers. For example, carotid sinus sensitivity is considered an indication if bradycardia leading to symptoms can be documented. Alternating bundle branch block indicates severe disease of the distal conduction system. Congenital AV block is still one more indication, particularly if the escape rate is slow.

Tachyarrhythmias: antitachycardia pacemakers

Often pharmacologic therapy is not desirable, particularly in a young individual or for women of childbearing age who wish to become pregnant. In other cases, arrhythmias may be refractory to drug therapy. For some of these individuals, antitachycardia pacing may be beneficial. Antitachycardia pacing involves sensing circuitry and programmed algorithms to pace the tachycardia back to sinus rhythm. Sensing involves rate detection, e.g., a heart rate higher than 150 bpm and maintenance of this heart rate for a certain time interval. Then the pacemaker may be programmed to discharge at certain preset rates and with specific pacing intervals. The stimuli may involve single, double or triple extrastimuli, as well as overdrive or underdrive burst pacing. These cycles may be repeated, each time, decrementing or incrementing the specific intervals. Once sinus rhythm is restored, the pacemaker returns to the monitoring mode.

Antitachycardia pacemakers have been approved for atrial arrhythmias and may be useful for atrial flutter and for certain paroxysmal supraventricular tachycardias. They have not yet been approved for ventricular arrhythmias. One of the major concerns in terminating sustained ventricular tachycardia is that the arrhythmia may be accelerated and deteriorate into ventricular fibrillation. Consequently, the use of an antitachycardia pacemaker for ventricular tachycardia without the backup protection of an AICD may be hazardous. If ventricular fibrillation would occur with the defibrillator present, that device would be activated and defibrillation back to sinus rhythm would occur. This combination has the advantage of minimizing defibrillator shocks for ventricular tachycardia, prolonging battery life, but at this time necessitates two separate devices. In the future, it is likely that these units will be combined.

Automatic cardioverter defibrillators

This device was invented by Michael Mirowski and has been successful in reducing the yearly incidence of sudden death in patients with recurrent ventricular tachycardia or ventricular fibrillation from 25–40% to 2%.

Current indications include patients at risk for recurrent sudden cardiac arrest who are refractory to or who cannot tolerate drug therapy. Patients inducible into sustained ventricular tachycardia at electrophysiology study who do not respond to pharmacologic therapy are also candidates. Patients who have survived ventricular fibrillation (not associated with acute MI) who are noninducible at electrophysiology study merit consideration. Indications for AICDs are expanding although not all indications have yet been approved for reimbursement by third-party payers.

One device has been approved and other manufacturers are developing similar models. Basically the device contains a sensing circuit connected to endocardial or epicardial electrodes. Another set of electrodes is attached to the heart and delivers an internal shock after the sensing circuit recognizes a malignant ventricular arrhythmia. Recognition may occur via rate detection alone or in combination with analysis of morphology of the arrhythmia. The defibrillating electrodes usually consist of two patches over the right and left ventricles or a spring electrode at the junction of the superior vena cava and right atrium and a left ventricular patch. Newer designs have involved testing of three ventricular patches and further attempts at refining the original idea of a single catheter with electrodes in the atrium and ventricle.

The surgical implantation of these devices is relatively uncomplicated and consequently this discussion will be limited. The sensing and defibrillating electrodes are connected to a pulse generator that is implanted in a subcutaneous abdominal pocket. The newer pulse generators are projected to last 3–4 years and be capable of delivering up to 300 discharges. These devices have been the most successful of any treatment for patients with risk of sudden cardiac death. Surgery for resection of an arrhythmia zone is potentially more hazardous and cannot be offered to many patients due to various technical factors. Nevertheless, surgery for patients with discrete aneurysms who have sustained ventricular tachycardia may derive major benefit from electrophysiologically guided resection, whether it be by subendocardial excision, cryoablation, or laser therapy.

APPROACH TO THE PATIENT

Presentation

The initial presentation of coronary artery disease may be angina, acute MI, or sudden cardiac death. Thus, the patient with only angina is indeed the fortunate one. As the importance of coronary risk factors becomes more widely appreciated, greater numbers of patients with asymptomatic coronary artery disease may be identified through appropriate diagnostic tests and corrective measures instituted. Consequently, it is imperative that the physician be cognizant of potentially modifiable problems such as hyperlipidemia, hypertension, and smoking.

Risk factors

As implied above, *prevention* is more desirable than active treatment for the disorder once established. Nevertheless, prevention, which requires effort and life-style modification, is often difficult to accomplish. Unfortunately, it is unlikely that we will see the eradication of coronary artery disease or the need for coronary artery surgery or angioplasty in our lifetime.

Family history of premature coronary artery disease: When several generations of the family experience MI before the age of 55 years, there is a significant chance that subsequent generations may also be at risk. Often contributory factors include familial lipid disorders, hypertension, and habits such as smoking or diet. It is important to evaluate patients early, i.e., in their youth, as atherosclerosis is a process that develops over a lifetime. It is possible that proper nutrition, avoidance of cigarette smoking, and treatment of hypertension may delay or otherwise alter the progression to overt coronary artery disease. It is important to involve patients in their health care but at the same time avoid irrational fear of early death, which can become psychologically disabling.

Hyperlipidemia: Not only have we learned that elevated serum cholesterol is detrimental, but reduction in serum cholesterol values with diet and lipid-lowering drugs results in decreased cardiovascular morbidity. Initial therapy consists of weight reduction and an appropriate diet low in saturated fats. Unfortunately a subject often neglected in the training of physicians is nutrition. However, there is no longer any excuse because maintaining a desirable lipid profile should be considered part of the standard medical regimen after CABG surgery or angioplasty (Tables 1-18 and 1-19). If diet therapy alone is ineffective, one must consider therapy with bile-binding resins, fibric acids, niacin or HMG-Coenzyme A (CoA) reductase inhibitors, as is appropriate (Table 1-20).

Hypertension: Long described as the "silent killer," hypertension contributes to the risk of coronary artery disease. As demonstrated by the Framingham study, multiple risk factors are additive in contributing to cardiovascular morbidity. Hypertension and hyperlipidemia together accelerate atherosclerosis. Hypertension also places the patient at risk for cerebrovascular disease and renal failure. Various drug regimens are available

Table 1-18   Risk Levels for Elevated Serum Cholesterol

	Moderate risk	High risk
Age 20–29	200 mg/dL	220 mg/dL
30–39	220	240
≥40	240	260

Table 1-19   Estimation of Low-Density Lipoprotein (LDL) Cholesterol

$$LDL^\star = \text{Total cholesterol} - \text{High-density lipoprotein (HDL)} - \frac{\text{Triglycerides}^\dagger}{5}$$

$\star$LDL $\geq$ 160 mg/dL is indicative of moderate to highly increased risk of coronary artery disease.

$\dagger$Valid when triglyceride level is not severely elevated (<400).

Note: Decisions to treat patients with pharmacologic therapy are based on the level of LDL cholesterol, the presence of multiple cardiac risk factors, the demonstration of ischemic heart disease, and the failure of diet alone. It may be more difficult to increase the HDL level. Low HDL levels also provide an index of increased risk.

Table 1-20   Drug Therapy for Elevated Cholesterol and Triglycerides

1. **Cornerstone of therapy**
   Proper diet and nutrition
   Exercise
   Weight loss of overweight
2. **Drugs that increase LDL receptors**
   Bile acid sequestrants: By interfering with the enterohepatic circulation of bile and decreasing the absorption of bile acids, more cholesterol is converted into bile acids. Consequently, hepatic cholesterol decreases and stimulates the synthesis of LDL receptors, thereby decreasing plasma LDL.
   Cholestyramine   14–24 g/day in divided doses
   Colestipol   15–30 g/day in divided doses
   These agents are limited by adverse gastrointestinal side effects, including constipation and flatulence.
   HMG-CoA reductase inhibitors: By interfering with the synthesis of cholesterol by the liver, decreased levels stimulate the synthesis of LDL receptors, resulting in a reduction of LDL cholesterol by 30% to 40%.
   Lovastatin 20–80 mg od. This drug is generally well tolerated and quite effective. Follow-up is necessary.
   Pravastatin and Simvastatin are expected to be released soon.
3. **Drugs that decrease the production of lipoproteins**
   Nicotinic acid (Niacin): Interferes with the synthesis of very low-density lipoproteins (VLDL) and subsequently their breakdown into LDL.
   Start with 100–200 mg tid and gradually increase dose to 500–1000 mg tid. Prescribing an aspirin before the first dose mediates some of the side effects, such as flushing, which are partially mediated through prostaglandins.
   Fish oils: Inhibit synthesis of VLDL triglycerides by the liver. At the time of writing, the American Heart Association does not recommend fish oils for routine or prophylactic treatment of hyperlipidemias. Nevertheless fish oil therapy may be useful for selected patients with elevated triglyceride levels.
4. **Drugs that increase triglyceride-rich lipoproteins**
   Fibric acid derivatives: Promote the breakdown of triglyceride-rich lipoproteins by enhancing the activity of lipoprotein lipase. Cholesterol secretion into bile is also increased and bile acid synthesis is reduced, increasing the lithogenicity of bile.
   Gemfibrozil 600 mg bid
5. **Drugs that promote LDL clearance**
   Probucol: Results in an alteration in the structure of LDL, allowing increased clearance from the circulation, but also reduces HDL cholesterol.
   Probucol 500 mg bid

for the treatment of high blood pressure and the drug of choice may depend on the presence of associated factors, such as ischemia, as well as potential adverse effects of the drugs themselves.

Smoking: Little doubt remains that cigarette smoking is detrimental to patients with ischemic heart disease and contributory to chronic lung disease and lung cancer. Even passive smoking (i.e., being in a room with a smoker) can be harmful, because inhalation of smoke in the air can produce the same results. Nicotine is a vasoconstrictor and the carbon monoxide produced binds more firmly to hemoglobin than does oxygen. Continued smoking after angioplasty increases the risk of restenosis. Thus, a patient should stop smoking, particularly if coronary artery disease has been established and if invasive intervention has been performed.

Diabetes mellitus: It is well known that diabetic patients are at risk for coronary artery disease and in fact demonstrate severe diffuse disease that makes surgery (i.e., anastomosis of a vein or artery graft to the native vessel) extremely difficult. Diabetics are reported to have "small vessel" disease with small arteries and arterioles affected by the atherosclerotic process. It remains somewhat controversial whether "tight" control of the serum glucose level will significantly reduce vascular complications of diabetes, but recent work seems to indicate potential benefit. One important factor for the physician to remember is that diabetics may have a defective anginal warning system and not experience chest pain. Quite often a "silent" MI will appear on the ECG. Assessment of the diabetic patient may require more routine noninvasive diagnostic studies to evaluate the presence of asymptomatic ischemia.

Obesity: Obesity is a risk factor in that it contributes to elevated blood pressure and serum cholesterol levels. Exercise is important for maintaining cardiovascular fitness but should be performed after discussion with the patient's physician if coronary artery disease is present or suspected. A patient who cares about body image and cardiovascular fitness is more likely to comply with dietary guidelines and take medications if and when appropriate.

Symptoms of coronary artery disease

Classic angina pectoris: This symptom has been described as a sense of choking or strangling accompanied by a pressure or weight on the chest. Most often the sensation is substernal, occasionally radiating to the jaw, teeth, shoulder, arm, or fingers. Sometimes the patient will complain of a numbness in the extremities. Other associated symptoms include dyspnea, cold diaphoresis, nausea, dizziness, or a feeling of "imminent doom." Initially the symptoms are exertional, but as the problem progresses, they may occur at rest. Usually, stopping the activity results in relief of symptoms, as does sublingual nitroglycerin. When asked to describe the symptoms, the patient may gesture with a clenched fist (Levine's sign). The author has observed some patients to twist the fist and the knuckles have become white. There is little doubt they have angina. Patients with angina often may be able to describe when discomfort first occurred (e.g., last winter, shoveling snow). Precipitating factors often include physical exertion, emotional stress, exposure to cold, heavy meals (i.e., overeating), or sexual relations.

Atypical angina: Some patients may describe angina in different terms such as a sharp pain, dull ache, or "grabbing" sensation. Often the ability of a patient to provide a classic description is related to the educational background and the ability to articulate. Sometimes the discomfort will appear in an atypical location. Some patients may describe only a feeling of breathlessness or undue fatigue. These descriptions may represent an "anginal equivalent."

Asymptomatic (silent) ischemia: This syndrome is defined by myocardial ischemia occurring in the absence of typical or atypical chest discomfort. Proposed explanations have included subthreshold stimuli for pain, a high pain threshold, or impaired pain sensation. Despite the absence of pain, the consequences to the myocardium may be the same as painful ischemia and include infarction, ischemic myopathy, or sudden cardiac death. Transient left ventricular dysfunction may be the first manifestation of ischemia, followed later by ECG changes and finally pain in some cases. The patient must be aware of the possibility of silent ischemia because the warning to stop activity causing ischemia is absent.

Medical evaluation

In addition to obtaining a careful history and performing a comprehensive physical examination, specific diagnostic tests may be indicated. More often than not, the physical examination will be unrevealing, possibly indicating an S_4 gallop at most. Exercise testing with or without radionuclide techniques will provide diagnostic and prognostic data. Coronary arteriography and left ventriculography may be necessary. These tests will be described in the next chapter.

For the patient with valvular heart disease, the approach will be different. There may be a history of heart murmur or rheumatic fever. The symptoms may be different, with dyspnea more likely than pain. The physical examination may be diagnostic and can be confirmed by further echocardiogram–Doppler studies.

As part of the total approach, analysis of total, LDL, and HDL cholesterol as well as triglycerides is important for assessing lipid disorders. Determination of renal function (blood urea nitrogens, creatinine, electrolytes) is important if the patient is scheduled for cardiac catheterization or to assess the long-term effects of hypertension or congestive heart failure. Patients with heart failure will often demonstrate evidence of hepatic enzyme elevation. The serum glucose and hemoglobin values will provide an index to the degree of control of diabetes.

Psychologic aspects of undergoing cardiac surgery

All too often, this aspect of patient care is overlooked. Concerns such as insurance, nursing assistance, return to work, or driving are more likely to be addressed than the patient's fear of the procedure or confrontation of mortality. Patients may become apprehensive and anxious prior to the procedure, particularly the night before. Every physician can recall patients who have suffered MI or sudden death immediately before surgery. There is little doubt that emotional factors may have been at least partly contributory (e.g., provoking an adverse physiologic response such as sympathetic nervous system stimulation or catecholamine release in addition to the underlying severe coronary artery disease). Addressing this issue is important, as may be the appropriate administration of sedatives, especially the night before the procedure. The patient and family do better when they understand the details of the procedure and what to expect once it is completed. Presenting clear and detailed information in a hopeful tone while at the same time indicating the risks (but not in an alarming tone) is necessary and appropriate.

One other problem encountered is postoperative depression, often a result of coming to grips with accepting the illness, realizing what tests have been performed, and accepting one's own mortality. When warned beforehand about the possibility of depression, it may be easier to deal with when it occurs. The family's support at this time may be helpful.

SUGGESTED READING

Many of these textbooks have been updated in later editions.

Cardiac surgery

Glenn WWL, Bave AE, Geha AS, Hammond GL, Laks H. *Thoracic and Cardiovascular Surgery.* 4th ed. Norwalk, CT: Appelton-Century Crofts; 1983.

Kirklin JW, Barratt-Boyes BG. *Cardiac Surgery.* New York: John Wiley & Sons; 1986.

Schwartz SI, Shires GT, Spencer FC, Storer EH. *Principles of Surgery.* 4th ed. New York: McGraw-Hill; 1984.

Cardiology

Braunwald E. *Heart Disease.* 3rd ed. Philadelphia: WB Saunders; 1988.

Hurst JW, Logue RB, Rackley CE, et al. *The Heart.* 5th ed. New York: McGraw-Hill; 1982.

In addition to standard textbooks on cardiology, the reader may wish to consult some of these subspeciality texts.

Ellestad MH. *Stress Testing.* Philadelphia: FA Davis; 1986.

Feigenbaum H. *Echocardiography.* 4th ed. Philadelphia: Lea & Febiger; 1986.

Grossman W. *Cardiac Catheterization and Angioplasty.* 2nd ed. Philadelphia: Lea & Febiger; 1980.

King SB, Douglas JS. *Coronary Arteriography and Angioplasty.* New York: McGraw-Hill; 1985.

Vlietstra RE, Holmes DR. *PTCA*. Philadelphia: FA David; 1986.

Vlay SC, ed. Manual of cardiac arrhythmias. Boston: Little, Brown & Co, 1988.

Valvuloplasty

Cribier A, et al. Percutaneous transluminal balloon valvuloplasty of adult aortic stenosis: report of 92 cases. *J Am Coll Cardiol*. 1987; 9:381–386.

Holmes DR. Balloon valvuloplasty for aortic stenosis. *Hosp Pract*. January 15, 1990:69–77.

Mckay RGP. Balloon valvuloplasty for treating pulmonic, mitral and aortic valve stenosis. *Am J Cardiol*. 1988; 61:102G.

Palacios IF, et al. Followup of patients undergoing percutaneous mitral balloon valvulotomy: analysis of factors determining restenosis. *Circulation*. 1989;79:573.

Powers ER. Balloon valvuloplasty for mitral stenosis. *Hosp Pract*. May 30, 1990:37–46.

Richenbacher WE, Myers JL, Waldhausen JA. Current status of cardiac surgery: a 40 year review. *J Am Coll Cardiol*. 1989;14:535–544.

Other Reading

Bonow RO, Dodd JT, Maron BJ, et al. Long-term serial changes in left ventricular function and reversal of ventricular dilatation after valve replacement for chronic aortic regurgitation. *Circulation*. 1988; 78:1108–1120.

Cardiovascular Surgery 1988, Part I. *Circulation*. 1989;80:I-1–279.

CASS, Principal Investigators, et al. The National Heart, Lung and Blood Institute Coronary Artery Surgery Study. *Circulation*. 1981;63 (suppl I):1–81.

CASS, Principal Investigators, et al. CASS A randomized trial of cornary artery bypass surgery: survival data. *Circulation*. 1983;68:939–950.

European Coronary Surgery Study Group. Long-term results of prospective-randomized study of coronary artery bypass surgery in stable angina pectoris. *Lancet*. 1982;2:1173–1180.

Hwang MH, Hammermeister KE, Oprian C, et al. Preoperative identification of patients likely to have left ventricular dysfunction after aortic valve replacement. *Circulation.* 1989;80(suppl I):65–76.

Levison JR, Akins CW, Buckley MJ, et al. Octogenarians with aortic stenosis. Outcome after aortic valve replacement. *Circulation.* 1989;80(suppl I):49–56.

Nishimura RA, McGoon MD, Schaff HV, Giuliani ER. Chronic aortic regurgitation: indications for operation—1988. *Mayo Clin Proc.* 1988;63:270–280.

Siemienczuk D, Greenberg B, Morris C, et al. Chronic aortic insufficiency: factors associated with progression to aortic valve replacement. *Ann Intern Med.* 1989; 110:587–592.

State-of-the-Art Symposium on Coronary Arterial Surgery. *Circulation.* 1989;79:I-1–192.

Veterans Administration Coronary Artery Bypass Surgery Cooperative Study. Eleven-year survival in the Veterans Administration randomized trial of cornary bypass surgery for stable angina. *N Engl J Med.* 1984;311:1333–1339.

Cardiac Diagnostic Techniques

Stephen C. Vlay, M.D.

2

This chapter discusses the most widely used cardiac diagnostic techniques: exercise testing, radionuclide studies, echocardiography and Doppler cardiography, ambulatory electrocardiographic (ECG) monitoring, cardiac catheterization, and electrophysiology study. The intention of this chapter is to familiarize the reader with the most important aspects of the diagnostic studies used in the decision-making process for the cardiac surgical candidate. The key points are noted but by no means should the reader consider the review to be comprehensive. For further details, the reader is encouraged to consult other volumes in this series or standard reference textbooks which deal specifically with these subjects.

EXERCISE TESTING

Exercise testing attempts, under controlled conditions, to simulate the cardiac workload and stresses experienced by the patient during activities of daily living. It is used to make a diagnosis or assess the severity of coronary artery disease, to evaluate the response to medications or procedures (angioplasty, bypass surgery [CABG]), to assess the degree of cardiovascular fitness, and to evaluate arrhythmias or in certain cases, heart failure. The specific indications are outlined in Table 2-1.

The procedure is widely available and can be performed with a minimum of expensive equipment (as compared with an invasive laboratory). Certain standards established by the American Heart Association must be followed (Schlant RC, Blomquist CG, Bradenburg RO, et al.: Guidelines for Exercise

Table 2-1 Indications for Stress Testing

1. *To establish or exclude a diagnosis of coronary artery disease in:*
   a. An individual with known cardiac risk factors
   b. A symptomatic individual with typical or atypical chest discomfort
   c. An individual in a high risk profession (e.g., airline pilot) in whom there is a suspicion of coronary heart disease
   d. A previously sedentary individual with some cardiac risk factors prior to starting an exercise training program
2. *To establish the physiologic severity of coronary artery disease in a patient with:*
   a. Known coronary artery disease
   b. Remote myocardial infarction (MI)
   c. Recent MI prior to discharge (low level test)
   d. Recent MI prior to returning to full activity (full exercise test at 6 wk after MI)
3. *To judge the response to:*
   a. Anti-ischemic therapy
   b. CABG surgery
   c. Percutaneous transluminal coronary angioplasty
   d. Other specific therapy directed at arrhythmias, heart failure
4. *To evaluate:*
   a. Arrhythmias
   b. Certain patients with heart failure (compensated)

Table 2-2 Contraindications to Stress Testing

Unstable angina
Severe ischemia at rest
Acute MI
Critical left main coronary artery stenosis
Critical aortic stenosis
Obstructive hypertrophic cardiomyopathy
Acute myocarditis
Decompensated congestive heart failure
Uncontrolled severe hypertension
Patients with advanced heart block or uncontrolled ventricular tachyarrhythmias (however, stress testing may be a necessary part of the evaluation and may be safely performed by physicians skilled and experienced in the management of certain rhythm disorders)

Table 2-3   End Points in Stress Testing (When to stop the test)

1. Progressive angina
2. Ischemic ST segment response (a positive test)
3. Hypotension
4. Other signs of decompensation (cold, clammy sensation, nausea)
5. Development of:
    a. Ventricular tachycardia (some physicians would terminate exercise with ventricular couplets)
    b. Atrial tachyarrhythmias
    c. Severe hypertension
    d. High degree heart block
6. Dyspnea
7. Fatigue
8. Achievement of maximal heart rate or exercise capacity

Table 2-4   Complications of Stress Testing

Death (mortality rate 0.5–1.0/10,000 tests)
Ventricular fibrillation
MI

Testing. *Circulation* 1986:74:653A–667A). Contraindications are listed in Table 2-2, and end points are summarized in Table 2-3. Complications are noted in Table 2-4, with commonly used protocols described in Table 2-5.

Indications of a stress test positive for ischemia

The most worrisome finding on exercise testing is the demonstration of global ischemia at an early stage of exercise. One notices horizontal or downsloping ST segment depression, in both anterior and inferior leads, that exceeds 1.0 mm below the baseline ST segment. Upsloping ST depression is a nonspecific finding. The greater the magnitude of the ST depression, the more likely it is to represent a true positive and severe ischemia. If the baseline ST segment is markedly abnormal (e.g., left ventricular hypertrophy, left bundle branch block [LBBB], Wolff-Parkinson-White [WPW] syndrome, digitalis or other drug-induced changes), the ST segment cannot be interpreted and radionuclide imaging is necessary.

If the ST segment changes are accompanied by hypotension,

Table 2-5   Commonly Used Exercise Protocols

Bruce Protocol

(3-minute stages with increases in speed and grade)

Stage	Speed (mph)	Grade (%)
1	1.7	10
2	2.5	12
3	3.4	14
4	4.2	16
5	5.0	18
6	5.5	20

Modified Bruce protocol

(3-minute stages, starting slower and lower rises in grade which may be desirable after MI)

Stage	Speed (mph)	Grade (%)
0	1.7	0
½	1.7	5
1	1.7	10
2	2.5	12
3	3.4	14
4	4.2	16
5	5.0	18

Naughton protocol

(2-minute stages, constant speed, slow (2.5%) rises in grade)

Stage	Speed (mph)	Grade (%)
1	3	0
2	3	2.5
3	3	5.0
4	3	7.5
5	3	10
6	3	12.5

Balke Protocol

Speed constant at 3.3 mph, gradual increase in grade starting at zero, 2-minute stages

Ellestad protocol

Stage	Speed (mph)	Grade (%)	Min
1	1.7	10	0
2	3.0	10	3
3	4.0	10	5
4	5.0	10	7
5	6.0	15	10
6	7.0	15	12
7	8.0	15	14

the likelihood of left main or severe triple vessel disease increases. Some patients with severe disease may become symptomatic within the first stage and the exercise test must be stopped before diagnostic ECG changes occur or imaging can be performed. To determine the extent of disease in this situation, cardiac catheterization must be performed. In the patient with ST changes, the longer they persist after exercise is completed, the more likely they represent severe ischemia.

Arrhythmias may occur during exercise but are not always related to ischemia. Some are related to catecholamine sensitivity and others may be related to specific electrophysiologic mechanisms. Nevertheless, they deserve evaluation.

Radionuclide imaging enhances the interpretation of the stress test. Regional areas of transient ischemia during exercise are identified. The more numerous and extensive the defects, the greater the amount of myocardium (and multiple coronary arteries) involved. Occasionally patients with left main disease will not demonstrate segmental defects due to the extent of jeopardized myocardium. If the left ventricular dysfunction occurs as a result of exercise, the ventricle may appear dilated and abnormal thallium uptake in the lung may occur.

If the radionuclide technique used is technetium-labeled blood pool imaging, ischemia may be visualized as either global or regional dysfunction. The left ventricular ejection fraction (EF) may be depressed at rest and fall further with exercise. Regional areas may contract abnormally and may be compared with the rest image.

Bayes' theorem

The possibility that the result of a test is a true finding is a function of the information obtained and the incidence of disease in that population. Thus, the chance that ST depression on an exercise test represents myocardial ischemia is different in a 28-year-old woman with mitral valve prolapse and no risk factors than in a 56-year-old hypertensive male smoker with hypertension and an elevated cholesterol level. The former is likely a false positive finding and the latter is likely a true positive. Thus, the interpretation of a test must account for the likelihood that disease is indeed present in the population.

Sensitivity and specificity

Sensitivity is a measure of identifying those patients with a diagnostic stress test out of all those who really have myocardial ischemia.

$$\text{Sensitivity} = \frac{\text{True positive}}{\text{True positive} + \text{False negative}}$$

Sensitivity can be increased by accepting a smaller degree of ST segment depression as a diagnostic test, but one risks the chance of more false positive studies.

Specificity measures the reliability that the test really identifies those with disease and, in fact, does not mistakenly identify those who are normal.

$$\text{Specificity} = \frac{\text{True negative}}{\text{True negative} + \text{False positive}}$$

The *predictive value* considers the fact that the diagnostic stress test reflects the presence of myocardial ischemia.

$$\text{Predictive value} = \frac{\text{True positive}}{\text{True positive} + \text{False positive}}$$

The *predictive accuracy* determines the truth of both the true positives and the true negatives.

$$\text{Predictive accuracy} = \frac{\text{True positive} + \text{True negative}}{\text{All tests}}$$

True positive = Patient has myocardial ischemia and diagnostic ECG changes on exercise test.

False positive = Patient has suggestive or diagnostic ECG changes on exercise but does not have myocardial ischemia.

True negative = Patient does not have myocardial ischemia. There are no diagnostic ECG changes on exercise test.

False negative = Patient has myocardial ischemia but diagnostic ECG changes on exercise test are absent.

RADIONUCLIDE TECHNIQUES
Thallium scintigraphy

To enhance the sensitivity of the exercise tests, thallium scinti-graphy may be performed (Table 2-6). In the body, thallium is handled like potassium and is taken up by areas of viable myocardium. Areas of permanent scar (MI) or temporary poor perfusion (myocardial ischemia) appear as cold spots or defects on the scan. Thallium is injected intravenously at peak exercise and imaged on a high-resolution low-energy collimator and scintillation camera. The amount of thallium extracted by the myocardium during its first pass through the heart is greater than 85%. Its half-life is 73 hours. Just as thallium is taken up by the myocardial cell, it also washes out. Areas of myocardium that were temporarily ischemic and since recovered may now extract thallium that washed out and continued to circulate. Thus, repeat imaging several hours after exercise when myocar-dium is no longer ischemic may demonstrate filling-in of the perfusion defect. Consequently, when a patient undergoes a thal-lium stress examination, imaging is performed twice, once im-mediately afterward and then 3–4 hours later in the so-called redistribution phase. Furthermore, in patients with severe ischemia at rest, double-dose delayed thallium imaging may be able to differentiate this condition from permanent scar tissue.

The image is analyzed qualitatively and quantitatively for areas of homogenous and heterogeneous perfusion. Areas that fill in on delayed imaging are considered to have been temporar-ily ischemic. Areas that remain poorly perfused represent perma-nent scar or may be related to some of the reasons listed in Table 2-7 for false positive results. Computer-assisted quantitative analysis of a good quality image increases both the sensitivity

---

Table 2-6   Indications for Stress Thallium Examinations

1. Nondiagnostic routine exercise test
2. Noninterpretable baseline ECG segments
   a. Left ventricular hypertrophy
   b. LBBB
   c. Nonspecific ST-T wave changes
   d. ST-T wave changes related to digitalis or other drugs
   e. WPW syndrome
3. Localization of area of jeopardized (ischemic) myocardium

Table 2-7   Explanations for False Positive Stress Thallium Perfusion

1. Limitations of collimator
2. Problems with data acquisition (improper patient positioning)
3. Interpretation error
   a. Breast shadow read as ASMI
   b. Apical thinning read as apical MI
   c. Septal abnormalities in patients with LBBB
   d. Decreased sensitivity in left circumflex coronary artery narrowings

(85%) and specificity (80%) to greater than 90%. *Caveat:* If the quality of the material to be analyzed is compromised at any point in the imaging process (from positioning the camera, the patient, computer error, interpretation error), the information obtained may be worthless. The physician must have confidence in the quality control of the radionuclide laboratory.

One factor that may further limit the ability to interpret the exercise test is the inability of the patient to exercise adequately due to arthritis or claudication, preventing achievement of an adequate workload (low heart rate and blood pressure). Even thallium scintigraphy may not demonstrate the defect. Two other possible methods can be used. The first uses temporary pacing to increase the heart rate. The second uses dipyridamole, a vasodilator, which may redistribute blood flow unequally and demonstrate regional areas of myocardial ischemia. Thallium scintigraphy is then performed in the usual manner. Dipyridamole can be administered either intravenously or orally (with a higher dose) but does have the risk of hypotension (possibly resulting in significant ischemia) or other effects such as bronchoconstriction. The administration of aminophylline can counteract these problems. Patients chronically taking aminophylline preparations are not candidates for dipyridamole thallium imaging since aminophylline blocks the vasodilatation.

Other radionuclide techniques that have not yet achieved wide application include tomographic perfusion imaging and positron emission tomography. Single photon emission computed tomography theoretically should allow precise localization of coronary artery narrowings and areas of myocardial ischemia but has associated drawbacks such as artifact from patient motion.

Blood pool imaging

For noninvasive assessment of myocardial function and contractility, radionuclide imaging is used to generate myocardial images in systole and in diastole (Table 2-8). The patient's red blood cells are labeled with technetium 99m and injected back into the patient. Imaging can then be performed immediately with first-pass imaging or by gated–equilibrium imaging (data acquisition over 5–10-minute periods). The isotope has a half-life of 6 hours.

The first-pass approach collects data from the first circulation of the isotope through the heart. Each ventricle may be visualized separately as the isotope first passes through the right and then the left ventricle. With the gated method, end diastole is timed by the onset of the QRS complex. Since multiple images are collected over time, better resolution of the images is obtained although separation of the right and left ventricles is not ideal.

As with thallium imaging, technical problems limit the study and include improper positioning of the camera, suboptimal labeling of the red blood cells (leading to higher background activity), and arrhythmia which makes proper gating difficult. When these problems are minimal, good quality images provide sufficient data to calculate an accurate left and right ventricular EF. Since the images represent the blood pool and not the structures of the heart, the different chambers can be differentiated. On the right side, the superior vena cava, right atrium, right ventricle, and pulmonary artery are separated; on the left side, the left atrium, left ventricle, and aorta can be distinguished. Dilatation of any chamber can easily be appreciated.

In addition to calculation of EF, regional areas of contractility can be evaluated qualitatively in the same manner as the angiographic ventriculogram. Motion can be graded as normal, hypokinetic, akinetic, or dyskinetic. Regional areas of

Table 2-8   Indications for Stress Radionuclide Ventriculography and Stress Echocardiography

1. Evaluate regional wall motion abnormalities at rest and their response to exercise
2. Evaluate the response of global function as measured by EF to exercise

dysfunction correlate with areas of ischemic or infarcted myocardium or may represent focal cardiomyopathic processes.

Blood pool imaging may be performed at rest and with exercise, allowing comparison of EF and global and regional contractility. In general, the patient with normal left ventricular function will increase the EF with exercise and those with dysfunction will decrease or remain the same. Certainly, these are broad guidelines and exceptions occur. The older patient may be less capable of a large increase in EF due to hemodynamic changes associated with the aging heart.

The severity of valvular regurgitation may be estimated from the data obtained during blood pool imaging. In the absence of regurgitation (or shunting) the stroke volume of the left ventricle should equal that of the right ventricle. By calculating a ratio of right:left ventricular stroke counts, a regurgitant index may be derived to estimate the degree of regurgitation.

ECHOCARDIOGRAPHY AND DOPPLER EXAMINATION

Echocardiography

Few other techniques in medicine provide as much vital information without any apparent risk to the patient as echocardiography and Doppler examination, which can be performed at the bedside as well as in the laboratory. With echocardiography, data can be obtained by M–mode to record echo motion while the transducer is moved. Although no longer the predominant technique, it provides a wealth of information about chamber size, wall thickness, valvular structure, and to a lesser extent about ventricular motion. With the two-dimensional technique, one can even better appreciate mitral valve prolapse, assess global and regional left ventricular motion, describe valvular structures, and delineate intracardiac structures such as thrombus or masses including tumor or vegetations. Today, transesophageal echocardigraphy is being introduced. The Doppler examination adds physiologic flow data to the echo technique and allows calculation of flow as well as valve areas. Valvular regurgitation is quantitated and may be qualitatively demonstrated by color enhancement techniques.

In addition to diagnosis, echocardiographic techniques may be used to follow a particular lesion over time or to judge the response to surgery (e.g., revascularization, valve repair or replacement). The techniques are used in conjunction with other noninvasive techniques such as ambulatory ECG recording and exercise testing to provide a comprehensive assessment of the patient's cardiac condition. Often the information gathered will indicate the need for further invasive studies such as cardiac catheterization. Furthermore, the catheterization correlation with the data obtained noninvasively is excellent. The purpose of this section is not to describe echocardiographic or Doppler techniques but rather to point out how and when to best use them. As previously noted, they are easily accomplished and safely performed. However, financial expenditure is a consideration and the techniques should not be misused.

Coronary artery disease

Echocardiography evaluation of coronary artery disease centers on analysis of global and regional left ventricular function. Occasionally, the left main coronary artery ostium can be visualized, but not often enough and not with sufficient definition to make this a routine part of the examination. Other limitations center on the ability to visualize the endocardium, which may be difficult in an obese patient or one with a very thick chest wall. Without adequate visualization of the thickening and relaxation of the endocardium, it is difficult to comment on function.

Global function can be assessed and EF calculated, although a gated blood pool scan (MUGA) may be better suited for this latter task. Regional motion may be assessed in a manner similar to left ventriculography, characterizing different degrees of contractile abnormalities as akinesis (no motion), hypokinesis (weak motion), dyskinesis (paradoxical motion as seen in aneurysm), or normokinesis (normal motion). Some have calculated the amount of asynergy as a percentage of acontractile segments.

Echocardiography can be performed at rest and also with exercise in those individuals suitable for this technique. Just as the routine exercise test can reflect ischemia by evaluating ST segment changes or thallium imaging by perfusion changes, exercise echocardiography can detect exercise-induced regional contractile abnormalities. Thus, this technique may dynamically demonstrate ischemia and confirm a suspected diagnosis.

When a patient has global left ventricular dysfunction, one suspects extensive ischemic heart disease or a nonischemic cardiomyopathy. Localized regional dysfunction is most often related to myocardial ischemia or infarction. Echocardiography may not only define a discrete aneurysm but also may demonstrate thrombus. Thus, the echocardiogram can confirm the diagnosis of coronary artery disease and indicate areas of jeopardized myocardium, both of which may influence the decision to perform surgery or attempt bypass of a specific coronary vessel. Although left ventriculography is necessary before aneurysm resection, the echocardiographic demonstration of thrombus may indicate the need for extra caution.

The echocardiogram may be particularly useful for evaluating complications of MI. It may easily demonstrate left ventricular aneurysm, pseudoaneurysm, rupture of a papillary muscle (with acute mitral regurgitation), or ventricular septal defect. Furthermore, the ease of performance provides vital information quickly.

Cardiomyopathy

Most nonischemic cardiomyopathies do not require surgery but are often diagnosed in patients initially thought to be candidates for a cardiac surgical procedure. Occasionally these patients will require another type of intervention, such as a pacemaker or automatic internal cardioverter defibrillator (AICD). Obviously, it is important for the surgeon to know the underlying disorder.

Hypertrophic cardiomyopathy: will be recognized by thickened ventricular walls, often with asymmetric septal hypertrophy. In addition there may be systolic anterior motion of the anterior mitral leaflet and midsystolic closure of the aortic valve. Hypertensive cardiomyopathy may result from many years of hypertension, is usually concentric, and must be distinguished from the hypertrophic variety.

Dilated congestive cardiomyopathy: is characterized by a dilated, poorly contractile left and right ventricle. Often the atria are also enlarged. Certain cardiomyopathies may be localized to the right ventricle, such as in arrhythmogenic right ventricular dysplasia, often referred for refractory ventricular arrhythmias.

Infiltrative cardiomyopathy: may be characterized by small ventricular size, often ventricular hypertrophy, and often generalized hypokinesis. One of the most common varieties is amyloid, whose speckled appearance on echocardiography may suggest the diagnosis.

Restrictive cardiomyopathy: reflects difficulty with ventricular relaxation, in which the ventricles cannot fill normally. Although the left ventricle may have minimal findings, the left atrium, right ventricle, and right atrium may be dilated due to elevated left ventricular filling pressures.

Infectious etiologies: of cardiomyopathy such as Chaga's disease in South America represent a major problem for the population. In Chaga's disease, the echocardiogram may display an apical aneurysm.

Valvular heart disease

The greatest benefit to the cardiac surgeon from this noninvasive technique may be seen in patients with valvular disease. In addition to visualizing endocardium and chamber size, valvular leaflets can be characterized in terms of mobility, redundancy, and calcification. Doppler measurements of gradient, cardiac output, and flow across a valve allow calculation of valve area. Degrees of valvular stenosis and regurgitation correlate well with measurements obtained at the time of cardiac catheterization.

Mitral stenosis: The echocardiogram in mitral stenosis reveals a decreased EF slope as well as concordant motion of the anterior and posterior mitral leaflets. The leaflets may be thickened. On two-dimensional study, doming of the mitral valve is noted, as well as a reduction in the valve orifice itself. The rate of diastolic filling of the left ventricle is reduced.

Doppler examination involves measuring the velocity of flow across a valve, which is increased in stenotic lesions. Using the Bernoulli equation, it is possible to calculate the pressure gradient (Table 2-9). Cardiac output is estimated by measuring cross-sectional area at the level of the aortic annulus using the two-dimensional echo and the time-velocity integral (stroke distance) from the Doppler spectral recording. The valve area is calculated by measuring the time in milliseconds required for the diastolic pressure gradient across the mitral valve to fall to half its initial valve (pressure half-time) (see Table 2-9). Correlation with data obtained at cardiac catheterization is excellent,

---

Table 2-9   Common Doppler Measurements

$$\text{Mitral valve area in cm}^2 = \frac{220}{\text{Pressure half-time (msec)}}$$

$$\text{Aortic valve area} = \frac{\text{Area of LVOT} \times \text{Velocity flow at LVOT}}{\text{Velocity flow at aortic valve}}$$

Modified Bernoulli equation for measuring pressure gradient:
$P_1 - P_2 = 4V^2$
V = Peak velocity of blood flow across obstruction

CO = (Flow velocity integral) (Cross-sectional area) (HR)
The equation may be simplified as follows:

$$CO = \frac{(\text{Velocity}) (\text{Ejection time})}{2} \times .785 \text{ (Aortic annular diameter} \times \text{Heart rate)}$$

---

but certainly depends on the quality of data obtained at the echo-Doppler examination.

Aortic stenosis: In aortic stenosis, the echocardiogram reveals thickness of the leaflets, often intense calcification. Opening of the valve is restricted. Systolic doming may be appreciated on the two-dimensional study in patients with a congenital bicuspid valve. Many patients will also have left ventricular hypertrophy.

Doppler examination may overestimate the severity of aortic stenosis because it is the peak rather than the mean gradient that is usually measured. The aortic valve area is calculated using data from the two-dimensional echo measurement of the left ventricular outflow tract and the Doppler-obtained velocities at both the aortic annulus and valve orifice (see Table 2-9).

As with mitral stenosis, the multiple sources of error in making Doppler measurements and calculations are beyond the scope of this presentation.

Mitral regurgitation: The Doppler examination is superior to the echo in evaluating mitral regurgitation. The echo may reveal an enlarged left ventricle and left atrium, but the Doppler will demonstrate regurgitant flow and the resultant turbulence. By measuring flow from various points in the left atrium, the clinician can estimate the degree of mitral regurgitation. Color flow techniques demonstrate the regurgitant flow graphically.

Aortic regurgitation: Aortic regurgitation may occasionally be missed on physical examination but may be nicely demonstrated by echo and Doppler. Characteristically the echocardiogram will show diastolic fluttering on the mitral valve on M-mode. If the left ventricular diastolic pressure is elevated, the mitral valve may close early. In aortic regurgitation, the left ventricle becomes dilated.

Doppler examination reveals the diastolic jet in the left ventricle, again graphically enhanced by color flow. Severity may be measured by quantitating the area of diastolic flow and comparing it to systolic flow.

Other valvular lesions: Echocardiography may be used in a similar fashion to evaluate tricuspid stenosis. Doppler may be particularly useful to document tricuspid regurgitation.

Patients with endocarditis may occasionally have visible vegetations on the affected valves, particularly if involved by certain organisms. Flail leaflets as a result of endocarditis or MI can be observed to "flail" on the two-dimensional echo examination.

Prosthetic valves can be visualized and observed over time to demonstrate normal motion or to document paravalvular leaks, vegetations, or other valve dysfunction.

Mitral valve prolapse is a common finding at echocardiogram due to its frequency in the population but is not a problem referred to the surgeon unless severe valve dysfunction occurs.

Pericardial disease

The echocardiogram is frequently used to evaluate the possibility of pericardial effusion. It may be necessary to differentiate pericardial effusion from pleural effusion. Occasionally the patient with pericardial tamponade is evaluated prior to pericardiocentesis. However, it should be remembered that the pulmonary artery catheterization revealing diastolic equilibration and hemodynamic compromise may be the diagnostic procedure of choice. In patients with constrictive pericarditis, the echocardiogram may demonstrate a variety of findings although none may be pathognomonic.

AMBULATORY ELECTROCARDIOGRAPHIC RECORDING

While the standard 12-lead ECG provides information about rhythm and ST segments at a fixed point in time, the 24- or 48-hour recording provides dynamic information over a period of time. It may reveal sustained or nonsustained arrhythmias, heart block, or ischemia. Ongoing ischemia despite medical therapy may indicate a need for further therapy, possibly even revascularization.

It is important for the physician to be aware of serious arrhythmias prior to cardiac surgery, whether they be atrial, ventricular, or preexcitation. In some cases, additional procedures may be necessary and may include ablation of a tachycardia zone, implantation of an AICD or pacemaker, or interruption of an accessory bypass tract.

The procedure is fairly simple. It involves attachment of chest electrodes connected to a recorder usually the size of a small transistor radio. The patient wears the recorder over the shoulder for 1–2 days, after which time the information is retrieved. Endless loop event recorders are also available in which the patient is able to trigger the recorder when the arrhythmia occurs, thus capturing it for transmission to a central station.

Depending on the results, the patient may or may not require further evaluation, such as electrophysiology study. Today another technique is now available, the *signal-averaged ECG*. This technique analyzes multiple ECG signals obtained through a special filter and specifically looks at the terminal portion of the QRS segment. The presence of late and low amplitude signals indicates an increased risk of serious ventricular arrhythmias. Depending on the clinical situation, it may be appropriate to have some of these patients undergo electrophysiologic evaluation.

CARDIAC CATHETERIZATION

Commonly and routinely performed, cardiac catheterization involves measurement of intracardiac pressures, oxygen saturations, cardiac output, and calculation of hemodynamic variables in addition to coronary arteriography and left ventriculography. Although the procedure carries certain risks, they should not deter any patient who really needs the procedure from having it performed. Generally patients are informed of a 0.1%–0.2% risk of a major complication including death, MI, cerebrovascular accident, or injury to a blood vessel or the heart (i.e., perforation). The risk for a patient with critical aortic stenosis or left main obstruction may be higher and for patients with only minor disease, the risks are much lower. Even for the most critically ill patient, cardiac catheterization usually will merit the risk, particularly if it permits a lifesaving therapeutic procedure such as angioplasty or cardiac surgery.

Hemodynamic evaluation

Measurement of the intracardiac pressures permits an assessment of cardiac function in addition to allowing calculation of valve areas in patients with obstructive lesions. Intracardiac pressures will be elevated in valvular stenosis and similarly in left ventricular or right ventricular failure. This subject will be discussed in detail in Chapter 3. Calculation of the systemic vascular resistance may permit the administration of certain medications such as vasodilators in heart failure which may improve the overall efficiency of the heart. A fixed pulmonary vascular resistance may be an ominous sign in patients with advanced mitral stenosis. Measurement of oxygen saturations permits calculation of the cardiac output by Fick principle (provided oxygen consumption is also simultaneously measured). This result may be compared with the cardiac output obtained by thermodilution measurements or green dye curves. Oxygen step-ups may indicate atrial or ventricular septal defects.

Cardiac catheterization

For the patient with ischemic heart disease, coronary arteriography is the "gold standard" for establishing the location and severity of coronary artery narrowings (Table 2-10). Coronary arteriography may be performed by either the femoral artery (Judkins technique) or brachial artery (Sones technique) approach. The selection of technique depends on the preference of the center as well as the severity of peripheral vascular disease. If the iliac arteries are occluded or if the aorta is extremely tortuous, it may not be possible to advance the catheters to the ostia of the coronary arteries, or the tortuosity may not allow manipulation of the catheter. In this situation, the brachial artery approach will be necessary. Contraindications to cardiac catheterization are listed in Table 2-11.

Table 2-10 Indications for Coronary Arteriography and Cardiac Catheterization

1. Establish a diagnosis of coronary artery disease in patients with nondiagnostic noninvasive studies
2. Determine the severity and location of coronary artery narrowings in patients with known coronary artery disease on the basis of history or previous exercise test particularly when coronary angioplasty or CABG surgery is anticipated
3. Characterize the coronary artery anatomy in patients with unstable angina in whom exercise testing is contraindicated
4. Evaluate patients after MI
   a. Particularly if thrombolytic therapy has salvaged myocardium but in whom a residual eccentric high grade narrowing is suspected
   b. When continued ischemia suggests the presence of other critically narrowed coronary arteries
   c. To assess the severity of disease particularly in a young individual (controversial if no residual ischemia)
   d. If they experience complications such as:
      i. Ventricular septal defect
      ii. Rupture of papillary muscle leading to acute mitral regurgitation
      iii. Cardiogenic shock
      iv. Congestive heart failure related to a potentially correctible lesion such as a discrete aneurysm
   e. If chest pain continues without a diagnosis
5. Evaluate patients with cardiogenic shock in the acute phase of MI who might benefit from acute angioplasty
6. Evaluate recurrent angina or ischemia in patients who have previously undergone coronary angioplasty or CABG surgery
7. Establish a diagnosis in survivors of sudden cardiac arrest
8. Evaluate the coronary anatomy in patients who require valvular sugery
9. Make a diagnosis of vasospastic angina in patients with suspicious symptoms but nondiagnostic nonivasive studies (provocative study with ergonovine)
10. Evaluate the possibility of coronary artery disease in asymptomatic patients with markedly abnormal noninvasive studies suggesting silent myocardial ischemia
11. Evaluate suspected left main stenosis
12. Evaluate atypical symptoms or noninvasive studies suspicious for ischemia in individuals in high-risk populations (e.g., pilots)
13. Evaluate potentially correctible causes of heart failure
14. Evaluate other types of potentially correctible cardiac disorders such as atrial septal defect, hypertrophic cardiomyopathy, or other congential heart disease
15. Evaluate the possibility of a coronary artery anomaly

Table 2-11   Contraindications to Coronary Arteriography

1. Prior anaphylactic reaction to contrast media unless desensitized or premedicated with the assistance of an allergy consultant
2. Absolute refusal of patient to undergo recommended or necessary therapeutic procedure such as cardiac surgery or angioplasty
3. Very advanced degree of physical debility
4. Very severe chronic disease such as cancer with poor prognosis
5. Failure to obtain informed consent

Femoral artery approach: The femoral artery is percutaneously entered via direct arterial puncture and a guidewire advanced into the aorta. The coronary catheter may be directly advanced over the guidewire or a femoral artery sheath inserted. The sheath permits easier access, particularly when multiple catheters are necessary. A guidewire is still used to facilitate advancement of the catheter into the aortic arch. Various preformed catheter shapes are available for cannulating not only the native coronary artery but also for saphenous vein or internal mammary artery grafts. Depending on the degree of tortuosity or dilatation of the aorta, one particular shape may be more advantageous. Most commonly, the Judkins shape of catheter is used. The Amplatz shape catheter is also useful but may require more caution because it may advance down the coronary artery if not manipulated properly. After the coronary arteriograms are completed and the procedure finished, the catheter and sheath are removed, with hemostatis achieved by direct compression.

Brachial artery approach: Access to the brachial artery is achieved by cutdown in the antecubital fossa. The operator must be skilled in arteriotomy and repair. Uncommonly, brachial artery catheterization may have a higher complication rate if the artery is more atherosclerotic (often these are the patients whose severe peripheral vascular disease did not permit the femoral approach), making it easier to dissect, and more difficult to repair. Once access is achieved, the catheter is advanced with a guidewire into the aortic arch. Using the Sones catheter, cannulation of both coronary ostia and entry into the left ventricle are possible, avoiding the need for catheter exchange.

Often more technical skill manipulating the catheter is necessary than with the Judkins approach. After the catheterization is completed, the catheter is withdrawn and the arteriotomy repaired.

Coronary arteriogram: Because this cineangiogram will determine the diagnosis and therapy, appropriate views of the arteries are necessary. One must endeavor to obtain all the necessary shots to avoid having the cardiac surgeon asking for more views (necessitating a second procedure). The coronary arteries must be separated from one another to avoid overlap. Angulated views are now routinely obtained with each catheterization. To best visualize the left main coronary artery, a shallow right anterior oblique (RAO) and a caudal left anterior oblique (LAO) view should be used. The left anterior descending artery is visualized best on cranial RAO, cranial LAO, and lateral views. The diagonal arteries are separated from the left anterior descending artery on the cranial RAO and LAO views. Left circumflex marginals are often best demonstrated with a caudal RAO projection. The right coronary artery and its posterior descending and posterolateral branches are viewed in RAO, LAO, and lateral views. When arteries are totally or partially occluded, one should look for collateral flow from other patent arteries. Often this means panning the camera to the appropriate segment of myocardium to look for late filling. In patients with grafts to the coronary arteries, views of the entire length of the graft as well as the anastomotic site are necessary. Several projections are required.

Coronary arteriography is a procedure that requires technical skill and clinical judgment. The injections must fill the arteries adequately, but not too long because of a risk of causing arrhythmias, heart block, or ischemia. The proper views and angulations must be achieved. Care must be taken to avoid injuring the coronary artery or dissecting an atherosclerotic plaque.

Left ventriculography

The left ventriculogram represents the "gold standard" for global and regional left ventricular function. It is routinely obtained in a biplane projection (both RAO and LAO views). In addition to function, the degree of mitral regurgitation, if any, can be judged. One must be cautious, however, if ventricular ectopy occurs during the ventriculogram because this may cause regurgitation not present under ordinary circumstances.

In some patients with critical left main disease, the left ventriculogram may not always be performed because it adds risk and cardiac surgery will be necessary in any event. Noninvasive evaluation of left ventricular function with a radionuclide ventriculogram may suffice.

Aortography

In some patients with valvular regurgitation, an aortic root injection is necessary to evaluate the degree of aortic regurgitation. In addition to making a decision about valve replacement, the presence of aortic regurgitation may necessitate cardioplegia directly down the coronary artery during surgery rather than an injection into the root. Aortography may also help visualize previous bypass grafts.

ELECTROPHYSIOLOGIC TESTING

The electrophysiology study is a safe invasive procedure designed to assist in the diagnosis of cardiac arrhythmias and to guide pharmacologic therapy. It may be wiser to obtain knowledge about the exact mechansim of the arrhythmia and the response to drugs than to proceed with empiric therapy. Pacemaker electrodes are percutaneously advanced to positions in the right atrium, right ventricle, across the bundle of His, and occasionally the coronary sinus. Baseline conduction is measured and provocative stimulation of the atria and ventricles is performed.

Arrhythmia induction provides correlation with out-of-hospital arrhythmias and allows assessment of the mechanism. Pharmacologic therapy can be administered intravenously with acute observation of the response. Responders may be discharged on oral preparations of successful intravenous drugs. Patients who fail to respond to initial drug therapy may require additional trials of other agents or may be candidates for antitachycardia pacemakers or AICDs, depending on the arrhythmia. Certain patients with bradyarrhythmia or heart block may be candidates for permanent single chamber or dual chamber pacemakers.

In patients with serious life-threatening ventricular arrhythmias, the physician must be aware that CABG surgery

Table 2-12	Indications for Electrophysiologic Study

1. Ventricular fibrillation or sustained ventricular tachycardia not associated with acute MI
2. Severely symptomatic supraventricular tachycardia refractory to pharmacologic therapy
3. Severely symptomatic patients with preexcitation syndromes (such as WPW syndrome) who are at risk for sudden cardiovascular collapse
4. Symptomatic patients in whom sustained ventricular tachycardia may be suspected but not documented
5. Diagnosis of wide complex tachycardia or other unknown arrhythmia
6. Patients with syncope after all other possibilities (including neurologic, vascular, and metabolic) have been excluded
7. Documentation of conduction disturbance in symptomatic patients in whom the diagnosis has not been made by ambulatory ECG recording
8. Serial drug testing for refractory arrhythmia
9. Selected patients with complex ventricular ectopy or nonsustained ventricular tachycardia in the pressence of serious underlying heart disease in whom empiric therapy with type 1 antiarrhythmic drugs is potentially hazardous
10. Selected patients with an abnormal signal-averaged ECG

alone for coronary artery disease will not correct the arrhythmia. These patients must be fully evaluated prior to surgery so that the appropriate adjunct procedures can be performed. The indications of electrophysiologic study are listed in Table 2-12.

The risks are minimal and are outweighed by the benefits. Physicians should not hesitate to recommend the procedure when appropriate. Failure to adequately treat ventricular arrhythmias may negate any benefit achieved from any other cardiac surgical procedure.

SUGGESTED READING

Many of these textbooks have been updated in later editions.

Cardiac surgery

Glenn WWL, Bave AE, Geha AS, Hammond GL, Laks H. *Thoracic and Cardiovascular Surgery.* 4th ed. Norwalk, CT: Appelton-Century Crofts; 1983.

Kirklin JW, Barratt-Boyes BG. *Cardiac Surgery.* New York: John Wiley & Sons; 1986.

Schwartz SI, Shires GT, Spencer FC, Storer EH. *Principles of Surgery.* 4th ed. New York: McGraw-Hill; 1984.

Cardiology

Braunwald E. *Heart Disease.* 3rd ed. Philadelphia: WB Saunders; 1988.

Hurst JW, Logue RB, Rackley CE, et al. *The Heart.* 5th ed. New York: McGraw-Hill; 1982.

In addition to standard textbooks on cardiology, the reader may wish to consult some of these subspecialty texts.

Ellestad MH. *Stress Testing.* Philadelphia: FA Davis; 1986.

Feigenbaum H. *Echocardiography.* 4th ed. Philadelphia: Lea & Febiger; 1986.

Grossman W. *Cardiac Catheterization and Angioplasty.* 2nd ed. Philadelphia: Lea & Febiger; 1980.

King SB, Douglas JS. *Coronary Arteriography and Angioplasty.* New York: McGraw-Hill; 1985.

Vlietstra RE, Holmes DR. *PTCA.* Philadelphia: FA David; 1986.

Vlay SC, ed. Manual of cardiac arrhythmias. Boston: Little, Brown & Co, 1988.

Valvuloplasty

Cribier A, et al. Percutaneous transluminal balloon valvuloplasty of adult aortic stenosis: report of 92 cases. *J Am Coll Cardiol.* 1987;9:381–386.

Holmes DR. Balloon valvuloplasty for aortic stenosis. *Hosp Pract.* January 15, 1990:69–77.

Mckay RGP. Balloon valvuloplasty for treating pulmonic, mitral and aortic valve stenosis. *Am J Cardiol.* 1988;61:102G.

Palacios IF, et al. Followup of patients undergoing percutaneous mitral balloon valvulotomy: analysis of factors determining restenosis. *Circulation.* 1989;79:573.

Powers ER. Balloon valvuloplasty for mitral stenosis. *Hosp Prac.* May 30, 1990:37–46.

Richenbacher WE, Myers JL, Waldhausen JA. Current status of cardiac surgery: A 40 year review. *J Am Coll Cardiol.* 1989;14:535–544.

Other Reading

Bonow RO, Dodd JT, Maron BJ, et al. Long-term serial changes in left ventricular function and reversal of ventricular dilatation after valve replacement for chronic aortic regurgitation. *Circulation*. 1988; 78:1108–1120.

Cardiovascular Surgery 1988, Part I. *Circulation*. 1989;80:I-1–279.

CASS, Principal Investigators, et al. The National Heart, Lung and Blood Institute Coronary Artery Surgery Study. *Circulation*. 1981;63 (suppl I):1–81.

CASS, Principal Investigators, et al. CASS A randomized trial of cornary artery bypass surgery: Survival data. *Circulation* 1983;68:939–950.

European Coronary Surgery Study Group. Long-term results of prospective-randomized study of coronary artery bypass surgery in stable angina pectoris. *Lancet* 1982;2:1173–1180.

Hwang MH, Hammermeister KE, Oprian C, et al. Preoperative identification of patients likely to have left ventricular dysfunction after aortic valve replacement. *Circulation*. 1989;80(suppl I):65–76.

Levison JR, Akins CW, Buckley MJ, et al. Octogenarians with aortic stenosis. Outcome after aortic valve replacement. *Circulation*. 1989; 80 (suppl I):49–56.

Nishimura RA, McGoon MD, Schaff HV, Giuliani ER. Chronic aortic regurgitation: indications for operation—1988. *Mayo Clin Proc*. 1988;63:270–280.

Siemienczuk D, Greenberg B, Morris C, et al. Chronic aortic insufficiency: factors associated with progression to aortic valve replacement. *Ann Intern Med*. 1989; 110:587–592.

State-of-the-Art Symposium on Coronary Arterial Surgery. *Circulation*. 1989;79:I-1–192.

Veterans Administration Coronary Artery Bypass Surgery Cooperative Study. Eleven-year survival in the Veterans Administration randomized trial of cornary bypass surgery for stable angina. *N Engl J Med*. 1984;311:1333–1339.

HEMODYNAMIC EVALUATION

William E. Lawson, M.D.

3

An understanding of hemodynamic data and their proper interpretation is vital for the preoperative assessment of the cardiac surgery patient. Hemodynamics complement the anatomic information obtained by cardiac catheterization to yield a more complete knowledge of both the pathophysiology and functional significance of cardiac lesions. Perioperative management of the cardiac surgery patient depends on knowledge of and proper use of this information.

BACKGROUND

Pressures in the heart are generally measured by fluid-filled catheters connecting to fluid-filled transducers coupled to electrical strain gauges. The use of a fluid-transmitting medium can cause problems with temporal delay and signal fidelity. Higher fidelity and virtually instantaneous (speed of light) transmission can be obtained with catheter tip transducers (Millar instruments) but at an increased cost and set-up time.

Several general caveats apply to ensuring accurate and reproducible pressure measurements.

1. An appropriate zero reference level (most commonly mid chest level with the patient supine) must be chosen and the scale should be calibrated using a manometer. Pressures are usually recorded in mm Hg (1 mm Hg = 13.6 mm H_2O).
2. An appropriate time and amplitude scale for display, analysis, and recording is chosen. Too small an amplitude scale will result in information being lost off screen; too large an

amplitude scale decreases the accuracy of pressure measurements. Similarly, slow time scales are often appropriate for peak, nadir, and mean measurements but will not allow accurate assessment of transvalvular gradients. A calibration signal (zero pressure, standardized pressure, and time interval) routinely recorded prior to and immediately after recording pressures allows confirmation of the reliability of recordings.

3. Because of the effect of breathing on intracardiac pressures, obtained measurements are usually averaged over two to three respiratory cycles. However, in instances of marked respiratory variation, pressures are usually recorded at end expiration.

Several technical considerations allowing optimization of pressure recording fidelity also must be observed.

1. Eliminate unnecessary stopcocks.
2. Minimize connector pressure tubing length.
3. Flush lines thoroughly, tapping and inspecting for air bubbles (a damped pressure recording is most commonly due to blood or air in the system).
4. Check that all connections are tight, but do not overtighten and risk stripping the threading.
5. Pressures are recorded preferably before obtaining blood samples or filling the catheter with contrast.
6. The catheter should probably be at least 6F in size. Although catheter length choices are limited, shorter is better for pressure measurements.

Measurement of pressures in the patient intubated on positive end–expiratory pressure (PEEP) requires special discussion and consideration. Although some authorities have advocated taking the patient off PEEP and placing him on 100% O_2 for the duration of making pressure measurements, the patient is often too ill for this to be a realistic option. The use of PEEP makes it mandatory to check Swan-Ganz catheter tip position. In the supine position under normal conditions most of the lung is in West's zone III. In zone III both arterial and venous pressures exceed alveolar pressure. The pulmonary capillary wedge (PCW) pressure most accurately reflects the left atrial pressure when measured in zone III because there is a continuously open fluid–filled channel between the PCW and left atrium at this level. In zone I, alveolar pressure exceeds arterial and venous pressures, resulting in collapse of the connecting vasculature. In zone II, alveolar exceeds venous, but not arterial pressure, resulting in partial collapse of the connecting vasculature. With PEEP, the alveolar pressure is increased and a catheter tip that was in zone III may now be in zone I or II. Zone III pressures will be obtained if the catheter tip is placed at or below the level of the left atrium (on cross-table lateral chest x-ray). A PEEP of less than 10 cm H_2O generally has no significant effect on measured PCW pressure.

THE PATIENT WITH CORONARY ARTERY DISEASE

Hemodynamic evaluation of the coronary artery disease patient for revascularization may include both right and left heart catheterization. Right heart catheterization allows measurement of intracardiac pressures and cardiac output, enabling risk stratification by hemodynamic subsets and appropriately targeted therapy. Risks associated with right heart catheterization have lessened with increased experience with the technique, its complications, and catheter improvements. Table 3-1 lists the major risks of right heart catheterization. The particular risks vary with the route and duration of monitoring. The femoral vein route poses the greatest risk of infection, thrombosis, and pulmonary embolism. The jugular vein approach is associated with a risk of carotid artery perforation. The subclavian vein

Table 3-1   Swan-Ganz Catheterization

Major risks	Incidence
Atrial and ventricular arrhythmias	30–60% (usually not requiring therapy)
Right bundle branch block	3–6%
Pneumothorax	1–6% (highest with subclavian vein)
Hemorrhage	Highest with subclavian vein
Pulmonary infarction	1.3%
Septicemia	0.5–1.0% (highest with femoral vein)
Thrombosis, pulmonary embolism	Highest with femoral vein
Pulmonary artery rupture	0.1–0.2%
Hemorrhage	Greatest risk with subclavian approach

Table 3-2   Normal Pressures (mm Hg)

Right atrium	a/v wave	2–10/2–8
	mean	2–8
Right ventricle	peak systole/end diastole	15–25/2–8
Pulmonary artery	peak systole/ end diastole	15–25/4–12
	mean	8–16
PCW	a/v wave	4–10/4–15
	mean	4–12
Left ventricle	peak systole/end diastole	90–150/4–12
Aorta	peak systole/end diastole	90–150/60–90
	mean	70–110

approach has the notable risks of pneumothorax, hemothorax, and less commonly brachial plexus trauma. With a significant bleeding diathesis the antebrachial approach is probably the safest.

Right heart catheterization is generally performed under fluoroscopy or continuous pressure monitoring using a flow-directed balloon tipped (Swan-Ganz) catheter. Models available range from a simple end-hole catheter allowing oximetry and pressure measurement to multiple port and thermistor versions allowing simultaneous measurements in several chambers, pacing, and thermodilution cardiac outputs.

During right heart catheterization the right atrial, right ventricular, pulmonary arterial, and PCW pressures are recorded. Table 3-2 shows normal values. The pressure waveforms of the respective atria, ventricles, and great vessels (aorta and pulmonary artery) are generally similar in morphology, though left-sided pressures are normally higher than their respective right counterparts (Figure 3-1). Peak systolic and end-diastolic pressures are recorded as the systolic and diastolic pressure, respectively.

The right and left atria normally show three positive pressure deflections (the a, c, and v waves) and two negative pressure deflections (the x and y descents) during each cardiac cycle. The a wave is caused by atrial contraction. The following c wave is caused by atrioventricular (AV) (mitral/tricuspid) valve closure. The x descent results from subsequent atrial relaxation and descent of the AV valve annulus. The v wave occurs next due to atrial filling while the AV valve is closed. The y descent

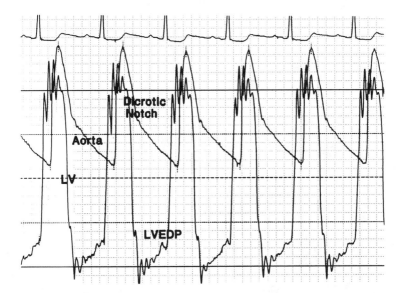

Figure 3-1: Simultaneous recording of LV (left ventricular) and aortic pressures in a normal patient. Note the time delay in pressure transmission from LV to distal aorta. Note timing of the LVEDP (left ventricular end-diastolic pressure) at end diastole and Dicrotic Notch at end systole.

follows and reflects early atrial emptying following AV valve opening. In the right atrium the a wave normally exceeds the v wave; the opposite is true in the left atrium (reflecting differing right and left ventricular compliances).

While the right atrial and PCW (left atrial) pressures are usually recorded as mean values, a knowledge of the normal and abnormal waveform morphology may be helpful (Table 3-3). For instance, papillary muscle dysfunction resulting in acute mitral regurgitation might be demonstrated as a filling in of the normal *x* descent with a large cv wave with preservation of the *y* descent. Analysis of right atrial and PCW waveforms can also be helpful in detecting atrial activity (presence of a waves) and assessing its relation to ventricular contraction. For instance, large "cannon" a waves are seen in the right atrium when atrial contraction occurs with a closed tricuspid valve (during ventricular systole) and may be demonstrated with complete heart block and ventricular premature complexes.

The right and left ventricular pressure waveforms (see

Table 3-3   Atrial Pressure Morphology (Common Abnormalities)

a wave	Increased	AV valve stenosis
		Ventricular hypertrophy
	Decreased	Postoperatively following cannulation of the right atrium during heart surgery
	Loss	Atrial fibrillation
x descent	Decreased	Postoperatively following cannulation of the right atrium during heart surgery
		Atrial fibrillation
	Loss	AV valve regurgitation; filling in by cv wave
v wave	Increased	AV valve regurgitation
y descent	Increased	AV valve regurgitation
		Congestive heart failure
		Constrictive pericarditis
	Decreased	AV valve stenosis
		Ventricular hypertrophy

Figure 3-1) can be divided into systolic and diastolic components. Systole begins with the closure of the AV (tricuspid/mitral) valve. This is followed by a rapid rise in pressure during isovolumic contraction ending with semilunar (aortic/pulmonary) valve opening and systolic ejection. Diastole begins with closure of the semilunar valve, terminating systolic ejection and beginning isovolumic relaxation. The ventricular pressure continues to fall as the AV valve opens and rapid filling of the ventricle ensues. Ventricular pressures rise gradually with early rapid and slower mid-diastolic filling. Diastasis may be reached with slow heart rates, compliant ventricles, and constrictive physiology. Diastole ends with atrial systole giving a booster kick to ventricular filling (a wave on right atrial or PCW pressure tracing) just prior to AV valve closure.

The arterial (pulmonary/aorta) waveform is characterized by a rapid initial rise in pressure coincident with semilunar valve opening and systolic ejection. Systolic ejection is terminated with semilunar valve closure (recorded as the dicrotic notch) and is followed by a slow decline in pressure to end diastole.

In the patient without cardiovascular or pulmonary disease the mean right atrial pressure is useful in evaluating intravascular volume status and ventricular preload. However, in the cardiac surgery patient the mean right atrial pressure (in the absence of significant tricuspid valve disease) is more commonly used to monitor right ventricular end-diastolic pressure and filling.

The pulmonary artery pressure is useful in assessing the degree of pulmonary hypertension. Mean pulmonary artery pressure may be obtained as an electrical mean or alternatively calculated as pulmonary artery diastolic pressure plus ⅓ the pulse pressure (PAS − PAD). The pulmonary artery diastolic pressure is usually in close agreement with the PCW in the absence of pulmonary disease. If the pulmonary artery diastolic pressure exceeds the mean PCW by more than 4 mm Hg, it signifies an elevated pulmonary vascular resistance and pulmonary disease. The mean PCW may exceed the pulmonary artery diastolic pressure when a large v wave is present (usually with mitral regurgitation).

The PCW pressure is typically recorded with the inflated Swan-Ganz balloon floated to a wedge position (occluding the pulmonary artery branch) so that the pressure waveform detected is a direct transmission of left atrial pressure across the pulmonary bed. Proper wedging of the balloon can be confirmed by slowly withdrawing blood for oximetry from the port distal to the inflated balloon (discard the first 10–15mL of blood withdrawn). A true PCW will have an oxygen saturation greater than or equal to arterial saturation (i.e., greater than 95%). The electrical mean of at least three to five cycles of PCW pressure is taken as the mean PCW, in the absence of marked respiratory variation. If marked respiratory variability is present, the PCW mean is usually calculated during lightly held end expiration (Figure 3-2).

An elevated mean PCW pressure is a reliable measure of the severity of pulmonary vascular congestion, as well as being an accurate predictor of perioperative pulmonary edema. An elevated PCW pressure may modify the choice of anesthesia (e.g., nitrous oxide might be avoided during anesthesia induction). Postoperatively both an elevated mean PCW pressure and prominent v waves may be sensitive indices of myocardial ischemia or infarction.

The PCW pressure normally reflects left ventricular end-diastolic pressure (LVEDP). It is not uncommon, however, for the LVEDP to significantly exceed the mean PCW pressure

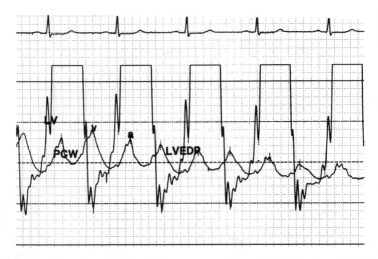

Figure 3-2: Normal, simultaneous recording of LV (left ventricular) and PCW (pulmonary capillary wedge) pressures. Note "a" and "v" waves on PCW caused by atrial and ventricular contraction respectively. Note absence of diastolic pressure gradient across the mitral valve.

when left ventricular compliance is decreased from conditions such as ischemia or hypertrophy. With acute severe aortic insufficiency, left ventricular pressure may exceed left atrial pressure by mid diastole, closing the mitral value prematurely and resulting in a "reverse" transmitral gradient.

The mean PCW pressure does not accurately reflect the LVEDP in the presence of significant mitral valve disease. Mitral regurgitation may result in giant v waves as left ventricular blood leaks into the left atrium during systole (Figure 3-3). The actual v wave size is a function of many factors including afterload, regurgitant volume, left atrial size and compliance, preload, and heart rate. A v wave greater than twice the mean PCW pressure usually indicates mitral regurgitation. The absence of a large v wave does not, however, exclude mitral regurgitation. Larger than normal v waves may also be noted with decreased left ventricular compliance and increased flow volumes (such as in a ventricular septal defect [VSD]).

In mitral stenosis a pressure gradient is present across the mitral valve during diastole. The more severe the stenosis, the greater the transmitral diastolic gradient and the longer it will

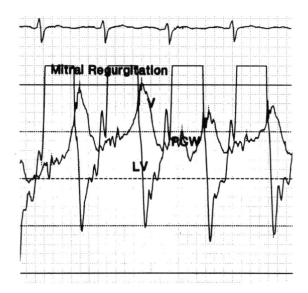

Figure 3-3: Mitral regurgitation. Simultaneous recording of PCW (pulmonary capillary wedge) and LV (left ventricular) pressures. Note the delayed large "v" waves in the PCW tracing detected as the mitral regurgitation is transmitted across the pulmonary vascular bed.

take during diastole for left atrial and left ventricular pressures to equalize (diastasis). This can be differentiated from mitral regurgitation, where a large gradient may be noted in early diastole, by the delayed time course of gradient diminution with mitral stenosis.

Cardiac output

The Fick principle is commonly used to measure cardiac output. The Fick principle states that the amount of a substance released or extracted by an organ is the product of blood flow and the arteriovenous difference (a − v) in concentration.

The *Fick oxygen consumption method* is a direct application of this method. The amount of O_2 extracted by the lungs is measured using a Douglas bag or more commonly by a polarographic oxygen sensor cell and a hood (Waters instruments metabolic rate meter). Pulmonary artery and systemic artery oxygen contents are measured to determine the amount of oxygen extracted by the lungs. In the absence of shunts the pulmonary blood flow equals the cardiac output. Low cardiac outputs are most accurately determined by this technique because the $(a - v)$ O_2 is increased, decreasing the relative error of measurement of the $(a - v)$ O_2 difference.

$$\text{Cardiac output} = O_2 \text{ consumption}/ (a - v)\ O_2 \text{ difference}$$

Example: Given: O_2 consumption of 200 mL O_2/min
Hemoglobin (Hb) of 10 g/dL
Pulmonary artery saturation of 70%
Arterial saturation of 100%
Calculate the cardiac output.

1. O_2-carrying capacity of blood = Hb × 13.6
   10 × 13.6 = 136 mL O_2/L blood
2. Oxygen content of arterial blood = carrying capacity × saturation
   136 × 100% = 136 mL O_2/L blood
3. Oxygen content of mixed venous (pulmonary artery) blood
   136 × 70% = 95 mL O_2/L blood
4. $(a - v)$ O_2 difference = arterial − venous O_2 content
   136 − 95 = 41 mL O_2/L blood
5. Cardiac output = O_2 consumption/ $(a - v)$ O_2 difference
   200/ 41 = 4.9 L/min

Cardiac output is also commonly measured by the *indicator dilution* method, which is an application of the Fick principle. A known quantity of an indicator is injected at a specific site. Continuous downstream monitoring of indicator concentration in the blood is performed and recorded as a time-concentration curve. This time-concentration plot shows an initial time delay between indicator injection and its first arrival downstream. This is followed by a gradual rise and then a decline in indicator concentration. If recirculation (second time around) takes place, a second rise in concentration will be noted, interrupting the first-pass fall in concentration. The formula for the indicator dilution cardiac output method is:

$$\text{Cardiac output} = \text{Indicator amount}/\text{Mean indicator}$$
$$\text{concentration} \times \text{Duration of first pass}$$

In the absence of significant recirculation (as in the *thermodilution* technique) the area under the time-concentration curve is equal to the mean first-pass indicator concentration × the

Table 3-4   Cardiac Output Methods

	Error	Accuracy lessened
Fick O_2 consumption	10%	High cardiac output
Thermodilution	5–10%	Low cardiac output
		Tricuspid insufficiency
Indocyanine green dye	5–10%	Low cardiac output
		Tricuspid insufficiency

first-pass duration. This area may be calculated by planimetry; more commonly computer analysis is used. Higher cardiac outputs result in smaller time-concentration areas (i.e., the indicator is more dilute, with a faster transit time).

The thermodilution technique overestimates cardiac outputs in low flow states (cardiac output under 3.5 L/min) and with significant tricuspid insufficiency because of the loss of the cold indicator (due to increased warming of the cold injectate by the body) with slow transit times. The smaller area under the time-concentration curve will falsely and consistently increase the calculated cardiac output.

When significant recirculation is present, as in the *indocyanine green dye* indicator technique, a second rise in indicator concentration is seen. To eliminate second-pass effects the time-concentration curve is first replotted on semilog paper. The fall in first-pass concentration from its peak is linear on the semilog replot and can be extrapolated to yield the time to zero first-pass concentration. The planimetered area under this constructed first-pass curve equals the mean first-pass indicator concentration × the first-pass duration.

Severe valvular regurgitation and low cardiac outputs can make it impossible to accurately separate the first-pass curve from subsequent indicator recirculation (there is insufficient dye concentration decline after initial peak to allow extrapolation of the first pass concentration decline before recirculation occurs). Intracardiac shunts will also interfere with this technique, causing early recirculation. Table 3-4 summarizes the error rates and accuracies of the methods.

Derived indices and hemodynamic subsets

The four major determinants of left ventricular function are preload, afterload, contractility, and heart rate. Preload is reflected in the filling pressure (PCW or LVEDP) which correlates

---

Table 3-5   Derived Indices

Cardiac output	CO	
Cardiac index	CI	= CO/Body surface area (BSA)
Stroke volume	SV	= CO/Heart rate
Stroke volume index	SVI	= SV/BSA
Pulmonary vascular resistance	PVR	= (mean PA − mean PCW) × 80/CO
Systemic vascular resistance	SVR	= (mean BP − mean RA) × 80/CO
Stroke work	SW	= SV × (mean BP − mean PCW) × .0136
Stroke work index	SWI	= SVI × (mean BP − mean PCW) × .0136

Normal values	
CI =	$2.6–4.2 \ \text{L/min/m}^2$
SVI =	$30–65 \ \text{mL/beat/m}^2$
PVR =	$20–130 \ \text{dynes sec cm}^{-5}$
SVR =	$700–1600 \ \text{dynes sec cm}^{-5}$
SWI =	$30–90 \ \text{g} \cdot \text{m/m}^2$

---

with end–diastolic volume. Afterload is calculated as the resistance to flow using the general formula (Table 3-5):

$$\text{Resistance} = \text{Pressure difference/Flow}$$

The pressure difference is the drop in pressure across the specific vascular bed. The flow equals the cardiac output in the absence of shunts. A conversion factor of ×80 is used to convert the resultant resistance units to dynes sec cm^{-5}.

> Example: A patient has the following measurements made:
>
> | | | | |
> |---|---|---|---|
> | BP | 150/90 mm Hg | CO | 5 L/min |
> | RA mean | 5 mm Hg | PCW mean | 12 mm Hg |
> | PA | 25/10 mm Hg | | |
>
> What are his systemic and pulmonary vascular resistances?

1. Systemic vascular resistance = [Mean BP − mean RA] × 80/CO
   Mean BP = End-diastolic BP + ⅓ pulse pressure
   $$90 + 20 = 110$$
   SVR = [110 − 5] × 80/5 = 1680 dynes sec cm^{-5}
2. Pulmonary vascular resistance = [Mean PA − mean PCW] × 80/CO
   Mean PA = End-diastolic PA + ⅓ pulse pressure
   $$10 + 5 = 15$$
   PVR = [15 − 12] × 80/5 = 48 dynes sec cm^{-5}

The amount of blood ejected with each heart beat, the stroke volume, can be figured by dividing the cardiac output by the heart rate. Both the cardiac output and the stroke volume are commonly normalized for the patient's size by dividing by the body surface area (BSA). This yields the cardiac index (L/min/m^2) and the stroke volume index (mL/beat/m^2).

Example: Given: CO = 5 L/min   Heart rate = 50 bpm
BSA = 2.0 m^2
Calculate the stroke volume, stroke index, cardiac index.

1. Stroke volume $= \dfrac{\text{Cardiac output}}{\text{Heart rate}}$ or $\dfrac{5000 \text{ mL/min}}{50 \text{ bpm}} = 100$ mL/beat

2. Stroke index $= \dfrac{\text{Stroke volume}}{\text{BSA}}$ or $\dfrac{100 \text{ mL/beat}}{2.0 \text{ m}^2} = 50$ mL/beat/m^2

3. Cardiac index $= \dfrac{\text{Cardiac output}}{\text{BSA}}$ or $\dfrac{5 \text{ L/min}}{2.0 \text{ m}^2} = 2.5$ L/min/m^2

Although left ventricular function can probably best be evaluated using pressure-volume loops, this technique is not practical in the clinical setting. Cardiac work is instead calculated and followed as an index of left ventricular function. Work is calculated as the force expended × the distance moved. Left ventricular stroke work (LVSW) and left ventricular stroke work index (LVSWI; normalized for patient size by dividing by the patient's BSA) are calculated using the following formulas (mean BP is commonly used as a substitute for mean LV systolic pressure):

$$LVSW = SV \times [\text{mean BP} - \text{mean PCW}] \times .0136 \text{ g·m/beat}$$

$$LVSWI = SV \times [\text{mean BP} - \text{mean PCW}] \times .0136/BSA \text{ g·m/m}^2/\text{beat}$$

While calculation of the left ventricular work is clinically useful and reflects the area under the left ventricular pressure-volume curve, reducing the information contained in the left ventricular pressure volume loop to a single number is a significant simplification. The mean PCW of the ventricle on which the cardiac work is performed is recaptured by plotting the LVSWI (y axis) against the PCW (x axis). A shift upward and to the left reflects improved left ventricular performance. A shift downward and to the right reflects decreased contractility.

The left ventricular volume at which the cardiac work is performed is, however, lost in calculating the LVSWI. For instance, a patient with a compensated congestive cardiomyopathy, where the left ventricular volume is grossly increased and the ejection fraction markedly decreased, could demonstrate a normal stroke volume and calculated LVSWI. Because of the increase in left ventricular volume, however, wall tension and myocardial oxygen demand are markedly higher than in the normal patient. While this presents a difficulty in comparing patients, the LVSWI finds its greatest utility in the individual patient, where it is used to track left ventricular performance and follow the effect of interventions.

Example: Serial hemodynamic readings are taken. Calculate LVSWI. Is left ventricular function improving? Which therapy is best?

	Rest	Inotrope	Vasodilator + Diuretic
Heart rate	100 bpm	100 bpm	80 bpm
Cardiac index	1.8 L/min/m²	2.5 L/min/m²	3.2 L/min/m²
Mean BP	90 mm Hg	90 mm Hg	70 mm Hg
Mean PCW	20 mm Hg	20 mm Hg	10 mm Hg

1. Stroke volume index = Cardiac index/Heart rate (mL/bpm/m²)
   SVI =   18   25   40
2. LVSWI = SVI × [mean BP − mean PCW] × .0136 (g·m/m²/beat)
   LVSWI =   17   24   33
3. Left ventricular function is improving with best results on the combination of a vasodilator and diuretic.

Perhaps the best measure of left ventricular function is peak dp/dt. The peak rate of change in left ventricular pressure (peak dp/dt) normally occurs during isovolumic contraction. Because peak dp/dt is achieved before aortic valve opening, it is afterload independent. The effect of preload is also small. To decrease catheter and fluid transmission effects on the pressure curve a transducer-tipped catheter should be used to make recordings for dp/dt analysis. The dp/dt is an accurate measure of left ventricular contractility, increasing when contractility increases and decreasing when it falls. Analysis of dp/dt is of lessened usefulness in the presence of mitral regurgitation (isovolumic contraction is no longer isovolumic due to leakage of blood into the left atrium) and when significant dyssynchrony of contraction is present (left bundle branch block commonly; at times with ischemic heart disease). The right ventricular peak dp/dt occurs after pulmonic valve opening and is thus afterload dependent.

THE PATIENT WITH VALVULAR HEART DISEASE

The normal cardiac valve offers minimal impediment to forward flow. With progressive stenosis of the valve, a pressure gradient develops. For any given valve area the gradient will be increased by increasing the transvalvular flow. Smaller valve areas will result in higher gradients if flow is maintained. An equation for this relationship was developed by Gorlin and Gorlin.

$$\text{Valve area (cm}^2) = \frac{\text{transvalvular flow}}{C \times 44.3 \times \sqrt{\text{Mean gradient}}}$$

$$C = \text{constant} = 1 \text{ for the aortic, pulmonic, tricuspid valves}$$
$$= 0.85 \text{ for the mitral valve}$$

Mitral stenosis

In the patient with mitral stenosis progressive stenosis results in a transvalvular gradient of increasing magnitude and duration in diastole. This gradient is exacerbated by any condition increasing transmitral flow (i.e., exercise, tachycardia, pregnancy, hyperthyroidism, fever). The pulmonary artery pressures and pulmonary vascular resistance increase with worsening mitral stenosis, but in a somewhat unpredictable fashion. The resultant pulmonary vascular disease may result in a "second stenosis" and must always be evaluated in patients with mitral stenosis. As the mitral stenosis becomes severe, resting cardiac output is decreased, adding low output symptoms to the antecedent symptom of dyspnea on exertion.

Evaluation of the patient with mitral stenosis requires a careful right and left heart catheterization, measurement of cardiac output, and angiography to rule out associated aortic or mitral insufficiency. After passing the Swan-Ganz catheter to the PCW position and before recording the transmitral gradient, it is mandatory to confirm the PCW position with a "wedge" saturation (should be greater than 95% or in excess of the arterial saturation). The right and left heart transducers are commonly switched back and forth to confirm the gradient and to verify proper transducer calibration. Cardiac outputs should be measured in close temporal proximity to the pressure measurements. Simultaneous PCW and left ventricular pressure tracings are recorded at fast recording speed for at least 5 cycles in sinus rhythm or 10 cycles in atrial fibrillation.

If the cardiac output and PCW pressure are low, the patient exercises and the measurements are repeated to improve the accuracy of the valve area calculation. Because of the time delay in pressure transmission across the pulmonary bed from the left atrium, the Swan-Ganz pressure tracing will lag behind actual left atrial pressure. This is usually corrected by shifting the PCW to the left, lining up the v wave peak with the descending limb of the left ventricular pressure curve.

Both associated aortic and mitral insufficiency will affect the transmitral gradient in mitral stenosis. With aortic insufficiency, diastolic filling of the left ventricle through the incompetent aortic valve will decrease the transmitral gradient by increasing the left ventricular diastolic pressure. The result is an

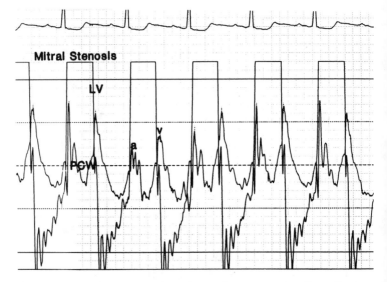

Figure 3-4: Mitral stenosis patients demonstrate a diastolic pressure gradient across the mitral valve between simultaneous LV (left ventricular) and PCW (pulmonary capillary wedge) tracings. Note "a" and "v" waves on the PCW tracings result from atrial and ventricular contraction respectively. The mean diastolic pressure gradient is used in the Gorlin formula to calculate the mitral valve area.

underestimation of mitral stenosis severity. If there is coexistent mitral regurgitation, the transvalvular flow exceeds the forward flow calculated from the cardiac output, resulting in an increase in the measured transmitral gradient. The severity of the mitral stenosis is thus overestimated when mitral regurgitation is present. If the aortic valve is competent, transmitral flow in patients with combined mitral stenosis and regurgitation may be more accurately calculated using properly validated ventricular volumes (total flow = forward + regurgitant flow = end-diastolic volume − end-systolic volume).

To calculate the mitral valve area (Figure 3-4) the PCW and left ventricular pressure tracings are first aligned using tracing paper (most computer systems will do this). The diastolic separation between the curves is measured as an area (usually by planimetry) and converted to a mean gradient by dividing by the duration of diastole. This is repeated for each of the selected cycles and the results are averaged to obtain a mean gradient. The sum of the diastolic filling periods of the measured cycles is divided by the sum of the total cycle times and multiplied by 60 to give the diastolic filling period in sec/min. The mitral valve flow is calculated as the cardiac output divided by the diastolic filling period. The Gorlin equation as modified for the mitral valve is:

$$\text{Mitral valve area} = \frac{\text{Mitral valve flow}}{38 \times \sqrt{\text{Mitral gradient}}}$$

Example: Calculate the mitral valve area given the following:
CO = 4.5 L/min
Diastolic filling period = 36 sec/min
Mean transmitral gradient = 16 mm Hg

1. $\text{Mitral valve area} = \dfrac{\text{Mitral valve flow}}{38 \times \sqrt{\text{Mean mitral gradient}}}$
   Mitral valve flow = 4500 mL/min / 36 sec/min = 125 mL/sec
   Mitral valve area = 125 / 38 × 4 = 0.8 cm^2

A commonly used simplification of the Gorlin formula was proposed by Hakki for calculating valve areas in patients with mitral or aortic stenosis. This simplified formula is:

$$\text{Valve area} = \text{Cardiac output (L/min)} / \sqrt{\text{Pressure gradient}}$$

This formula was further modified by Angel who recommended dividing the Hakki formula result by 1.35 when the heart rate was less than 75 bpm in mitral stenosis or greater than 90 bpm in aortic stenosis.

Aortic stenosis

The evaluation of the patient with aortic stenosis (Figure 3-5) is in many respects similar to the methodology used in calculating the mitral valve area. After careful calibration the peripheral arterial pressure (usually from the femoral artery sheath) is recorded simultaneously with the central aortic pressure. The left ventricular pressure is next recorded simultaneously with the peripheral artery pressure. Transducers may be switched to confirm the gradient and proper calibration. The left ventricle to aorta pullback is also recorded to confirm the previously documented gradient and to look for Carabello's sign (with severe aortic stenosis the catheter is itself significantly obstructive and the peripheral systolic pressure may rise by more than 5 mm Hg on catheter withdrawal).

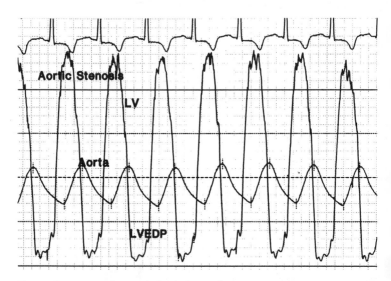

Figure 3-5:   Aortic stenosis patients demonstrate a pressure gradient between the LV (left ventricle) and aorta in systole. The average (mean) gradient determined by planimentry of the area between the curves is used in the Gorlin formula to determine the aortic valve area. LVEDP (left ventricular end diastolic pressure) may rise with associated aortic insufficiency or LV failure.

The cardiac output is measured in close temporal proximity to the pressure recordings. Careful simultaneous pressure recordings are made of the left ventricle and PCW to exclude accompanying mitral valve disease. Left ventricular and aortic angiography are desirable to exclude, or if present, to quantify aortic or mitral insufficiency. If the cardiac output and the transaortic pressure gradient are low, exercise may be performed and pressures repeated to improve the accuracy of the valve area calculation.

The presence of aortic insufficiency increases aortic valve flow and thus the transaortic gradient. Aortic insufficiency will result in an overestimate of aortic stenosis severity. An attempt to correct for the increased volume is possible in the presence of a competent mitral valve and accurate, standardized volumetric information (total transaortic flow = end-diastolic volume − end-systolic volume from the left ventricular angiogram).

A common source of confusion is the difference between the various described aortic pressure gradients. These include the mean gradient, the peak-to-peak gradient, and the peak instantaneous gradient. The mean gradient is the quantity properly used in the Gorlin formula. The peak-to-peak gradient is an estimate of the mean gradient derived by subtracting the peak left ventricular systolic pressure from the peak peripheral artery systolic pressure (these peaks do not occur at the same time). The peak instantaneous gradient is derived from the superimposed left ventricle and peripheral artery curves as the maximum systolic separation occurring at the same instant of time. With worsening aortic stenosis all these pressure gradients tend to become closer together.

To calculate the aortic valve area, the peripheral artery and left ventricular pressures are first traced and superimposed (i.e., the arterial tracing, which lags behind central pressure, is aligned with the beginning of its upstroke on the ascending limb of the left ventricle tracing). The area between the systolic pressure curves is measured by planimeter and the mean gradient calculated by dividing by the systolic ejection period. This is repeated for each of the selected cycles and the results are averaged to give a mean gradient. The sum of the systolic ejection periods of the selected cycles is divided by the sum of the total cycles and multiplied by 60 to yield the systolic ejection period in sec/min. The aortic valve flow is calculated as the cardiac output divided by the systolic ejection period. The Gorlin equation for the aortic valve is:

$$\text{Aortic valve area (cm}^2) = \frac{\text{Aortic valve flow}}{44.3 \times \sqrt{\text{Mean gradient}}}$$

Example: Calculate the aortic valve area given:
  Mean aortic gradient = 81 mm Hg
  CO = 5 L/min
  Systolic ejection period = 25 sec/min

1. Aortic valve flow = Cardiac output/Systolic ejection period
         = 5000 mL/min/25 sec/min = 200 mL/sec
2. Aortic valve area = Aortic valve flow/ 44.3 × $\sqrt{\text{Mean gradient}}$
         = 200 mL/sec/44.3 × $\sqrt{81}$ = 0.5 cm^2
3. Hakki's simplified formula: Valve area = Cardiac output/$\sqrt{\text{Gradient}}$
         Aortic valve area estimate = 5.0/$\sqrt{81}$ = 0.55 cm^2

Valvular regurgitation

The hemodynamic effects of valvular regurgitation depend on multiple factors, including chronicity, size of regurgitant orifice, afterload, size and compliance of the receiving chamber, and heart rate. Angiographic quantitation is generally based on the degree and duration of opacification of the receiving chamber and is semiquantitated on a scale of 1+ to 4+. Quantitation of aortic insufficiency (with a competent mitral valve) or mitral insufficiency (with a competent aortic valve) can be performed using a combination of ventriculographic volumes and the forward cardiac output (usually from Fick oxygen consumption or thermodilution). The total stroke volume is figured as the difference between ventriculographic end–diastolic and end–systolic volumes. The forward stroke volume equals the cardiac output divided by the heart rate. The regurgitant stroke volume, then, is just the difference between the total and forward stroke volumes. The regurgitant fraction is calculated as the regurgitant volume divided by the total stroke volume. Cardiac output may fall with both acute aortic and mitral insufficiency and a decreased forward stroke volume is often partially compensated for by tachycardia. Progressive dilation of the left ventricle with chronic insufficiency may lead to an increase in the forward stroke volume and a decrease in the heart rate required to maintain cardiac output.

Total stroke volume = End-diastolic volume − End-systolic volume
Forward stroke volume = Cardiac output/ Heart rate
Regurgitant stroke volume = Total − Forward stroke volume
Regurgitant fraction = Regurgitant stroke volume/ Total stroke volume

Acute aortic insufficiency is associated with a rapid rise in left ventricular diastolic filling pressure and tachycardia. With severe acute aortic insufficiency the left ventricular diastolic pressure may reach and exceed the PCW pressure by mid diastole, resulting in premature closure of the mitral valve. With chronic aortic insufficiency the left ventricle may become massively enlarged (cor bovinum) with an associated bounding, collapsing pulse (increased systolic and pulse pressures, decreased diastolic pressure). The LVEDP characteristically remains markedly elevated over the PCW pressure. Use of the intra-aortic balloon pump is contraindicated by aortic insufficiency.

Acute severe mitral regurgitation is characterized by large v waves in the PCW (v waves more than twice the mean PCW) and sometimes even pulmonary artery tracing as well as a marked elevation in mean PCW and pulmonary pressures. The LVEDP is characteristically substantially lower than the mean PCW when significant acute mitral regurgitation is present (due to the large v waves). With chronic mitral regurgitation the left atrium dilates and tends to buffer the lungs from exposure to the high v waves and high mean PCW characteristic of significant acute mitral regurgitation. Mitral regurgitation severity is highly influenced by afterload. Systolic unloading with the intra-aortic balloon pump or reduction of the systemic resistance with drug therapy are both effective maneuvers in reducing the severity of mitral regurgitation.

CARDIOVASCULAR SHUNTS

The detection, localization, and quantitation of cardiovascular shunts can be challenging. Detection is aided by a strong index of suspicion. The routine oximetry performed during catheterization may alert one to the presence of a shunt. Arterial saturation is normally greater than 95%. A lower than normal saturation may be seen with physiologic right-to-left shunting due to alveolar hypoventilation or oversedation. Failure to correct the abnormally low arterial saturation with 100% oxygen, however, is presumptive evidence of a right-to-left shunt.

Routine right heart *oximetry* can alert one to the presence of a left-to-right shunt. A pulmonary artery saturation of greater than 80% warrants a fuller saturation run. Small right-sided step-ups may be noted due to incomplete mixing of blood, particularly in the more proximal chambers. As the blood becomes progressively better mixed, the maximum expected difference in oxygen saturation step-up between chambers decreases. The maximum expected step-ups in oxygen saturation over the proximal chamber are:

Right atrium over vena cava	7%
Right ventricle over right atrium	5%
Pulmonary artery over right ventricle	3%

If a greater than expected step-up is confirmed on serial sampling, a left-to-right shunt is present. A full oxygen saturation run is performed to localize the level and quantitate the degree of the shunt. Oximetry is performed in close temporal sequence on samples from the right or left and main pulmonary artery, the right ventricular outflow tract, the body of the right ventricle, the right ventricular inflow, the high, mid, and low right atrium, the superior and inferior vena cava, the left ventricle, and the aorta.

If the left ventricular and arterial saturations are greater than 95% (i.e., no evidence of desaturation), the shunt can be assumed to be left-to-right unidirectional. The magnitude of the left-to-right shunt can be calculated as the difference between pulmonary and systemic blood flow (Qp − Qs) using the Fick oxygen consumption technique.

$$Qp = \text{Oxygen consumption/ } (a - v)O_2 \text{ difference}$$
$$= \text{Oxygen consumption/ (Pulmonary vein } O_2 \text{ content } - \text{ Pulmonary artery } O_2 \text{ content)}$$
$$= \text{Oxygen consumption/ (Left ventricle } O_2 \text{ content } - \text{ Pulmonary artery } O_2 \text{ content)}$$
$$Qs = \text{Oxygen consumption/ } (a - v)O_2 \text{ difference}$$
$$= \text{Oxygen consumption/ [Arterial } O_2 \text{ content } - \text{ Mixed venous (mv) } O_2 \text{ content]}$$

Expressing the pulmonary and systemic flow as a ratio, Qp/Qs, eliminates the need to measure oxygen consumption because it will factor out, yielding the following equation:

$$Qp/Qs = \text{Arterial } O_2 \text{ content} - MV\ O_2 \text{ content}/\ LV\ O_2 \text{ content} - PA\ O_2 \text{ content}$$

The Qp/Qs ratio is important physiologically. Small left-to-right shunts with ratios less than 1.5 may be followed medically. Large shunts with flow ratios of greater than or equal to 2.0 require surgical repair. The management of intermediate shunts between 1.5 and 2.0 depends on factors such as the relative surgical risk or development of pulmonary hypertension.

Example: Calculate the left-to-right shunt and the Qp/Qs ratio in a patient with the following: O_2 consumption = 250 mL O_2/min, Hb 15 g, arterial saturation 98%, PA saturation 80%, superior vena cava (SVC) saturation 60%, inferior vena cava (IVC) saturation 65%.

1. O_2-carrying capacity = Hb $\times$ 13.6
    = 15 $\times$ 13.6 = 204 mL O_2/L
2. O_2 content = O_2 sat. $\times$ O_2 carrying capacity
    Arterial O_2 content = .98 $\times$ 204 = 200 mL O_2/L
    PA O_2 content = .80 $\times$ 204 = 163 mL O_2/L
    SVC O_2 content = .60 $\times$ 204 = 122 mL O_2/L
    IVC O_2 content = .65 $\times$ 204 = 133 mL O_2/L
3. MV O_2 = [3 $\times$ SVC O_2 content + IVC O_2 content]/ 4
    = ([3 $\times$ 122] + 133) /4 = 125 mL O_2/L
    MV O_2 is calculated in this patient from a weighting of the SVC and IVC oxygen contents because of the left-to-right shunt in a more distal chamber (i.e., the right atrium or ventricle in the case of an ASD or VSD, respectively).
4. Qp = Oxygen consumption/ Arterial O_2 content $-$ PA O_2 content = 250/ [200 $-$ 163] = 6.76 L/min
5. Qs = Oxygen consumption/ Arterial O_2 content $-$ MV O_2 content = 250/ [200 $-$ 125] = 3.33 L/min
6. Left-to-right shunt volume = Qp $-$ Qs = 3.43 L/min
    Qp/Qs ratio = 2.0

If there is evidence of a bidirectional shunt (i.e., the arterial saturation is less than 95%) the following formulas are used to calculate the right–left and left-to-right shunts.

$$\text{Left-to-right} = \frac{Qp(MV\ O_2 \text{ content} - PA\ O_2 \text{ content})}{(MV\ O_2 \text{ content} - PV\ O_2 \text{ content})}$$

$$\text{Right-to-left} = \frac{Qp \, (PV \, O_2 \text{ content} - \text{Arterial } O_2 \text{ content}) \, (PA \, O_2 \text{ content} - PV \, O_2 \text{ content})}{(\text{Arterial } O_2 \text{ content} - MV \, O_2 \text{ content}) \, (MV \, O_2 \text{ content} - PV \, O_2 \text{ content})}$$

The major problem with detection of shunts by oximetry is the insensitivity of the technique for small shunts. The minimal shunt that can be reliably detected at the great vessel level has a Qp/Qs of 1.3. At the atrial level a shunt has to have a Qp/Qs of at least 1.5 to be reliably detected.

Using the *indicator dilution* technique shunts as small as 2% to 3% of systemic blood flow can be detected by appropriate choice of injectate and sampling sites. If the indicator is injected into or proximal to the chamber from which the shunt originates, downstream sampling will yield an abnormal time-concentration with a low peak concentration and distorted slope indicative of early recirculation (e.g., injection into the left ventricle and sampling in a peripheral artery in a patient with a VSD and left-to-right shunt). If the indicator is injected distal to the originating chamber with sampling further downstream, the time-concentration curve will be normal (e.g., injection into the left ventricle and sampling in a peripheral artery in a patient with an ASD and left-to-right shunt). The minimal shunt detectable by the indicator dilution technique used in this fashion is approximately 25%.

Smaller shunts may be detected by the early appearance of indicator when the indicator is injected into or proximal to the originating chamber and sampling is performed at or distal to the receiving chamber (e.g., injection into the left ventricle and sampling in the pulmonary artery in a patient with a VSD and left-to-right shunt). If sampling is performed proximal to the receiving chamber, the curve will be normal (i.e., in the prior example if sampling had been performed in the right atrium, a normal curve would have been demonstrated). Injections distal to the originating chamber with sampling proximal, at, or distal to the receiving chamber will yield a normal-appearing curve. The minimal shunt detectable by the indicator dilution technique used in the above fashion is 2% to 3%. The relation of indicator and sampling sites to originating and receiving chamber locations in the detection of a shunt is summarized in Table 3-6.

The sensitivity of the technique can be at times enhanced

Table 3-6   Detection of Shunts by Indicator Dilution

	Sampling site		
	Distal to the originating chamber	Proximal to the receiving chamber	At or distal to the receiving chamber
Injector site (relative to the originating chamber)			
Into or proximal to	**Abnormal curve**	Normal	**Early detection**
Distal to	Normal	Normal	Normal
Sensitivity	**>25%**		**2–3%**

by altering right and left heart filling independently (i.e., inspiration, expiration, strain, and release phases of Valsalva). The use of an indicator normally filtered out by the lungs may also prove useful in demonstrating right-to-left shunting (i.e., detection of the indicator in the left heart would indicate the lungs are bypassed).

As can be appreciated, by carefully combining the correct sites of sampling and injection very small shunts can be accurately detected. Valvular regurgitation can potentially confound accurate localization of the shunt by allowing admixture of the indicator with blood from chambers proximal to the receiving and originating chambers.

The indicator dilution method has also proven useful in the quantitation of shunts. A discussion of this methodology is, however, beyond the scope of this synopsis.

The patient with a central left-to-right shunt will have an increased pulmonic blood flow. Pulmonary hypertension due to pulmonary vasoconstriction and progressive pulmonary vascular disease commonly supervenes as the patient ages. Compensatory right ventricular hypertrophy develops in response to the pulmonary hypertension. Measurements of pulmonary vascular resistance made at this juncture are markedly increased, both absolutely and in comparison to the systemic vascular resistance. The ratio of PVR:SVR is a commonly used index of the potential reversibility of pulmonary hypertension after surgical repair. A ratio greater than 0.75 indicates severe pulmonary vascular disease and a high operative risk. Particularly when seen with a small (less than 1.5:1) shunt, operative repair is probably contraindicated in this setting. When the PVR:SVR ratio exceeds 1.0 the patient is considered inoperable.

The marked elevation in PVR leads to either a stiff, non-compliant right ventricle or right ventricular failure and potential shunt reversal (right to left with attendant desaturation, cyanosis). When this occurs, the patient is said to have developed an Eisenmenger physiology.

It is important in the setting of a central shunt with pulmonary hypertension to evaluate the potential reversibility of the elevated PVR. This is done by administration of 100% O_2 and repeated calculation of pulmonary flow and resistance. In children an α adrenergic blocking agent (tolazoline) is often used to evaluate potential pulmonary vascular hyperreactivity as a contributing factor to the pulmonary hypertension. A significant fall in the PVR by either of these methods may make the patient an operative candidate.

In summary, hemodynamic evaluation is an integral part of the evaluation of the cardiac surgical patient. The information obtained may be vital to a proper understanding of the pathophysiology and assessment of cardiac structure and function. Diagnosis, prognosis, and therapeutic management may all be contingent on a knowledge of and proper interpretation of hemodynamics.

SUGGESTED READING

Angel J, Soler-Soler J, Anivarro I, Domingo E. Hemodynamic evaluation of stenotic cardica valves. II. Modification of the simplified formula for mitral and aortic valve area calculation. *Cathet Cardiovasc Diagn.* 1985; 11:127–138.

Caraballo BA, Barry WH, Grossman W. Changes in arterial pressure during left heart pullback in patients with aortic stenosis: a sign of severe aortic stenosis. *Am J Cardiol.* 1979; 44:424–427.

Goldenheim PD, Kazemi H. Cardiopulmonary monitoring of critically ill patients. *N Engl J Med.* 1984; 311:717–720, 776–780.

Grossman W (ed). Cardiac catheterization and angiography. 3rd ed. Philadelphia: Lea & Febiger; 1986.

Hakki AH, Iskandrian A, Bemis C, et al. A simplified valve formula for the calculation of stenotic cardiac valve areas. *Circulation.* 1981; 63:1050–1055.

Matthay MA, Chatterjee B. Bedside catheterization of the pulmonary artery: risks compared with benefits. *Ann Intern Med*. 1988; 109:826–834.

O'Quin R, Marini JJ. Pulmonary artery occlusion pressure: clinical physiology, measurement, and interpretation. *Am Rev Respir Dis*. 1983; 128:319–326.

Yang SS, Bentivoglio LG, Maranhao V, Goldberg H. From cardiac catheterization data to hemodynamic parameters. 3rd ed. Philadelphia: FA Davis; 1988.

Pulmonary Function Evaluation

Mark Greco, M.D.
Adam Hurewitz, M.D.

4

Advances in intraoperative technique and postoperative management have reduced mortality and morbidity associated with cardiac surgery. As a result, higher risk patients are now considered for surgery when previously they may have been excluded. Among the high-risk groups now considered are patients with chronic pulmonary diseases.

The most common perioperative complications in all cardiac surgical patients tend to be respiratory, even in the absence of underlying pulmonary disease. In patients with preexistent pulmonary diseases the risk of respiratory complications may be even greater. In this chapter we will focus on recognizing patients at risk for pulmonary complications, optimizing preoperative function, and treating postoperative respiratory complications.

RECOGNIZING THE PATIENT AT RISK

Preoperative risk factors are well described for patients requiring upper abdominal surgery or thoracotomy. These procedures pose significant risks of postoperative respiratory complications when compared with other operations requiring general anesthesia. Even patients requiring lower abdominal incisions have a substantially lower incidence of postoperative respiratory problems than those patients with upper abdominal incisions. Few studies, however, have examined perioperative respiratory evaluation and care in cardiac surgery patients.

Some important differences do exist for these patients.

First, most patients now receive a midline thoracic incision in place of a lateral thoracotomy. Also, with improvement in cardiac function postoperatively, a parallel improvement in lung function can also be expected. However, although no loss of functional lung parenchyma occurs in the cardiac surgery patient, alterations in chest wall mechanics, impaired clearance of secretions, abnormal lung defense mechanisms, and aspiration may compound the already marginal lung function and place the patient at high risk for postoperative pulmonary complications including atelectasis, pneumonia, and respiratory failure.

Can we define a group of patients, preoperatively, who are at high risk for these complications, and if so, can anything be done to reduce these risks? The answer to both questions is yes when considering the group of patients with chronic lung disease. Of this group, specific diseases seen with some frequency include emphysema, chronic bronchitis, and asthma. Several modalities are available to identify these patients at risk and these will now be discussed.

History and physical examination

The pulmonary history and physical examination in the preoperative period are important in two regards. First, they complement other tests in defining both the character and the severity of the pulmonary disorder. Second, exacerbations in symptoms such as those caused by superimposed infection or bronchospasm may be recognized and corrected. Since most physicians are comfortable with specific aspects of the pulmonary history and physical, we will focus upon just two important risk factors: cigarette smoking and obesity.

Smoking: Many authors have documented increased perioperative morbidity in patients who smoke as compared to those who do not. A higher incidence of fever, productive cough, and abnormal chest findings have been found in smokers as compared to nonsmokers undergoing a variety of elective surgical procedures. Laszlo and coworkers reported a 53% incidence of postoperative complications in smokers as compared with a 22% incidence in nonsmokers. These complications included changes in the quality and quantity of sputum, new radiographic findings, fever, and abnormal physical findings on chest examination. Many of these changes were attributed to abnormal tracheobronchial clearance resulting from alterations

101

in ciliary function and mucous hypersecretion. Clearance rates may remain abnormal for weeks to months following the cessation of smoking. An increase in bronchial reactivity, alterations in pulmonary surfactant production, and impairment of the immune response within the lung are also seen. The latter includes depressed neutrophil chemotaxis, decreased immunoglobulin levels, abnormal T-cell activity, and abnormal macrophage function. No study has fully documented improved clearance mechanisms or decreased postoperative respiratory morbidity when smoking is halted shortly before surgery.

However, cigarette smoking has a second, more rapidly reversible effect, namely a reduction in oxygen carriage. Carbon monoxide levels in blood can become significantly elevated in smokers, often reaching levels of 5% to 10%. The carbon monoxide competes with oxygen for hemoglobin-binding sites and reduces the amount of hemoglobin available for oxygen binding as well as the amount of oxygen released to the tissues. Both anemia and a lower cardiac output further contribute to reduced oxygen-carrying capacity and oxygen delivery, respectively. Since carbon monoxide is cleared from the blood within about 12 hours, even brief abstinence from smoking may be of benefit.

Obesity: Of the various systemic disorders that promote respiratory complications following surgery, obesity is one of the most common. Obesity is defined as weight that exceeds 130% of the ideal body weight. A direct reduction of lung volumes in proportion to the degree of obesity can be expected, particularly if the obesity is central rather than peripheral. The most striking reduction is of the expiratory reserve volume (ERV) and functional residual capacity (FRC). These changes result in a reduction of ventilation to dependent portions of the lung, perhaps because of airway closure or a predominantly intercostal mode of inspiration. The consequence is basal atelectasis and hypoxemia. The changes in ventilation are exaggerated in the supine and lateral decubitus positions and the effects of anesthesia and incisional pain further enhance the reduction in these lung volumes. Another problem of the severely obese is obstructive sleep apnea, caused by the mechanical interaction of obesity and reduced airway muscle tone during sleep. These patients can develop profound nocturnal apnea resulting in hypercapnia and life-threatening hypoxemia. When the patient is intubated, the apnea is eliminated and may only become evident in the immediate postextubation period. It is therefore important to ask the obese patient about excess daytime sleepiness, snoring, or frequent automobile accidents and, even more important to ask the spouse about irregular breathing episodes observed during the night. Although nasal continuous positive airway pressure (CPAP) masks have become an effective means of treating these patients, the fundamental treatment is weight reduction. If possible, this should be insisted on prior to accepting a patient for elective surgery. If uncertainty exists about a diagnosis of sleep apnea, preoperative nocturnal monitoring is advisable.

Laboratory data

Arterial blood gas: Arterial blood sampling relays important information about the three important functions of the respiratory system: oxygen carriage in blood, carbon dioxide excretion, and acid–base regulation. By contrast, clinical signs are notoriously unreliable indicators of pulmonary gas exchange functions.

Arterial oxygen tensions (Pa_{O_2}) and arterial oxygen saturation (Sa_{O_2}) are measures of oxygen transport in the lung. Oxygen tension indicates oxygen activity in blood, not the amount of oxygen in blood; oxygen diffusion from high to low activity accounts for passage of oxygen from alveoli (where $Po_2 = 100$ mm Hg) into tissues (where $Po_2 < 40$ mm Hg). Oxygen saturation, on the other hand, is directly proportional to oxygen content, in mL/dL. Normal oxygen saturation is 98% and oxygen content (in the absence of anemia) is 20 mL/dL. The relationship between Pa_{O_2} and Sa_{O_2} is alinear as expressed in the oxyhemoglobin dissociation curve. Furthermore, both the Pa_{O_2} and Sa_{O_2} vary with alveolar ventilation. Hyperventilation lowers the Pco_2 and simultaneously raises the Pa_{O_2}. By contrast, hypoventilation raises the Pco_2 and lowers the Pa_{O_2} by a similar amount.

To account for changes of Po_2 with changes of alveolar ventilation, an alveolar − arterial oxygen [(A − a)O_2] difference is calculated. In calculating (A − a)O_2, Po_2 is measured in arterial blood and alveolar Po_2 is calculated from the alveolar air equation:

$$Pa_{O_2} = P_iO_2 - \frac{Pco_2}{\text{Respiratory quotient}}$$

P_iO_2 is the inspired oxygen concentration (F_iO_2) multiplied by (barometric pressure $- 47$ mm Hg). At sea level, breathing room air, P_iO_2 is 150 mm Hg. PCO_2 is theoretically obtained from alveolar tensions although the arterial CO_2 tension is more readily measured and may be freely used in this equation. The respiratory quotient is the ratio of carbon dioxide production divided by oxygen consumption. With a normal diet, the respiratory quotient is 0.8 but with a carbohydrate diet rises to 1.0. Typical values include a PaO_2 of 105 mm Hg, a PaO_2 of 95 mm Hg and an $(A - a)O_2$ gradient of 10 mm Hg.

Although the $(A - a)O_2$ gradient effectively measures pulmonary oxygen exchange, neither it nor the PO_2 or the SaO_2 has been found to correlate with the incidence of postoperative morbidity in cardiac surgery patients. Whereas severe hypoxemia ($PaO_2 < 50$ mm Hg) is a contraindication to lung resection, cardiac surgery often results in improved oxygenation if the basis for the hypoxemia is cardiac disease. One such example is a resolution of pulmonary congestion following mitral valve replacement for tight mitral stenosis resulting in improved arterial oxygen tensions.

Pulmonary function testing: Pulmonary function testing is the most important method presently available for classifying the various types of lung disease. Specific diseases show characteristic patterns of altered lung volumes and expiratory flows. With bronchial asthma, the diagnostic pattern is a lower airway obstruction which resolves with bronchodilator therapy and exacerbates with bronchoprovocation. For other diseases, the pattern of pulmonary function abnormalities are not specific for a single disease but are indicative of a broad category of diseases. For example, a reduction of lung volumes associated with normal expiratory flow rates and a normal diffusion capacity is a useful marker for extraparenchymal restrictive diseases such as pleural effusions, obesity, or neuromuscular weakness.

In addition to their diagnostic value, pulmonary function tests permit a quantitative measure of the response to therapy. Just as the sphygmomanometer is routinely used to check responses to antihypertensive therapy, spirometry can and should be used to monitor changes of lung function over time. Such tests can be performed at the bedside, need not be expensive, and are safe to repeat on a daily basis if needed. The following section is a brief review of the commonly available pulmonary function tests which can be ordered in the patient considered for cardiac surgery. Particular attention will be devoted to the effort and strength demanded of the cardiac patient in performing each of these tests.

The two major components of pulmonary functions are the lung volumes and the flow rates. Other components, such as the diffusion capacity, helium mixing time, and inspiratory and expiratory muscle strength are valuable in certain conditions, depending on the pattern of changes of lung volumes and flow rates. In most lung diseases, measurement of certain lung volumes and inspiratory and expiratory flow rates by spirometry is sufficient; more complex testing methods are only rarely necessary.

Lung volumes: Spirometry is the standard method of measuring lung volumes (Figure 4-1). The tidal volume (V_T) is the amount of gas inspired and expired during quiet breathing. A typical value for V_T is 500 mL in a 70-kg man. The product of V_T and respiratory rate is the minute ventilation. In an average adult, minute ventilation ranges between 6 and 10 L/min. With extraordinary effort, minute ventilation can rise to more than 100 L. This maximal voluntary ventilation (MVV) is measured

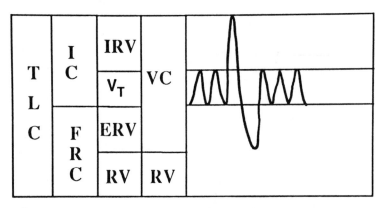

Figure 4-1   Lung volume versus time (spirogram) in the absence of forced expiratory effort. Vital capacity (VC) consists of the tidal volume (V_T), inspiratory reserve volume (IRV) and expiratory reserve volume (ERV). The volume of air remaining after forced expiration is the residual volume (RV). At maximal inspiration, the total lung capacity (TLC) consists of the VC + RV. At the end of a tidal volume expiration, the amount of air remaining in the lung is the functional residual capacity (FRC); the maximal volume of air which can be inspired from the FRC is the inspiratory capacity (IC).

by having the patient breathe deeply and rapidly for 15 sec and then extrapolating the volume to a 60-sec value. The MVV is particularly instructive because it consists of elements reflecting lung volume, expiratory flow, respiratory muscle strength, and motivation. Patients who lack either sufficient lung function or sufficient motivation to carry out this maneuver are at risk for perioperative respiratory complications.

The vital capacity (VC) is the volume of gas which can be exhaled after a maximal inspiration. In an average man, VC is about 5 L, whereas in women the value is somewhat lower. Since measurement of VC is effort dependent, accuracy varies with strength, alertness, and motivation. Reduction of VC is typical of restrictive lung diseases and many obstructive lung diseases. No disease and no amount of training are known to increase the VC; any values which exceed the predicted norms are due to individual variations of normal thoracic size.

Following a maximal expiratory effort, a residual amount of air remains within the lung and cannot be expelled, even with maximal expiratory effort. Residual volume (RV) is not measured by spirometry but can be measured with special techniques such as helium equilibration or body plethysmography. These techniques are available in most hospitals and some office practices and are safe and easy to perform.

At the end of a relaxed exhalation, the amount of air remaining in the lung is the functional residual capacity (FRC). This volume consists of the RV plus a potentially exhalable volume, the ERV. Helium equilibration or body plethysmography is needed to measure the FRC; however, unlike the RV, no patient effort is required. Thus, the FRC is the most reliable lung volume measurement since it does not depend on patient effort and strength. The FRC is also valuable because it reflects an equilibrium position of the respiratory system. At the FRC, lung deflation forces are precisely balanced by chest wall expansion forces. As a consequence, the respiratory system passively exhales to FRC in the absence of persistent inspiratory muscle effort. In restrictive lung diseases the FRC is reduced, typically to values which are less than 80% of predicted normal values. In obstructive lung diseases the FRC is often hyperinflated and may exceed 120% of the predicted normal values.

Inspiratory and expiratory flows: Obstructive lung disease is defined by a reduction of inspiratory and expiratory airflow. These reductions of airflow result from intraluminal, extraluminal, or bronchial wall abnormalities. Mucus plugging is the most common cause of intraluminal obstruction and accounts for inspiratory and expiratory obstruction associated with asthma and chronic bronchitis. Extraluminal obstruction is less common but accounts for expiratory obstruction in patients with emphysema. In these patients, loss of elastic elements of the lung reduces airway tethering and airway diameter, particularly during forced expiration. Other causes of airway obstruction include hypertrophy and contraction of airway smooth muscle; these represent the major cause of reduced inspiratory and expiratory flow in patients with bronchial asthma and asthmatic bronchitis.

Obstruction to airflow causes characteristic changes of flow versus volume loops (Figure 4-2). Lung volumes are recorded on the abscissa, with total lung capacity (TLC) at the far left and RV at the far right. Flows are recorded on the ordinate, with inspiratory flows below the abscissa and expiratory flows above the abscissa. In the normal loop, expiratory flow reaches a peak at volumes near TLC. During exhalation expiratory flow falls in a nearly linear fashion, reaching zero flow at RV. The peak of inspiratory flow occurs near the midinspiratory lung volumes.

By contrast, the obstructed loop can be seen by gross inspection to have reduced flows at any given lung volume. The concavity of expiratory flow is characteristic of obstructive lung diseases. The most important indicator of reduced expiratory flow is the one second forced expiratory volume (FEV_1). Normally, 83% of the entire VC can be exhaled within the first second of forced exhalation from TLC. Given the variability of normal, expiratory obstruction is defined when the FEV_1 is less than 75% of the forced vital capacity (FVC). Since reductions of the FEV_1 also occur with restrictive processes, the FEV_1/FVC ratio is a more specific indicator of obstruction. Other measures of obstruction such as reduced midexpiratory flows have also been described, but the FEV_1/FVC ratio is the best measure of clinically significant disease and is probably the only test of expiratory flow which need be examined. This ratio is readily obtained from either volume versus time spirograms or flow versus volume loops.

Diffusion capacity: Gas diffusion across the alveolar capillary interface is a passive process requiring no active transport mechanisms. The rate of diffusion of all gases such as oxygen

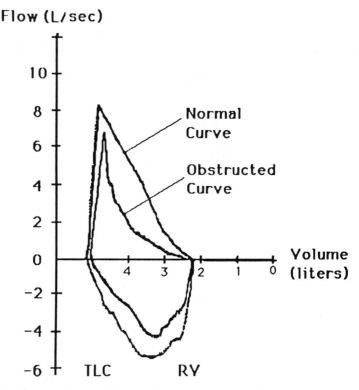

Figure 4-2 Flow vs lung volume loops during forced inspiratory and expiratory effort. The loops of both a healthy person and one with with obstructive lung disease are shown. Expiratory flows are plotted above the abscissa, inspiratory flows are below. In the expiratory portion of the normal curve, the relationship between lung volume and expiratory flow rates is linear; in obstructive lung disease the expiratory flow rates rapidly decrease at lower lung volumes, giving a characteristic concave appearance to the loop.

or carbon monoxide is more readily measured using carbon monoxide as the test gas. This rate is a function of the alveolar capillary surface, diffusion resistance of the tissues, blood flow, and the gradient of pressure of gases across the interface.

A reduced diffusion is characteristic of three diseases: interstitial lung disease, emphysema, and pulmonary vascular diseases. In the interstitial diseases, a reduction of carbon monoxide diffusion often precedes reductions of lung volumes and is a sensitive marker of the severity of disease. In emphysema, reduction of the diffusion capacity is characteristic and is not

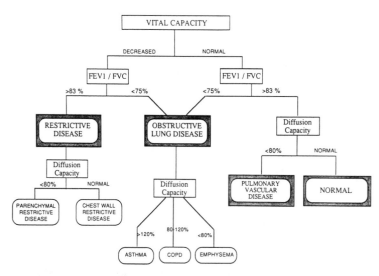

Figure 4-3 Algorithm for categorizing patients with lung disease based upon pulmonary function abnormalities. The two major disease categories are obstructive and restrictive lung disease. Restrictive lung diseases are characterized by reduced lung volumes (vital capacity) with normal expiratory flow rates (ratio of one-second forced vital capacity, FEV_1, to forced vital capacity, FVC). Restrictive disease of the lung parenchyma will also reduce the diffusion capacity; restriction in the chest wall (pleura, neuromuscular, etc) will not affect diffusion. By contrast, patients with obstructive lung disease will manifest a reduced FEV_1/FVC; the additional finding of a low diffusion capacity suggests emphysema. A low diffusion capacity in the absence of obstruction or restriction may be an indicator of pulmonary vascular disease.

seen in either asthma or bronchitis with obstruction. Finally, a reduction of the diffusion capacity in the absence of lung volume restriction or expiratory obstruction is compatible with pulmonary vascular diseases. Examples include pulmonary embolism and primary pulmonary hypertension. Artifactual reduction of diffusion can result from recent cigarette smoking or from anemia and both causes should be considered and corrected if an unexpected reduction of diffusion is detected.

Figure 4-3 presents an algorithim for pulmonary function test interpretation.

The preoperative chest radiograph: The preoperative chest x-ray not only serves as a baseline for comparison in the postoperative period, but also may identify occult disease such as pneumonia, pleural effusions, malignancy, and pneumothorax. It also serves a complementary role with other diagnostic tests both in diagnosis and postoperative management. For example, a chest radiograph which shows hyperinflated lungs, flattened diaphragms, and large bullae together with pulmonary function tests that show marked airway obstruction place the patient at high risk for barotrauma during mechanical ventilation. The x-ray may also help define the cause of restrictive pulmonary impairment such as a large pleural effusion, major atelectasis, or chest wall deformity such as kyphoscoliosis. Enlargement of the pulmonary arteries with peripheral oligemia is highly suggestive of pulmonary hypertension which may be confirmed with hemodynamic monitoring.

Comparison of the use of pulmonary function testing in predicting postoperative outcome in noncardiac versus cardiac surgery patients

One of the more widely accepted tests used to predict postoperative mortality and morbidity has been the MVV. Since this value depends on several factors including patient effort, lung function, and muscle strength, it may be one of the best indices of respiratory reserve and the best predictor of postoperative respiratory complications. An MVV less than 50% predicted or less than 28 L/min predicts a high probability of respiratory complications and death. Other parameters that have been used to predict perioperative risks and adverse outcomes are summarized in Table 4-1.

Not all patients with abnormal lung function develop postoperative complications. Features which distinguish these

Table 4-1 Pulmonary Function Parameters and Risk in Noncardiac Thoracic Surgery

Parameter	Risk value
FEV_1	<1 L
FVC	<1 L
Midmaximal Expiratory Flow Rate	<.6 L/sec
Maximum Expiratory Flow Rate	<100 L/min
$Paco_2$	>45 mm Hg

patients from those who do develop respiratory complications are not known. However, as a group, patients with the abnormalities listed in Table 4-1 are at greater risk than those who have more normal function. Several investigators have reported that preoperative treatment with bronchodilators, chest physiotherapy, cessation of smoking, and antibiotics for preoperative respiratory infection will significantly reduce morbidity and mortality in patients with abnormal lung function undergoing noncardiac surgery.

Cain and coworkers were among the first to examine whether preoperative pulmonary function testing predicted postoperative complications in the cardiac surgery patient. In their study, a prolonged stay in the ICU was the index of postoperative complications. Preoperative pulmonary function tests were abnormal in more than 90% of the patients studied. Most of these patients had reduced expiratory flows. Thirty percent of patients with abnormal pulmonary function tests had a complicated postoperative course. Seventy-five percent of these complications were attributed to pulmonary disease (i.e., atelectasis, pneumonia). These same investigators analyzed several parameters used previously to predict outcome in thoracic surgery patients. No difference in the postoperative course was identified in patients with an FEV_1 of less than 1.0 L or greater than 2.0 L; an FVC under or over 60%; or an MVV less than 40% and greater than 60% of predicted. The only effective predictor of postoperative morbidity was a $Paco_2$ which exceeded 45 mm Hg in patients with obstructive lung disease. This observation is consistent with previous studies in which hypercapnia predicted a poor outcome in patients undergoing thoracic surgery with or without lung resection. No reduction in total intensive care days resulted from treatment of patients with a FEV_1 less than 1.5 L who were treated with bronchodilators, intermittent positive-pressure breathing (IPPB), and chest physiotherapy. This is in contrast to several noncardiac thoracic surgery studies in which similar therapeutic interventions reduced postoperative complications. Cain and colleagues also found that the incidence of postoperative atelectasis did not depend on the preoperative pulmonary function but rather on the type of surgery performed. The repair of a thoracic aortic aneurysm not only produced the highest rate of atelectasis, but also the longest ICU stay. There was no significant difference in ICU stay between patients undergoing coronary artery bypass graft (CABG) surgery and valvular repair. Thus, it seems from this study that postoperative complications in patients undergoing cardiovascular surgery are determined more by the type of surgery rather than the preoperative pulmonary functions. Also, poor pulmonary function detected preoperatively does not necessarily predict a complicated postoperative course as it does in patients undergoing other thoracic surgery procedures. One exception is that preoperative hypercapnia in both the cardiac and noncardiac surgery groups consistently predicted increased postoperative respiratory morbidity and mortality, reflecting the extremely limited reserve.

Although much more information is needed, it seems from the available data that poor pulmonary function need not be a contraindication to cardiac surgery because at least one study so far has shown it to be an inadequate predictor in identifying those at risk for a complicated postoperative course as contrasted to patients undergoing noncardiac, thoracic surgery.

OPTIMIZATION OF PREOPERATIVE LUNG FUNCTION

A variety of measures are now available to optimize lung function preoperatively (Table 4-2). Although there is limited evidence that these therapeutic interventions will affect postoperative respiratory morbidity and mortality, most data from noncardiac surgery suggests at least a probable advantage.

Preoperative pulmonary function testing is most valuable in patients with obstructive lung disease because of the many effective bronchodilator medications presently available as well as the number of effective anti-inflammatory agents. The standard medications used to treat obstructive lung diseases are listed in Table 4-3. Some, such as theophylline or β-agonists are bronchodilators; that is, they promote a reduction of airway smooth muscle tone. Others, such as corticosteroids, are not direct bronchodilators, but promote a reduction of airway resistance indirectly, either by reducing airway inflammation or by improving overall β-adrenergic responsiveness.

Theophylline derivatives are bronchodilators, promote mucociliary clearance, increase respiratory drive to breathe, and improve diaphragmatic contractility. Side effects and toxicity are common, perhaps of particular concern in patients with cardiac disease since side effects include arrhythmias and tachycardia. Dosing varies from person to person and is ideally

Table 4-2   Optimization of Preoperative Lung Function in Patients with Obstructive Airway Disease

A. Patient education
  1. Review importance and need for postoperative coughing, deep breathing, and early mobilization
  2. Practice preoperative incentive spirometry and chest splinting techniques
B. Pulmonary function
  1. Maximize airway dynamics (see Table 4-3)
  2. Facilitate mucociliary clearance
    a. Hydration
    b. Bronchodilators
    c. Chest physiotherapy
    d. Treat airway infection when present
  3. Avoid smoking for at least 24 h prior to surgery
C. Systemic factors
  1. Maximize systemic oxygen delivery
    a. Optimize cardiac output if reduced
      i. inotropic agents
      ii. afterload reducing agents
    b. Raise hemoglobin concentration if anemic (>10 g/dL)
    c. Raise oxygen concentration to obtain Pa_{O_2} >60 mm Hg
  2. Correct nutritional disorders
    a. Weight reduction if obese
    b. caloric replenishment if underweight
      i. specific attention to K, PO_4, Mg
      ii. avoid excess carbohydrate load

adjusted according to changes of serum theophylline levels. Loading doses of 5–6 mg/kg have been recommended as have maintenance doses of 0.5-0.9 mg/kg/h. However, since metabolism varies with age, smoking history, congestive heart failure, other medications, and individual metabolic differences, such formulas are estimates and not necessarily safer than using estimated doses of 600–900 mg/d and then altering the dose according to the serum levels.

Inhaled β-agonists are more attractive as first-line therapy because they are well tolerated, work quickly, and are extremely effective. Like theophylline, β-agonists also have a positive effect on mucociliary clearance. Although absorption is minimal, systemic side effects such as cardiac rhythm disturbances (including sinus tachycardia, atrial and ventricular

Table 4-3 Pharmacologic Interventions in the Treatment of Obstructive Airway Disease

Aerosolyzed β-agonists	Dosage
Isoetharine (Bronchosol 1%)	0.25–0.5 mL/3 mL saline q4-6h
Metaproterenol (Alupent 5%)	0.3 mL/3 mL saline q4-6h
Albuterol (Ventolin .5%)	0.5 mL/2.5 mL saline q4-6h
Isoproterenol (Isuprel 1:200)	0.5 mL/3 mL saline q6h*
Methylxanthines	
Aminophylline	Loading: 5 mg/kg over 30 min
	Maintenance: 0.5–0.9 mg/kg/h according to levels†
Anticholinergics	
Atrovent	2 puffs q6-8h
Corticosteroids	
Methylprednisolone (Solumedrol)	20–100 mg IV q6h
Prednisone	1mg/kg/d with subsequent tapering

*Least β-selective and should be avoided, if possible, in patients with cardiac disease
†Downward adjustment in maintenance dose if congestive failure is present

arrhythmias) and tremulousness do occur, even with the newer β$_2$-selective agents.

The aggressive use of either the theophyllines or β-agonists in the perioperative period may induce cardiac arrhythmias, particularly when hypoxia or acidosis is present. Anesthetic induction with halothane is particularly problematic in patients using intravenous aminophylline since an increased incidence of tachyarrhythmias and ventricular arrhythmias have been reported, even when theophylline levels in serum are therapeutic. The use of enflurane or isoflurane may be more suitable, since both provide bronchodilation as does halothane, but arrhythmias are less common in patients currently taking theophylline.

Should maximal doses of β-agonists or theophylline prove insufficient to relieve serious bronchospasm or should the risks of arrhythmias be too great to permit the use of these medications, corticosteroids may be a better mode of therapy. The mode of action of corticosteroids for patients with obstructive lung diseases remains unknown, although several mechanisms have been postulated. These include primarily a reduction of airway inflammation and a bolstering of β-agonist sensitivity. Although the risks of serious side effects are substantial, the risks of arrhythmias are minimal and are further minimized by monitoring serum electrolytes. The major problems associated with corticosteroid therapy in the cardiac surgery patient include an impairment of wound healing, a reduction of respiratory muscle strength, and a suppression of cell-mediated immunity. These complications are minimized when corticosteroids are prescribed for brief bursts in either the pre- or postoperative periods.

POSTOPERATIVE CARE

Once the patient has undergone surgery, careful supervision of postoperative management is essential for patients with underlying pulmonary disease. Respiratory problems interfere with postoperative recuperation in 20% of cardiac surgery patients. The severity of complications varies from atelectasis and mucus plugging, which prolong the need for mechanical ventilation, to pneumonia and pulmonary edema, which severely reduce survival. Indeed, as many as 5% of the deaths in cardiac surgery patients are directly attributable to respiratory disease. The causes of respiratory failure in the postsurgical cardiac patient are listed in Table 4-4. Respiratory failure can occur transiently in the early postoperative period, usually implying a more benign etiology, or it can occur later in the postoperative course. Although the latter is more ominous, persistent respiratory failure can occur in either case.

Respiratory failure in the early postoperative period

In the first 6–12 hours following cardiac surgery, patients are rarely able to resume spontaneous ventilation. In most instances, this is a temporary failure of ventilation, due to persistent respiratory depression by anesthetic and analgesic medication. Other factors contributing to ventilatory failure in this early postoperative period are incisional pain and microatelectasis secondary to impaired cough and inability to sigh. The predominant factors leading to respiratory failure in this phase are extrapulmonic. The absence of serious lung injury permits this condition to resolve rapidly and spontaneously. Reduction in the dosage of anesthetic and analgesic medication has accelerated the rate of return to spontaneous breathing such that most patients are successfully weaned from mechanical ventilation within 24 hours. Attempts at

---

Table 4-4   Causes of Respiratory Failure in the Open Heart Surgery Patient

---

Neurologic

Persistent anesthetic/analgesic/sedative central nervous system depression

Iatrogenic suppression of ventilation

    Controlled ventilation with neuromuscular blocking agents and/or sedation

    Depression of respiratory drive by excess oxygen supplementation

    Depression of respiratory drive by excess mechanical ventilation

    Depression of respiratory drive by hyperinflation of lungs

Musculoskeletal

Diffuse respiratory muscle weakness

    Muscle fatigue from excess work of breathing

    Impaired muscle function

        Reduced oxygen delivery (hypoxia, low cardiac output)

        Electrolyte imbalance (low PO_4, low Mg, low K)

        Pharmacologically induced, e.g. aminoglycoside (gentamicin)

Conscious hypoventilation to minimize chest wall pain

Chest wall disorders

    Abdominal distention

        Aerophagia

        Ascites

        Obesity

    Pleural effusion / pneumothorax

Lung parenchymal injury

Airway disorders

    Bronchospasm

    Mucus plugging/atelectasis

Interstitial/alveolar disorders

    Cardiogenic pulmonary edema

    Adult respiratory distress syndrome

    Aspiration pneumonia

---

resumption of spontaneous breathing before 6 hours are occasionally tolerated but may prove unsuccessful because of small or absent tidal inspirations, a rising $Paco_2$, and a falling pH.

This example of relatively benign respiratory failure is difficult to distinguish from other more serious disorders in the early postoperative period. Several features suggest a benign course. A normal $(A - a)O_2$ gradient indicates an extrapulmonic cause of ventilatory failure rather than significant ventilation to perfusion inequality. Likewise, absence of parenchymal infiltrates on the chest radiograph also supports a more benign course and argues against diagnoses such as pneumonia, pulmonary edema, or lobar atelectasis. Lobar atelectasis is particularly common in the left lower lobe and the presence of a retrocardiac density or diminished visualization of the left hemidiaphragm are valuable clues to the presence of disease in this region.

In patients with underlying chronic obstructive pulmonary disease (COPD) these indicators of benign early respiratory failure must be modified. Prolongation of expiration and the presence of rhonchi or wheezes may simply reflect baseline findings. Also, expectations for establishing desirable arterial blood gas values vary according to the preoperative values. Severe airway obstruction with preoperative hypercapnia is unlikely to improve following cardiac surgery; the ideal $Paco_2$ during weaning from mechanical ventilation should approximate that which was present prior to surgery. Attempts to maintain a lower Pco_2 during the early postoperative phase leads to depletion of bicarbonate buffer stores and the risk of uncompensated respiratory acidosis during spontaneous breathing trials.

Respiratory failure in the late postoperative period

Inability to wean the patient from mechanical ventilation or the new onset of respiratory failure 24 hours or more following surgery implies a more ominous underlying process which is likely to reduce survival. Progressive deterioration of respiratory function in the cardiac surgery patient usually indicates either cardiac failure or a serious underlying lung disease of either the airway or lung parenchyma. These patients will typically suffer from marked impairment of oxygenation but rises of Pco_2 are variable. In some instances progressive deterioration is not evident but attempts at weaning prove unsuccessful. This stable but unresolving type of respiratory failure is more commonly due to either central impairment of respiratory drive or peripheral neuromuscular and skeletal dysfunction. These patients are more likely to have a predominant failure of ventilation with elevated Pco_2 and minimal or no impairment of oxygenation. The following sections will review in more detail each of these categories of persistent respiratory failure.

Central impairment of respiratory drive: The capacity to fine-tune alveolar ventilation and maintain $Paco_2$ within a narrow range of baseline arises in two anatomically separate foci, the peripheral chemoreceptors and the central respiratory centers. Peripheral chemoreceptors are located in the carotid body and aorta and are sensitive to changes of Pao_2 and pH. Hypoxemia and acidosis are the two most powerful ventilatory stimuli and will cause either a larger V_T or a more rapid respiratory rate. The other major center of ventilation originates in central chemoreceptors, located in the brain stem. These centers respond primarily to acidosis and are inhibited by hypoxia. They are depressed by anesthetic and analgesic medication and account for much of the early postoperative inhibition of breathing. These brain stem centers are also susceptible to cerebrovascular injury, explaining some instances of postoperative impairment of ventilation. Should injury to the brain stem account for hypoventilation, conscious attempts to raise ventilation are usually successful but the patient will quickly revert to hypoventilation if subconscious drive is depended on. This is a valuable bedside test if the patient is alert and cooperative.

When evaluating a patient for impairment of central respiratory drive, a serum pH between 7.32 and 7.38 is desirable. This range of acidemia poses an adequate drive to ventilate with none of the risks of a more severe acidemia; attempts to maximize respiratory drive by inducing hypoxia are not appropriate. Clinical evidence of a central drive impairment include an elevated Pco_2, a reduced serum pH, and a relatively normal $(A - a)O_2$ gradient. These are characteristics of an extrapulmonary mechanism and do not help to distinguish a peripheral neuromuscular from a skeletal etiology (see below). Iatrogenic induction of normal or high oxygen tensions and an alkalotic pH reduce respiratory drive and account for a reduction of minute ventilation and an apparent failure to wean.

Peripheral neuromuscular and skeletal impairment: Extrapulmonary diseases are an important cause of respiratory failure in the open heart surgery patient. Peripheral neuropathies, myopathies, muscle fatigue, and skeletal disorders have all been observed in these patients. As with central ventilatory failure, respiratory acidosis with little impairment of oxygenation is characteristic.

Although peripheral neuropathies randomly occur, the only neuropathy which occurs in cardiac surgery patients with any frequency to warrant discussion is phrenic nerve palsy.

Phrenic nerve injury has been extensively described in cardiac surgery literature and occurs in up to 20% of CABG patients as determined by phrenic conduction studies. Markland and colleagues examined diaphragmatic function using transcutaneous phrenic nerve stimulation in 44 patients undergoing cardiac surgery. They found that only a small percentage of patients (5/44 or 11%) sustained phrenic nerve injury postoperatively. Total phrenic paralysis was found only in one patient. Interestingly, despite phrenic nerve injury, all patients were extubated by the second postoperative day.

Etiologies for phrenic nerve damage include hypothermic injury from cold cardioplegic solution and stretching of the nerve during sternal retraction and pericardial stretching. The duration of cardiopulmonary bypass affects phrenic nerve dysfunction, most likely reflecting prolonged exposure to these factors. Less common is a complete transection of the phrenic nerve. In instances of temporary dysfunction, impairment in diaphragmatic function may persist for several days to perhaps several months postoperatively. Symptoms range from exertional dyspnea following extubation to prolonged inability to wean from mechanical ventilation. In addition to the nonspecific findings of respiratory acidosis and minimal hypoxemia, these patients have an inspiratory paradox, visible at the bedside. This paradox consists of an inward displacement of the anterior abdomen during inspiration, as contrasted with the usual outward displacement with normal diaphragmatic function. A rapid inspiration (sniff test) exaggerates the paradoxical rise of the diaphragm during inspiration and can be visualized during ultrasound or flouroscopy. The diaphragm is elevated (either unilaterally or bilaterally) and linear atelectasis is common at the lung bases. Diaphragmatic function can be determined by measurement of the negative inspiratory force (NIF). This is an inexpensive bedside test which is a useful measure of inspiratory muscle strength. There is little to offer patients with phrenic nerve injury other than passive ventilatory support in the few instances where this is needed.

Respiratory muscle weakness is also relatively common in cardiac surgery patients. In most instances, a combination of factors act to either fatigue a previously healthy muscle or else to overload a previously fatigued muscle. Reduced oxygen delivery or serious electrolyte problems such as hypokalemia or hypomagnesemia create serious deficiencies in both contractile strength and endurance potential of the diaphragm and intercostal muscles. Severe malnutrition with protein deficiency also contributes to these deficiencies. Finally, in patients with COPD, such as those with emphysema, hyperinflation of the lungs and thorax places the diaphragm and other inspiratory muscles in a position of mechanical disadvantage. Flattening of the diaphragm reduces the radius of curvature of this muscle and reduces the capacity to generate effective contraction. Paradoxical motion of the abdomen during inspiration, described above for paralysis of the phrenic nerve, can also be seen with inspiratory muscle fatigue.

Skeletal disorders are uncommon causes of ventilatory failure in the cardiac surgery patient. This is an improvement resulting from predominant use of midsternal instead of lateral chest wall incisions.

Diseases of the airway or lung parenchyma: Most pulmonary diseases primarily affect either the airway or the lung parenchyma. Those which attack the airway produce a pattern of increased airway resistance referred to as *obstructive lung disease.* Those which primarily damage the lung parenchyma are collectively referred to as *restrictive lung diseases* and typically produce a generalized reduction of all lung volumes. The use of pulmonary function tests to distinguish between these two common types of pulmonary disease is rarely possible in the first few days after surgery and certainly not in patients who are intubated and mechanically ventilated. Other tests, however, are available to permit reasonably accurate diagnoses in the critically ill patient. The following section will briefly review some of the more common examples of obstructive and restrictive lung diseases with an emphasis on diagnosis in the critical care unit and on basic principles of therapy.

Asthma: Bronchial asthma is characterized by episodic bronchospasm and mucus plugging of the airways. Although asthma primarily affects adolescents and young adults, persistence of asthma throughout life is quite common and a small percentage of asthmatics develop initial symptoms late in life. Maximizing airway function is an important element of preoperative care in the asthmatic patient. The asthmatic typically has a much greater response to bronchodilator medication than the patient with either emphysema or obstructive bronchitis. A variety of bronchodilator medications are available and are most effective when delivered by the aerosol route. If necessary, corticosteroids can also be given, either by aerosol, orally, or systemically. Preoperative pulmonary functions indicate the severity of obstruction and the response to therapy. With vigorous preoperative care, airway obstruction can return to normal in the asthmatic patient.

In the postoperative period, clinical signs such as wheezing and prolonged expiration provide only a limited estimate of the severity of obstruction. Spirometry is not possible while the patient is mechanically ventilated but other indicators of airflow obstruction can be monitored. A reasonable estimate of airway obstruction can be obtained by recording changes of peak inflation pressure during mechanical ventilation and calculating airway resistance. A rise in peak pressure indicates either increased airway resistance or decreased total pulmonary compliance. Distinction between these two categories is facilitated by temporarily occluding the expiratory port at end inspiration. Peak inflation pressures will fall to a value referred to as the plateau pressure. The difference between the peak pressure and plateau pressure is a measure of airway resistance. Normally the difference is 5–10 cm H_2O; when airway resistance rises, the gradient between peak and plateau increases to 20–30 cm H_2O.

Postoperative therapy of bronchial asthma consists of bronchodilators and medications to improve mucus clearance and dissolve mucus plugs. Aerosolized bronchodilators such as albuterol are rapidly effective and can be given during mechanical ventilation. The duration of effect is variable, lasting up to 6 hours in stable patients or as little as 1 hour in severely bronchospastic patients. In addition to their effect on bronchospasm, adrenergic bronchodilators also enhance mucociliary clearance. Although most bronchodilator aerosols are relatively specific for bronchial adrenergic receptors, some cardiac stimulation is inevitable. When adrenergic medication is not tolerated or not fully effective, corticosteroids will usually effectively reduce airway resistance and also may improve responsiveness to adrenergic medication. Corticosteroids are not true bronchodilators but are extremely effective for patients with asthma, particularly those who are refractory to adrenergic bronchodilators. The onset of action is delayed for at least 6–12 hours but a marked improvement in both airway resistance and mucus plugging is usually evident within 24–48 hours. No evidence exists that oral agents are less effective than systemic but most physicians prescribe intravenous methylprednisolone in dosages which vary from 60 mg to 300 mg daily. Whether the higher dosages are more effective for patients with severe bronchospasm remains a focus of controversy and uncertainty. The role of theophylline in obstructive lung diseases is becoming more and more uncertain; the risks of toxicity are significant and the benefit observed is modest when theophylline is added to adrenergic bronchodilators.

Emphysema: Expiratory obstruction in emphysema is a result of progressive destruction of peripheral airways, alveoli, and pulmonary capillaries with loss of supportive elasticity of the remaining airways. Bronchospasm and mucus plugging are unusual and dyspnea is persistent rather than episodic. The thoracic cage is characteristically hyperinflated and breath sounds are diminished or absent. A higher than normal compliance permits the lung to be ventilated with unusually small inflation pressures; peak airway pressures in a patient with emphysema may rise to only 10–15 cm H_2O.

Since the primary pathologic element of emphysema is lung destruction rather than bronchospasm, edema, or mucus plugs, the benefits from adrenergic bronchodilators are limited. Anticholinergic bronchodilators (such as Atrovent) are more effective than adrenergic bronchodilators for emphysema patients and may soon be available in a liquid form for nebulization. Although oxygenation is impaired by severe emphysema, the response to supplemental oxygen is excellent.

In the postoperative period, emphysema interferes with weaning because of increased expiratory resistance, poor mechanical function of the respiratory muscles caused by hyperinflation, and a high incidence of generalized muscle weakness due to limited activity and reduced caloric intake. Despite these greater risks for overall postoperative complications, exclusion of emphysema patients for CABG or valve surgery based on data derived from upper abdominal surgery or thoracotomy data is not necessarily correct. Many patients with significant emphysema who might be excluded from consideration for thoracotomy for lung cancer have successfully undergone cardiac surgery.

Chronic obstructive pulmonary disease: COPD is a broad category which encompasses patients with expiratory obstruction who have neither the reversible features of asthma nor the extensive lung destruction characteristic of emphysema. These are patients with long histories of cigarette smoking and a chronic productive cough. Airways are edematous and inflamed and congested with copious and tenacious mucus. Rhonchi, or wheezes, are heard during auscultation of the lungs and the lung fields are hyperinflated on the chest radiograph. Hypoxemia and hypercapnia are often more severe than in emphysema. Postoperative respiratory complications are similar to those described for the patient with emphysema. Treatment is similar to that for the patient with asthma although the response is less substantial.

Atelectasis: Of the parenchymal lung diseases which occur in the postoperative period, atelectasis is probably the most common. Atelectasis is most likely when surgery has caused a postoperative reduction of lung volumes. This includes cardiac, thoracic, upper abdominal and, to a lesser degree, lower abdominal surgery. Segmental and subsegmental atelectasis occurrs in 80% of CABG patients, predominantly in the left lower lobe. Factors which predispose to atelectasis after thoracic and upper abdominal surgery include lung trauma during retraction, impaired mucociliary clearance, inadequate cough, and airway closure. These factors are directly attributable to effects of anesthesia, incisional pain, and nursing in the supine position as well as preoperative factors such as cigarette smoking, underlying lung disease, and obesity. As was mentioned previously, one additional factor which may contribute to left lower lobe atelectasis in the cardiac surgery patient is phrenic nerve dysfunction. However, in a recent study, it was shown that although atelectasis or infiltrates developed in the left lower lobe of 98% of patients undergoing open heart surgery (43/44 patients), only 5 (11%) had phrenic nerve dysfunction following surgery as assessed by transcutaneous phrenic nerve stimulation. Other factors pointing away from phrenic nerve injury as the sole cause of atelectasis include the still high incidence of atelectasis/infiltrate following surgery when cold cardioplegia was not used and the observation that the incidence of atelectasis is higher two or more days following surgery rather than immediately after.

According to Stein, aggressive respiratory therapy in the preoperative period has reduced the incidence of respiratory complications from 60% to 21% in COPD patients undergoing noncardiac surgery; such benefits in the cardiac population are not as clear. In the postoperative period, early mobilization, deep breathing exercises, incentive spirometry, and chest percussion, either alone or in combination, have been recommended to prevent atelectasis and to speed the resolution of established atelectasis. The impact of these measures on survival and their cost effectiveness have not been adequately determined in either the cardiac surgery or thoracic surgery patient. It seems reasonable, however, to recommend both early ambulation and some form of active lung expansion maneuver in the first few postoperative days since these measures are inexpensive, relatively free of risk, and probably contribute to improved lung expansion and mucus clearance. Bronchoscopy is rarely necessary except when atelectasis persists for several days and is associated with impaired gas exchange.

Pulmonary edema: Interstitial and alveolar edema is a common cause of hypoxemia and sudden respiratory decompensation in the cardiac patient. The usual basis is an elevated left atrial or left ventricular end-diastolic pressure; the pulmonary capillaries are structurally normal. This form of pulmonary edema is referred to as cardiogenic or cardiac. In some patients, a reduction of plasma oncotic pressure induces more edema than would be expected on the basis of the elevated intravascular pressure alone. Clinical features of cardiac edema include bibasilar rales, distended neck veins, leg edema, and cardiomegaly. Diagnosis is confirmed by measurement of pulmonary capillary wedge pressure and cardiac output. Treatment of cardiac edema includes a combination of diuretics to reduce vascular congestion, inotropic medication to improve cardiac contractility, and vasodilators to reduce cardiac afterload.

A more unusual cause of pulmonary edema is the adult respiratory distress syndrome (ARDS). The primary site of injury in this noncardiogenic pulmonary edema is the pulmonary capillary, principally as a consequence of an acute inflammatory reaction. Edema results from the increased capillary permeability to both water and proteins and causes reduced pulmonary compliance and interference with gas exchange. ARDS has been associated with sepsis, trauma, aspiration, and transfusion reactions. In the cardiac surgery patient, the pump oxygenator is an additional, although rare, risk factor. Pump oxygenators are believed to activate the circulating complement cascade, resulting in leukocyte agglutination and an intense inflammatory reaction within the pulmonary circulation.

Table 4-5   Cardiogenic and Noncardiogenic Pulmonary Edema

	Cardiogenic	Noncardiogenic
Underlying mechanism	Increased capillary hydrostatic pressure	Increased capillary permeability
Pulmonary wedge pressure	Elevated	Normal
Cardiac silhouette	Left ventricular enlargement	Normal heart size
Pleural effusions	Common	Rare
Therapy	Diuresis	PEEP
	Inotrope	Supportive therapy
	Vasodilator	Supplemental oxygen

This syndrome develops within hours of surgery when the pump oxygenator is implicated but may be delayed for 24–48 hours when other causes such as aspiration pneumonia or sepsis are implicated. In ARDS, left ventricular end-diastolic pressures are normal, the heart is not enlarged, and leg edema is less prominent than in cardiac edema. The lung edema, however, is often marked and rapidly progressive. The clinical picture consists of diffuse rales, rapidly progressive interstitial and alveolar infiltrates, and severe hypoxemia not corrected by supplemental oxygen therapy. The contrasting features of both forms of pulmonary edema are listed in Table 4-5.

The treatment of noncardiac edema is limited. Once the initiating process is brought under control (i.e., sepsis), therapy is largely supportive. Positive pressure ventilation, positive endexpiratory pressure (PEEP), and high inspired oxygen concentrations are necessary to maintain arterial and tissue oxygenation within acceptable limits. Diuretics reduce overall lung water by reducing pulmonary wedge pressures to low-normal values. No evidence exists that either corticosteroids or other pharmacologic agents reverse the permeability process itself. In essence, the principles of therapy are aimed at keeping the patient alive until the inflammatory process subsides spontaneously. Those patients who do survive regain relatively normal lung function within a year; unfortunately, the overall mortality rate of ARDS remains high, in some institutions exceeding 60%.

Pneumonia: Oropharyngeal aspiration of mouth secretions containing bacteria is believed to account for most instances of postoperative pneumonia. In some patients this occurs during induction of anesthesia but in others is a consequence of impaired pharyngeal reflexes associated with anesthetics and analgesic medication, tracheal intubation or other poorly characterized predisposing factors in patients who are critically ill. In patients who are in intensive care, oropharyngeal colonization shifts from predominantly gram-positive organisms to predominantly gram-negative bacteria within a matter of days. Pneumonia in these patients therefore requires broad-spectrum coverage for anaerobes as well as gram-positive and gram-negative aerobes.

Prior to oral feeding, aspiration from reflux of gastric contents is promoted by postoperative ileus and a distended abdomen; the presence of an endotracheal tube with an inflated cuff probably affords little or no protection against aspiration. The injury of gastric aspiration is initially a bronchial acid burn which subsequently evolves into an intense peripheral inflammatory response consistent with ARDS. Following a witnessed aspiration of oral or gastric contents, empiric antibiotic therapy is not routinely advised but rather can be deferred until evidence of a pneumonia occurs.

WEANING FROM MECHANICAL VENTILATION

With disappearance of anesthetic depressant effects in the early postoperative period, the process of weaning from mechanical ventilation can be initiated, despite the persistence of suboptimal lung mechanics. Weaning is more successful when postoperative analgesia is carefully titrated and when the patient is alert, cooperative, and free of significant dyspnea. In preparing a patient for weaning from mechanical ventilation, close monitoring is essential. Guidelines for weaning from mechanical ventilation and indicators of failure to wean are summarized in Table 4-6.

Gas exchange functions of the lung include the transport of oxygen from lung to blood and transport of carbon dioxide from blood to the lung. Although the normal arterial oxygen tension is 100 mm Hg, values exceeding 60 mm Hg permit SaO_2 to exceed 90%. Although SaO_2 can be monitored on a continuous basis with ear or finger oximeters, these devices vary from true SaO_2 values by as much as 4%. They, therefore, are more ideally suited for trending changes of saturation; more accurate measurements require arterial blood sampling.

Table 4-6   Criteria for Weaning from Mechanical Ventilation

	Difficult weaning	Ideal (normal)
Mental status	Cannot follow simple commands	Alert and cooperative
Neuromuscular drive/ respiratory muscles		
Peak inspiratory force	<-25 cm H_2O	>-60 cm H_2O
Tidal volume	<5 mL/kg	
Vital capacity	<10 mL/kg	
Respiratory rate	>30/min	10–15/min
Gas exchange		
Pao_2	<60 mm Hg ($Fio_2 > 0.4$)	>90 mm Hg ($Fio_2 = 0.21$)
$Paco_2$	>45 mm Hg	35–45 mm Hg
pH	<7.35	7.38–7.42
Parenchymal injury		
Auscultation	Signs of consolidation; rales	Clear breath sounds
Chest radiograph	Atelectasis, pneumonia, pulmonary edema	Clear lung fields
Peak airway pressure	>40 cm H_2O	<15 cm H_2O
Plateau airway pressure	>30 cm H_2O	<10 cm H_2O
Airway resistance		
Auscultation	Wheezing, prolonged expiration	Expiratory: inspiratory ratio $\sim$ 2:1
Peak-plateau airway pressure	>10–15 cm H_2O	5–10 cm H_2O

Alveolar ventilation is a measure of the bellows function of the lung and is best monitored by changes of $Paco_2$. The normal values for $Paco_2$ are 35–45 mm Hg, but the acceptable range is much larger in patients with COPD and chronic CO_2 retention. As a result, Pco_2 values which permit the arterial pH to remain between 7.35 and 7.45 are desirable. Transcutaneous CO_2 sensors have been effectively used for neonates but are not yet sufficiently reliable for noninvasive monitoring of Pco_2 in the adult. Continuous monitoring of end-tidal CO_2 is available as a guide to $Paco_2$ trends. The gradient between arterial and end-tidal Pco_2 is a measure of the alveolar dead space. In healthy people this gradient is therefore negligible whereas in patients with lung disease the gradient may rise to 20 mm Hg or more. The value of end-tidal Pco_2 monitoring is limited because the amount of dead space, and thus the difference from arterial values, can vary with changes of either pulmonary or cardiovascular function.

Several tests help to predict whether patients can sustain adequate gas exchange during weaning. Values of Sao_2 exceeding 90% prior to weaning are desirable although if the inspired oxygen concentration necessary exceeds 40% to 50%, the chances for weaning are reduced. Arterial pH values in the range of 7.35 to 7.40 indicate a satisfactory level of alveolar ventilation and acid–base balance during mechanical ventilation but do not reflect on the patient's independent capacity to do so. On the other hand, pH values less than 7.35 indicate inadequate ventilation even with mechanical ventilation support and predict a greater chance of failure to wean.

Respiratory muscle strength is evaluated by monitoring airway pressure during a maximum inspiratory effort. The NIF thus generated is ideally measured with a portable pressure gauge since the pressure gauges on most mechanical ventilators are not sufficiently adapted for measuring large negative pressures. Pressures of at least -30 cm H_2O indicate good muscle strength and potential for weaning; values of -20 cm H_2O or less indicate muscle weakness or poor cooperation and probable inability to wean.

Measurements of VC are also possible at the bedside and are another valuable predictor of the capacity to wean. Values larger than 10 mL/kg suggest adequate lung volumes, respiratory muscle strength, and patient effort.

When patients are found capable of weaning based on these various criteria of Po_2, Pco_2, NIF and VC, the chances for successful weaning are improved; however, as many as 50% of patients who fail to meet these standards are nonetheless successfully weaned, supporting the notion that weaning is presently as much an art as it is a science.

The usual prescription for weaning includes a gradual reduction of passive mechanical ventilation and a simultaneous increase of active spontaneous ventilation. In many centers this gradual return to spontaneous breathing is accomplished with a T-tube apparatus, commencing with 5 min of spontaneous breathing and progressing until spontaneous ventilation is tolerated for several hours. T-tube weaning requires continuous monitoring of patients for signs of fatigue or inadequate gas exchange. Since the T-tube apparatus does not include monitors of lung function, the signs of weaning failure include patient complaints of dyspnea, a rise in heart rate, a fall in systemic arterial pressure, or a documented impairment of arterial blood gases. To improve the capacity for monitoring during weaning, modern mechanical ventilators have a CPAP mode which when set to zero pressure (CPAP = 0) is nearly identical to T-tube weaning but takes advantage of the built-in monitors and alarms of the mechanical ventilator. Although the advantages of the internal alarm systems are substantial, these CPAP systems include flow valves which raise the resistance to inspiration by as much as 20%. At the present time, individual preferences dictate the use of T-tube or CPAP modes of weaning in most centers.

Although some patients are immediately weaned from passive mechanical ventilation to T tube or CPAP, many patients are weaned through an intermediate stage, intermittent mandatory ventilation (IMV). IMV delivers fixed positive-pressure V_{TS} from the mechanical ventilator at rates which can be progressively reduced; additional negative pressure breaths can be inspired by the patient as needed using the CPAP circuitry described above. In this manner, patients are able to determine a portion of their breathing but are also supplied with a guaranteed minute ventilation. IMV is distinct from the assist/control (A/C) mode for which inspiratory efforts from the patient trigger additional positive pressure inspirations at a preset V_T. The advantages and disadvantages of each of these modes of ventilation are summarized in Table 4-7.

If patients are unable to wean based on standard criteria or if they have already failed a weaning trial, passive ventilation is resumed until the patient's condition improves. Whether the respiratory muscles should be rested to avoid fatigue or stressed to improve performance remains controversial. Clearly if the failure of weaning is attributed to respiratory muscle weakness, a period of rest is indicated, using the A/C mode of ventilation rather than T tube, CPAP, or IMV. Ideally, in the A/C mode energy expenditure is limited to brief inspiratory efforts necessary to trigger the ventilator. If the inspiratory drive is suppressed by overbreathing the patient, the resultant elevated P_{O_2} and low P_{CO_2} may be sufficient to eliminate even this limited energy expenditure. If physiologic suppression of ventilation is

Table 4-7   Weaning from Mechanical Ventilation

Mode	FiO_2	Advantages	Disadvantages
T tube	variable	No added airway resistance Requires close supervision	No built-in alarms/monitors
CPAP=0	Variable	Takes advantage of monitor and alarm components of ventilator	Higher airway resistance than T-tube system; increased work of breathing
IMV	Variable	Monitors and alarms available Mixture of passive and active inspiration possible	High inspiratory resistance during spontaneous breathing
A/C	Variable	Permits patient to rest respiratory muscles *prior to* weaning	Limited exercise of respiratory muscles prior to weaning Impairs cardiac filling

IMV, intermittent mandatory ventilation; A/C, assist/control mode of mechanical ventilation; FiO_2, inspired oxygen fraction; CPAP, continuous positive airway pressure.

unsuccessful, similar results can be achieved by pharmacologic suppression of ventilation with sedation and, occasionally, muscle paralyzing agents such as pancuronium. This is the 'control' mode of mechanical ventilation and is most valuable for patients who are unable to wean and are fighting the ventilator. Such patients are wasting valuable energy stores, are anxious and uncomfortable, and are not efficiently ventilated. Control ventilation in these patients will often result in a substantial rise of Po_2 and a reduction of Pco_2. This mode, however, is appropriate only for patients who are not weaning, either because of altered ventilatory drive, musculoskeletal impairment, or active cardiopulmonary disease.

A recent modification of weaning with great promise is pressure support ventilation. In this mode, patients are able to establish their own rate and volume but the ventilator supplies a pressure boost which effectively reduces the work of breathing. Although the rationale for this mode is encouraging, there is insufficient data at this time to indicate if pressure support will reduce the duration of weaning, increase the percentage of patients weaned, or in any way improve survival.

In summary, weaning from mechanical ventilation is usually successful within 24 hours of surgery but is enhanced by measurement of a few essential parameters such as arterial blood gases, VC, and NIF. Attempts at weaning before these parameters fall within the desired range is occasionally successful but those who are extubated prematurely and then develop respiratory failure are placed in unnecessary jeopardy. Weaning is generally more successful when major systemic problems such as sepsis or malnutrition are corrected and acute and reversible lung diseases such as atelectasis or pneumonia are adequately treated. The ideal mode of weaning is a matter of choice, with some physicians preferring progressive periods of spontaneous breathing through a T piece and other physicians preferring IMV modes. Whichever is chosen, including the new form of pressure support ventilation, careful monitoring of patient function is essential.

Suggested Reading

Cain HD, Stevens PM. Preoperative pulmonary function and complications after cardiovascular surgery. *Chest*. 1979; 76:130–135.

Good JT, Woltz JF, Anderson JT, Dreisin RB, Petty TL. The routine use of positive end-expiratory pressure after open heart surgery. *Chest*. 1979; 76: 397–400.

Hodgkin JH, Dines DE, Didier EP. Preoperative evaluation of the patient with pulmonary disease. *Mayo Clinic Proc*. 1973; 48:114–118.

Hurewitz A, Bergofsky EH. The adult respiratory distress syndrome–physiologic basis for treatment. *Med Clin North Am*. 1981; 65:33–51.

Laszlo G, Archer GG, Darrell JH, Dawson JM, Fletcher CM. The diagnosis and prophylaxis of pulmonary complications of surgical operations. *Br J Surg*. 1973; 60:129–134.

Lell WA, Samuelson PN, Reves JG, Strong SD. Duration of intubation and ICU stay after open heart surgery. *South Med J*. 1979; 72:773–775.

Markland ON, Moorthy SS, Mahomed Y, King RD, Brown, JW. Postoperative phrenic nerve palsy in patients with open heart surgery. *Ann Thorac Surg*. 1985; 39:68–73.

Marvel SL, Elliot CG, Tocino I, Greenway LW, Metcalf SM, Chapman RH. Positive end-expiratory pressure following coronary artery bypass grafting. *Chest*. 1986; 90:537–540.

Mittman C. Assessment of operative risk in thoracic surgery. *Am Rev Respir Dis*. 1961; 84:197.

Morganroth, ML, Morganroth JL, Nett LM, Petty TL. Criteria for weaning from prolonged mechanical ventilation. *Arch Intern Med*. 1984; 144:1012–1016.

Pearce AC, Jones RM. Smoking and anesthesia: preoperative abstinence and perioperative morbidity. *Anesthesiology*. 1984; 61:576–584.

Pierson DJ. Weaning from mechanical ventilation in acute respiratory failure: concepts, indications, and techniques. *Respir Care*. 1983; 28:646–662.

Stauffer JL, Silvestri RC. Complications of endotracheal intubation, tracheostomy, and artificial airways. *Respir Care*. 1982; 27:417–434.

Stein M, Cassara EL. Preoperative pulmonary evaluation and therapy for surgical patients. *JAMA*. 1970; 211:787–790.

Tisi GM. Preoperative evaluation of pulmonary functions. *Am Rev Respir Dis*. 1979; 119:293–309.

Weisman IM, Rinaldo JE, Rogers RM, Sanders MH. State of the art–intermittent mandatory ventilation. *Am Rev Respir Dis*. 1983; 127:641–647.

Zwillich CW. Complications of assisted ventilation–a prospective study of 354 consecutive episodes. *Am J Med*. 1974; 57:161–170.

Renal Function Evaluation

Richard Barnett, M.D.

5

Acute renal failure (ARF) is observed in an estimated 2% to 7% of patients undergoing surgery requiring cardiopulmonary bypass. In this setting ARF is associated with an overall mortality rate of 35% to 50%. However, the mortality rate for cardiac surgery in patients with chronic renal failure (CRF) receiving maintenance dialysis is either not different or only marginally increased compared to cohorts with normal preoperative kidney function. It is not surprising that the kidneys, which normally receive 20% of the cardiac output, frequently mirror the potentially fatal depressions in myocardial, pulmonary, and systemic vascular function which may complicate cardiac bypass surgery. Appropriate preoperative evaluation of kidney function and management or even the prevention of ARF may favorably affect survival in these patients and will constitute a major focus of this chapter. Additionally we will also address the particular requirements of patients with CRF receiving maintenance dialytic therapy.

PREOPERATIVE EVALUATION

Preexisting renal failure is one of the most important predisposing factors for the development of severe ARF in patients undergoing coronary bypass surgery. A directed history, physical examination, and laboratory evaluation may target patients who will benefit from preoperative intervention (Table 5-1).

The medical history may not initially identify the individual

Table 5-1   Preoperative Renal Evaluation of the Cardiac Surgery Patient

History
   Preexisting renal failure
   Renal failure risk factors
      Congestive heart failure
      Hypertension
      Diabetes mellitus
      Peripheral vascular disease
      Obstructive uropathy
   Medications
Physical examination
   Blood pressure with orthostatics
   Fundoscopy
   Cardiopulmonary auscultation
   Edema or ascites
   Prostate size
Laboratory
   Creatinine, blood urea nitrogen
   Electrolytes, glucose, arterial blood gas*
   Ca, Po_4, Mg, uric acid
   Liver function tests, albumin
   Complete blood count
   Urinalysis
   24-h urine creatinine clearance*
   Renal sonogram,* renal scan*

*As needed.

with functional renal impairment. The patient should be specifically questioned about the presence of renal failure risk factors which in many cases are associated with altered myocardial performance. Congestive heart failure is seldom a cause of kidney impairment except when severe. Hypertension, which is important in the pathogenesis of left ventricular hypertrophy and coronary artery disease, may accelerate progressive nephron loss in many diseases promoting CRF. More frequently, coexisting hypertension and diabetes mellitus are involved in the pathogenesis of CRF and contribute to coronary artery disease. Peripheral vascular disease is often associated with renal vascular abnormalities resulting in kidney failure or hypertension. Coronary catheterization in these patients may dislodge atheromatous plaques, thereby precipitating ARF. Obstructive uropathy is a potentially reversible cause of CRF, more common in males, and may be a special consideration in patients with prostatic hypertrophy exposed to perioperative medications such as narcotic analgesics.

The value of establishing the varieties and doses of all prescription and over-the-counter medications is obvious to experienced clinicians. The antihypertensives and nonsteroidal agents, for example, may alone or in combination depress renal function. Other drugs such as digitalis depend on renal mechanisms for excretion and may accumulate if kidney function is acutely impaired. Diuretics may promote significant losses of electrolytes such as potassium and magnesium resulting in enhanced arrhythmogenic potential in addition to their well-known volume-depleting actions.

A thorough physical examination is essential in the evaluation of all patients with kidney disease. The key features in the preoperative evaluation of most cardiovascular surgery patients are outlined in Table 5-1. Conventional determination of blood pressure by cuff manometry should be supplemented with measurements of orthostatic changes in pressure or pulse rate, which may indicate effective volume depletion or the presence of autonomic neuropathy. Visualization of the fundi is markedly facilitated with standard mydriatics and can provide crucial information regarding the severity and chronicity of hypertension and diabetes. Examination of the heart and lungs for evidence of congestive heart failure or valvular abnormalities will often identify the patient with renal insufficiency consequent to diminished cardiac output. Such patients will frequently exhibit peripheral edema although other entities should be considered. These include right heart failure usually associated with chronic obstructive pulmonary disease, nephrotic syndrome and other hypooncotic states, urinary tract obstruction, and peripheral venous insufficiency. Vascular bruits are common in patients with extensive atherosclerotic disease who may not only be at risk for developing kidney failure secondary to renovascular abnormalities but are also more likely to sustain depression in renal function from atheroemboli.

Routine preoperative laboratory testing will provide valuable information regarding adequacy of kidney function. The serum creatinine is probably the most useful test for estimating kidney function, but its level depends on muscle mass in addition to the glomerular filtration rate (GFR). For example, after

---

Table 5-2   Renal Function Tests

1. **Glomerular filtration rate**

   A. Serum creatinine

   $$\frac{[(140 - \text{age}) \text{ wt kgl}^*}{72 \text{ (creatinine)}}$$

   *multiply $\times$ 0.85 if female

   B. Serum creatinine, 24–hour urine collection

   $$\frac{\text{urine creatinine (g/24 h)}}{\text{plasma creatinine (mg/dL)}} \times 70$$

2. **Fractional excretion of Na**

   $$\frac{\dfrac{\text{urine}}{\text{plasma}} (\text{Na}^+) \times 100}{\dfrac{\text{urine}}{\text{plasma}} (\text{creatinine})}$$

---

the fourth decade of life, GFR declines by approximately 1 mL/ min/y while creatinine remains within normal limits because of the proportional decline in muscle mass. This relationship is used in the derivation of formula 1A in Table 5-2. Individuals with more severe declines in muscle mass accompanying cirrhosis with malnutrition or progressive myopathies may exhibit normal creatinine despite GFRs less than 20 mL/min. When in doubt, the patient should be instructed to collect a 24–hour urine specimen to permit a more accurate determination of creatinine clearance. Use of the simplified version of the standard formula (see Table 5-2, formula 1B) depends on adequacy of collection. In general, urinary creatinine values much less than 1.2 g/24 h in men and 0.9 g/24 h in women should be viewed with suspicion if estimates of creatinine clearance by formulas 1A and 1B differ significantly.

In CRF, the blood urea nitrogen (BUN) is usually elevated in proportion to increases in creatinine. Marked depletion of effective vascular volume resulting commonly from diuretic-induced losses or, alternatively, poorly compensated congestive heart failure may be associated with an increase in BUN out of proportion to creatinine. In general, urea is reabsorbed along with sodium and its level is therefore especially elevated in sodium avid states associated with diminished effective vascular volume. However, urea synthesis is hepatic dependent and may be deceptively low in patients with liver disease.

Serum potassium (K^+) is depressed most often as a result of diuretics. Hyperkalemia is less commonly observed. Most individuals with CRF are able to maintain normal K^+ levels even at GFRs less than 10 cc/min. K^+ concentrations greater than 5 m Eq/L are often encountered in patients with tubulointerstitial abnormalities. These entities include individuals with chronic urinary obstruction and most frequently hyporeninemic-hypoaldosteronism. This latter entity is particularly frequent in individuals who have coexisting diabetes, hypertension, and moderate CRF. Other less common causes of altered K^+ levels may be encountered and their etiology should always be determined preoperatively.

Bicarbonate (HCO_3) levels reflect respiratory and metabolic abnormalities. Thus, a mildly depressed HCO_3 level is often more likely to represent respiratory alkalosis rather than metabolic acidosis. Elevated HCO_3 content is encountered in patients with diuretic-related metabolic alkalosis or alternatively associated with chronic lung disease and CO_2 retention. An arterial blood gas determination should resolve most of these uncertainties. Chloride usually balances changes in HCO_3 so that the anion gap ($Na - [Cl + HCO_3]$) remains within the normal range of approximately 8–16. An elevation of the anion gap is seldom observed in stable patients without advanced renal disease but its presence may suggest ongoing lactic or ketoacidosis.

Abnormalities in calcium (Ca^{++}) are uncommon but need to be evaluated preoperatively because of potentially adverse cardiovascular effects. Hypercalcemia is relatively rare except in patients with CRF receiving Ca and Vitamin D supplementation. Hypocalcemia most commonly results from hypoalbuminemia but may also be associated with CRF (usually in patients with hyperphosphatemia). Measurement of ionized Ca is a reasonable first step in patients with Ca abnormalities. Phosphorus (PO4) and magnesium (Mg) depletion can result from malnutrition or diuretic use and their plasma levels may not adequately reflect total body losses. Markedly increased uric acid levels may signify a cause of CRF or perhaps suggest a risk factor for developing contrast—induced ARF.

Anemia of chronic disease is observed in most cases of CRF

but gastrointestinal sources of blood loss should always be excluded. Urinalysis is a convenient method for identifying patients with renal or genitourinary abnormalities. Dipstick-positive proteinuria can be further quantitated with a 24-hour urine sample (in a 24-hour collection, measure creatinine simultaneously to ensure adequacy of collection). The presence of blood or protein in the urine should lead to a microscopic examination of a centrifuged specimen and in selected cases a urine culture. A renal sonogram is probably the most benign and cost-effective test for evaluating renal failure of unknown etiology. Renal size is usually reduced in CRF but may be normal or increased in ARF, diabetes mellitus, and other infiltrative diseases such as myeloma or amyloidosis. The urinary collecting system is ordinarily well-visualized by ultrasonography and is invaluable in excluding obstruction. Renal scan is an adjunctive test which provides functional information and can be helpful in diagnosing renovascular abnormalities.

Preoperative Management

Patients with underlying renal failure commonly have a variety of conditions that respond to effective preoperative management (Table 5-3). Congestive heart failure and volume depletion are usually correctable by conventional methods. In doubtful cases preoperative Swan-Ganz catheterization will guide diagnosis and management. In the late 1980s a wide range of therapeutic options existed for control of hypertension. The selection of oral agents should be tailored, if possible, to treat other medical conditions. Thus, the angiotensin converting enzyme inhibitors

Table 5-3   Preoperative Conditions in the Patient with Renal Failure

Congestive heart failure
Volume depletion
Hypertension
Diabetes
Electrolyte disorders
    Potassium
    Acid-base
    Phosphorous
    Magnesium
    Calcium

(ACEIs) and diuretics may benefit individuals with hypertension and congestive heart failure while coexisting hypertension and coronary ischemia may respond particularly well to β-blockers or calcium entry blockers. It should be noted that individuals with poorly controlled hypertension may experience transient worsening of preexisting renal dysfunction following the institution of an effective regimen. Modest decrements in GFR may be observed, but kidney function usually returns to normal within several weeks, thus emphasizing the desirability for early evaluation of such individuals. Patients requiring urgent or emergent surgery can be variably treated with oral, transdermal, or intravenous agents such as nitroprusside, β-blockers, enalapril, labetalol, and loop diuretics. These drugs have largely supplanted older intravenous medications including trimethaphan and methyldopa.

Effective preoperative management of diabetes mellitus may mitigate fluctuations in glycemic control resulting from the stress of the perioperative period. Large swings in plasma glucose values can alter intravascular volume consequent to an osmotic diuresis or via changes in plasma osmolality, promoting a shift of intracellular water to the extracellular and vascular compartments.

The influence of potassium on the cardiac conduction system and the relationship of this cation to glucose homeostasis and acid–base balance emphasize the need to correct abnormalities before surgery. Most hypokalemic patients undergoing cardiovascular surgery have diuretic losses accompanied by effective vascular volume depletion. Serum potassium concentration may not adequately reflect depletion of total body stores. Oral, and in some cases intravenous, supplementation should optimally be accomplished over at least several days and facilitated by the judicious use of a potassium-sparing diuretic. Correction of the volume depletion, which promotes secondary hyperaldosteronism, should mitigate further losses. Hyperkalemia is observed much less commonly but its etiology should be ascertained prior to surgery. Urinary tract obstruction associated with this abnormality may be encountered and treated primarily by relief of the obstruction. More commonly, hyporeninemic hypoaldosteronism is initially manifested in susceptible patients placed on a hospital-based sodium-restricted diet or medications that interfere with the renin-angiotensin-aldosterone system. These individuals usually respond to a diuretic often given with

$NaHCO_3$ to augment distal sodium delivery and maintain luminal electronegativity favorable for potassium secretion. Adrenal insufficiency as a cause of hyperkalemia is observed far less frequently, but potential deficient glucocorticoid production should be ascertained and hyperkalemia managed with hormone replacement and supplemental bicarbonate as needed. Kayexalate will bind potassium in the gut but should be used sparingly in the preoperative setting because its effectiveness often delays proper evaluation of the hyperkalemic patient.

Individuals with moderate to severe renal impairment frequently exhibit a variety of acid-base disorders. In most nondialysed patients metabolic acidosis need not be treated unless the serum HCO_3 concentration is less than 18 mEq/L. Oral $NaHCO_3$ or use of a HCO_3 precursor such as Shohl's solution (sodium citrate + citric acid) is an effective alternative to intravenous $NaHCO_3$. It is important to recognize that the serum HCO_3 may also be depressed consequent to a coexisting respiratory alkalosis. Interpretation of the arterial blood gas by use of a standard acid-base analysis may identify this possibility. It is important to avoid determining that "base deficit" equals "base requirement." Overzealous use of $NaHCO_3$ in a patient with a coexisting respiratory alkalosis may promote congestive heart failure, hypokalemia, tissue hypoxemia, and coronary vasoconstriction resulting from systemic alkalosis. Metabolic alkalosis often develops in CRF following the use of loop diuretics. Replacement of both volume and potassium losses will generally correct this abnormality.

Hyperphosphatemia may be encountered in individuals whose GFR is less than 25 mL/min. There is seldom a requirement for rapid correction of this disorder although institution of chronic binding therapy is a reasonable approach. Hypophosphatemia is occasionally observed in CRF patients receiving aluminum- or calcium-containing antacids. Given the adverse effects of this condition on musculoskeletal function, red blood cell integrity, and tissue oxygen delivery, phosphorous replacement to increase levels to greater than 2–3 mmol/L should be completed before surgery. Hypermagnesemia is infrequently encountered except in dialyzed patients but the hypomagnesemia seen in individuals on diuretics (usually with associated hypokalemia) or with malnutrition should respond to oral or intravenous replacement. Decreased magnesium levels may have adverse electrophysiologic consequences and promote hypocalcemia. Mild hypo- and hypercalcemia are commonly observed in CRF but rarely require acute intervention.

Intravenous contrast imaging and renal failure

Radiocontrast imaging is performed in the vast majority of patients undergoing cardiac surgery. The use of iodinated contrast agents has been linked to the development of ARF in 2% to 5% of cases in unselected series. Subsequent studies have identified preexisting renal failure as the most consistent abnormality associated with dye-induced ARF requiring dialysis. As many as half of all patients whose serum creatinine level is greater than 4 mg/dL, particularly those with diabetic nephropathy, will develop severe ARF. The contribution of other risk factors in the pathogenesis of dye-induced ARF such as volume depletion, advanced age, myeloma, and hyperuricemia is less clear. It has been our practice to initiate a saline-induced diuresis (a loop agent for congestive heart failure) the night before the study and to give 12.5–25 g of mannitol half an hour before contrast infusion. A postprocedure diuresis is maintained for an additional 8–12 hours with either saline or a loop diuretic. Other interventions including use of calcium entry blockers or newer non-anionic contrast substances have not been beneficial. The non-anionic dyes are not associated with a diminished incidence of ARF and should probably be reserved for individuals likely to develop congestive heart failure from the older, more hypertonic agents.

The onset of contrast-induced ARF is rapid, characterized by a variable sediment and low urine sodium; it is usually reversible within several days. Occasional patients may require dialysis support for several weeks. Nonetheless, despite the risk of renal failure, there is little rationale for delaying the expedient work-up in a patient with cardiovascular disease.

CARDIOPULMONARY BYPASS AND KIDNEY FUNCTION

The technical aspects of cardiopulmonary bypass are reviewed extensively in Chapters 10–12. The alteration in systemic and renal hemodynamics which occurs using this approach is ordinarily well tolerated. Interestingly in the absence of complications, duration of bypass may not alter the incidence of ARF. Renal blood flow may be diminished by more than 30% during bypass, but glomerular filtration is usually depressed to this extent only transiently. Research previously suggested that agents such as mannitol and furosemide confer protection against nephrotoxic and ischemic renal injury. As a result many centers have routinely used these agents perioperatively, although good controlled studies demonstrating their efficacy in this setting are lacking. At our center 12.5–25 g mannitol is added to the priming solution after initiation of bypass and supplemented hourly. Individuals undergoing repair of the aorta requiring cross-clamping above the renal arteries or those with preexisting renal dysfunction receive higher doses of mannitol to initiate and sustain a brisk diuresis. Postclamp or postbypass oliguria may be treated with successively increasing doses of furosemide or bumetanide (maximum 500 mg and 20 mg, respectively).

Attention to other factors may also limit the risk of ARF. Maximizing cardiac output by judicious volume replacement will tend to limit ischemic renal injury. Hemodilution, cold perfusion, and corticosteroids administered during bypass may be cytoprotective for a variety of organs including the kidney. The benefit of pulsatile versus nonpulsatile pump flow in reducing ARF has not been clearly demonstrated. Nephrotoxins such as methoxyflurane or perioperative aminoglycosides should be used sparingly if at all in patients with a history of CRF.

Postoperative acute renal failure

Acute renal failure is defined as the sudden deterioration of kidney function resulting from urinary obstruction, a diminution in perfusion, or severe renal parenchymal damage. The evaluation of the postoperative patient with ARF is geared toward excluding rapidly reversible causes (Table 5-4). Most ARF

Table 5-4   Initial Evaluation of Postoperative Acute Renal Failure

1. Rule out or exclude urinary obstruction
2. Exclude prerenal factors
3. Laboratory studies
   Serum: BUN, creatinine, electrolytes, liver function tests, creatine phosphokinase
   Urine: urinalysis and urinary sodium, potassium, chloride, creatinine, and osmolality
   Renal scan,* renal ultrasound*

---

*As needed.

associated with bypass surgery is observed within the first 1–2 days following surgery. A thorough preoperative evaluation will vastly facilitate the construction of a workable differential diagnosis and expedite the selection of a therapeutic regimen.

Perioperative period: Acute obstructive uropathy is unusual in the initial postoperative setting, but the response to treatment justifies a prompt evaluation. This entity should be strongly considered in the patient who develops sudden oligoanuria (less than 100 mL/d) without obvious hemodynamic compromise or active urinary sediment. Replacement, repositioning, or flushing of the Foley catheter can be curative as well as diagnostic. Bilateral acute ureteral obstruction is extremely rare in the postbypass setting and is generally easily diagnosed by renal ultrasonography.

In the early postoperative period, prerenal azotemia usually resulting from diminished cardiac output is the most frequently encountered readily reversible cause of kidney dysfunction. Urinary sodium, urinary osmolality, and a fresh spun microscopic urinalysis are extremely useful in confirming this diagnosis (see Table 5-4). Simultaneous measurements of urine and plasma creatinine and sodium levels are required to calculate the fractional sodium excretion (F_{ENa}) (Table 5-2), which may provide a more accurate index than urinary sodium alone. In prerenal states there is enhanced tubular reabsorption of both sodium and water. Thus a high urinary osmolality and a low F_{ENa} (<1%) and urine sodium (often accompanied by a high urine potassium secondary to aldosterone effect) are characteristically observed. Occasionally a developing metabolic alkalosis can promote an obligatory natriuresis and in these instances low urinary

Table 5-5   Urinary Studies in Evaluation of Acute Renal Failure

	Prerenal	ARF
Urinary sodium (mEq/L)	<20	>40
Fractional sodium excretion (F_{ENa})%	<1	>2
Urinary osmolality (mOsm/kg)	>500	<400
Urinary sediment	Benign	Brown casts
Urinary chloride (mEq/L)	<20	>40
Urinary/plasma creatinine	>40	<20
Urine/plasma osmolality	>2	<1

143

chloride (Table 5-5) and plasma BUN/creatinine greater than 20 are consistent with the prerenal state. Collectively this may be used to corroborate information obtained from Swan-Ganz catheterization. Thus, a reduced pulmonary capillary wedge (PCW) pressure and diminished cardiac output in the face of a low urinary sodium value should prompt the clinician to initiate volume repletion in the form of crystalloids or colloids, including blood products according to need. Frequently however, a low F_{ENa} is observed with nonelevated filling pressures and normal or even increased cardiac output. Under such circumstances it is reasonable to attempt "fluid challenges" with normal saline; 300–500 mL infused over 15–20 minutes may be repeated two or three times depending on the response. Measurements of cardiac output, PCW and systemic blood pressures, arterial blood gas, and urinary output are obtained to judge the adequacy of this response to volume challenge. If the patient demonstrates little change in these parameters, loop diuretics, mannitol or "renal dose dopamine," may be used to augment urine output. Patients manifesting low F_{ENa}, low cardiac output, high PCW pressure, poor oxygenation, and systemic hypotension have a very poor prognosis. Combination therapy including diuretics and afterload reduction (e.g., nitroprusside, ACEIs), inotropic agents, renal dose dopamine, and in some cases an intra-aortic balloon pump can be used. Reduced cardiac performance secondary to ongoing ischemia needs to be promptly addressed. Additional measures including plasma ultrafiltration will decrease PCW pressure and improve the oxygenation but may critically diminish cardiac output and end-organ perfusion, resulting in an increased anion gap lactic acidosis requiring vasopressors to maintain adequate blood pressure. On the other hand, patients with congestive heart failure who have low F_{ENa} and reasonable systemic blood pressures can often benefit from plasma ultrafiltration in the event that other maneuvers, including a loop diuretic given with 10 mg metolazone, are ineffective.

In the early postoperative period, a low F_{ENa} with seemingly adequate cardiac performance is encountered which does not respond to therapy despite further increases in cardiac output. This may be observed in early ARF despite a variable sediment although several other possibilities should be considered. Evolving septicemia is occasionally observed in the initial postoperative setting and should be avidly excluded. Vascular abnormalities which compromise renal perfusion including intracardiac shunts, arteriovenous fistulae, and aortic dissection involving both renal arteries are extremely uncommon but potentially correctable.

More than 48 hours postoperatively: ARF encountered after the first several days is usually the result of problems observed during or shortly after surgery. However, in this interval a variety of additional factors expand the differential diagnosis of ARF from that described in the previous section. Again, combining data from urine indices and Swan-Ganz monitoring is invaluable in evaluating and treating prerenal causes (Table 5-6). The common causes of prerenal azotemia, including congestive heart failure, true volume depletion, and sepsis, can usually be evaluated and appropriate therapy assessed by central hemodynamic monitoring. In the event the Swan-Ganz catheter has been removed and the patient is clinically stable, cautious volume challenges with efficacy measured by changes in arterial blood gases, blood pressure, and urine output is a reasonable initial approach. Alternatively, if the patient is exhibiting early congestive heart failure, diuretic or vasodilator therapy can be used. If these therapeutic "trials" fail to resolve the problem, replacement of the Swan-Ganz catheter can be invaluable.

The exclusion of prerenal and postrenal causes of renal failure should always be conducted in the work-up of ARF. Renal parenchymal injury may be exacerbated by either of these conditions and return of kidney function delayed by failure to institute appropriate measures. ARF not attributable to events in the perioperative period commonly results from nephrotoxic agents. The aminoglycoside antibiotics are probably

---

Table 5-6   Acute Renal Failure over 48 Hours Postoperatively

Prerenal azotemia
Urinary obstruction
Parenchymal renal injury
   Nephrotoxic
   Allergic interstitial
   Vasoactive agents
   Postischemic
   Renovascular
   Thromboemboli

---

the most frequent drug-related cause of ARF despite the widespread monitoring of levels. Intravenous contrast study should be avoided in the immediate postoperative period because it may cause ARF remarkable for low urinary excretion of sodium. Extensive muscle breakdown may promote rhabdomyolysis and renal failure associated with elevated creatine phosphokinase and a urine dipstick positive for blood with a relative paucity of erythrocytes on microscopic examination.

Allergic interstitial nephritis can result from the continuous use of virtually any drug although the penicillins and cephalosporins are perhaps among the more common offending agents. This entity is classically characterized by eosinophilia, eosinophiluria, a rash, and resolution following discontinuation of the drug. Careful review of the medication sheets will aid in deciding which of many agents should be removed.

A variety of medications have hemodynamic effects that may significantly impair renal perfusion. The antihypertensives and nonsteroidal agents can reduce kidney function in this manner. The ACEIs are major contributors to this entity by several mechanisms. Use of a shorter acting agent, such as captopril, in an initial dose of 6.25 mg or alternatively small frequent doses of IV enalapril, may minimize this problem in the postoperative period of cardiac bypass patients.

Postischemic ARF is more frequently encountered in the immediate postoperative period. Subsequent prolonged hypotension or cardiopulmonary arrest may result in ARF associated with evidence of other end-organ hypoperfusion. Abnormal liver function tests with marked elevation in the levels of serum transaminases and transient elevated anion gap metabolic acidosis may be the evidence that retrospectively supports this diagnosis.

Renal arterial or venous thrombosis are unusual causes of ARF in the late postoperative period but may induce unexplained hematuria or proteinuria. Since bilateral disease is usually required to promote significant renal dysfunction, renal scan may not delineate either entity. Findings on a renal ultrasound study correlated with Doppler flows may be suggestive. Angiography poses the major risk of contrast, but it is clearly the gold standard in the diagnosis of these disorders. Thromboembolic ARF is occasionally encountered in patients undergoing vascular surgery or catheterization who have extensive atherosclerotic disease. The appearances of ARF, eosinophiluria, a "fish net" rash, and distal emboli involving the lower extremities, are associated with this syndrome. There is at present no effective therapy for atheroembolic disease. The insertion or removal of an intraaortic balloon pump catheter has occasionally resulted in dislodgement of atheroemboli and the development of ARF.

Postoperative management: The preceding section focused on the evaluation of readily correctable causes of ARF. Persistent significant decreases in renal function will require modifications in the management of these individuals. Ultrafiltration or dialysis need not be used in the majority of cases if careful attention is paid to specific clinical parameters.

Nonoliguric ARF in which urine output exceeds 500 mL/d is generally managed more easily and has a better prognosis than oliguric ARF. Fluid intake should not exceed output (urine, stool, drainage tubes) by more than 500–1000 mL/d in patients with "normal" volume status who manifest established ARF. Despite the assiduous efforts of the ICU staff, intake and output sheets often do not adequately reflect ongoing losses. Daily weights are difficult to obtain in these patients but provide an invaluable tool for estimating appropriate intake. Hyponatremia is frequently observed in these patients, predominantly because the diminished GFR limits the ability to excrete a water load. However, pain, nausea, and stress can elevate vasopressin levels enough to impair water handling in patients even with normal renal function. Free water restriction, normal saline administration, and a loop diuretic may be variably used to treat hyponatremia. Hypernatremia is much less common but may ensue in patients with large hypotonic losses concurrently receiving saline or sodium-supplemented hyperalimentation solutions. Alteration in the sodium content of these solutions is usually sufficient to correct hypernatremia. The cause of hypernatremia in the individual with renal failure should be actively sought and therapy tailored accordingly. Sodium intake should obviously be restricted. Release of potassium from cells, which occurs commonly in acute metabolic acidosis, β-blockade, insulin deficiency, and rhabdomyolysis, may require emergent therapy. Renal excretion of potassium in ARF is often impaired, particularly in individuals with tubulo-interstitial disease but may be augmented by use of a loop diuretic. The emergent treatment of hyperkalemia with calcium, bicarbonate, insulin, and glucose is adequately detailed in standard medical and surgical texts. Of recent note is the use of aerosolized β-agonist bronchodilators which facilitate potassium uptake by cells. Their onset of action is within minutes and may persist for several hours. Resin binders, such as kayexalate, and hemodialysis are the methods of choice for removing large quantities of potassium.

The kidney ordinarily excretes 70–100 mEq nonvolatile acid each day. Net acid excretion is impaired in ARF and a decrease in serum HCO_3 levels of 1–3 mEq/d is often observed. After exclusion of coexisting respiratory alkalosis, base may be replaced when HCO_3 levels fall below 16–18 mEq/L. Bicarbonate may be provided as the sodium salt. With normal hepatic function it can also be infused as a precursor (acetate contained in alimentation solutions) or orally as a sodium citrate/citric acid preparation (Shohl's solution). Nasogastric suction of fluid less than pH 2 may be adjunctive therapy, which serves also to remove volume. Metabolic alkalosis is occasionally observed in ARF and is tolerated less well than metabolic acidosis. It may result from overzealous alkali supplementation, loop diuretic therapy, or aggressive nasogastric suction. The latter entity should only occur at low gastric pH. Thus, removal of 100 mEq acid by aspiration of 1 L of fluid with pH 1 generates 100 mEq HCO_3, pH of 2, 10 mEq, etc. An H_2-blocker will raise pH to 3 or greater (1 mEq H^+/L) and thus effectively prevent alkali generation via this route. Because HCO_3 excretion in ARF can be markedly reduced, metabolic alkalosis may be severe and can be treated by 0.1 N HCl infusion via a central vein or hemodialysis.

Calcium phosphate abnormalities are frequently observed in ARF but are not usually very significant. Hypocalcemia is usually modest and in such cases treated with calcium supplementation and vitamin D. Phosphate binding in the gut is best accomplished by the recently available calcium acetate preparation. Hypophosphatemia resulting from overzealous binding therapy is uncommon but may cause life-threatening hemolysis or rhabdomyolysis, while hyperphosphatemia is seldom an emergent entity. When in doubt, a situation occurring frequently on weekends/nights when automated Ca/PO_4 determination is not available, it is wise to err on the side of hyperphosphatemia. Modest hypermagnesemia is frequently seen and is well tolerated.

It should be obvious that many pharmacotherapeutics used in the perioperative setting directly impair renal function. The most common offending agents include antibiotics (particularly the aminoglycosides), antihypertensives (particularly the ACEIs), nonsteroidal agents, the immunosuppressive cyclosporine, and intravenous contrast agents. Renal dysfunction may also impair excretion of drugs or their metabolites, notably antiarrhythmic agents (e.g., digoxin, procainamide), antibiotics (e.g., aminoglycosides, vancomycin, and a variety of penicillins, cephalosporins), antihypertensives (captopril), cimetidine (ranitidine is less dependent on renal excretion), and a host of other pharmacotherapeutics. Fortunately several reference sources will guide use and dosage of the most frequently used drugs.

Hypertension is a common occurrence after bypass surgery, often resulting from volume overload, pain, or anxiety as well as enhanced systemic vascular resistance. It cannot be overstated how important effective analgesia is in mitigating hypertension in this setting; hypertension should be zealously treated. Increases in intravascular volume are usually suspected clinically or by central monitoring. Treatment of this condition with diuretics will usually not result in marked increases in BUN in contrast to their effect in volume depletion. Nondiuretic antihypertensive agents are effective but several points should be noted. By altering systemic vascular resistance or cardiac output, all agents may significantly impair renal perfusion. Consequently, unless the situation is emergent, very small doses of the shortest acting agents in a class should be used and the response monitored carefully. A rapid scan of the vital sign flow sheets will frequently demonstrate progressive renal dysfunction coincident with lowering mean arterial pressure, although other causes such as hemorrhage, cardiac dysfunction, and sepsis should also be considered. A compromise between the desired blood pressure (cardiovascular surgeon) and maximal renal perfusion (nephrologist) usually results in stabilization of renal function. ACEIs have been cited for promoting renal impairment out of proportion to changes in blood pressure as a result of preferential effects on the glomerular efferent arteriole. Small, gradually increasing doses are usually tolerated, but if in doubt, particularly in the setting of volume depletion, other oral or intravenous agents should be used.

Since the landmark study of Abel and coworkers, hypertonic glucose plus amino acid therapy has been used extensively in the management of the postoperative patient with ARF. Although it is the general impression that mortality, morbidity, and return of renal function are aided by this approach, studies in the past decade are not overwhelmingly supportive. Problems with patient selection may in part account for these results but fortunately significant increases in morbidity or mortality have not been noted. Consequently, we recommend early institution of hyperalimentation therapy for the cardiac patient with ARF in the postoperative setting. Sufficient calories and amino acids should be provided in a minimum infusion volume. In general, a basal requirement of 25–35 kcal/kg body wt/d should be provided and increased by 25% to 75% depending on the severity of postoperative complications. From 0.6 to 1.0/g protein/kg/d can be provided in the form of essential and nonessential amino acids. Measurement of nitrogen balance is the best way to estimate protein requirements (nitrogen can be converted to protein equivalent by multiplying by 6.25). However, use of nitrogen balance can be difficult when there are large daily fluctuations and losses from hemorrhage, gastrointestinal tract, wound sites, or dialysis. Nonetheless, it can be estimated by adding the nitrogen from change in BUN to 0.031 g/nitrogen/kg/d (from nonurea compounds). Thus, in a 70-kg patient (total body water approximately 42 kg) who has no urine or other substantial urea losses and whose BUN increased by 10 mg/dL in a day when protein intake is 0, then the protein catabolic rate is [100 mg/L × 42 L + 0.031 × 42] 6.25 = 34 g protein. Under optimal circumstances 34 g protein could be provided to this patient to achieve neutral nitrogen balance. Loss of nitrogen from urine hemodialysis and peritoneal dialysis must be considered to effectively use this approach. Additionally, protein requirements may increase significantly during an acute clinical deterioration associated with higher protein catabolism.

Enteral alimentation has been vastly simplified because of the wide variety of formulas presently available and should be used wherever possible. Although a large amount of calories and protein can be provided in a relatively small volume, an osmotic-induced diarrhea may result during rapid infusion rates. Changes in formula osmolality or infusion rate may be corrective.

As described previously, electrolyte monitoring should

result in manipulations of the specific alimentation regimen. Of note, hyperglycemia is frequently observed in these patients whose glucose tolerance may be impaired because of the effects of uremia and the presence of high levels of counterregulatory hormones. Insulin resistance is to be anticipated and rather large doses may be administered in the hyperalimentation formula or by an intramuscular or subcutaneous route.

The widespread availability of dialytic therapy in the past few decades has vastly altered the approach to the surgical patient with ARF. In most circumstances dialysis is initiated early in the course of ARF before heart failure, hyperkalemia, acidosis, pericarditis, or seizures warrant emergent measures. The advantages and disadvantages of three major types of renal replacement therapy are summarized in Table 5-7. Optimally, a cardiac surgery center should have substantial experience with each method, but institutional preferences often play the major role in selecting the specific modality. Hemodialysis is the most popular technique and is invaluable in managing catabolic post-operative patients requiring high clearances. Acute volume removal is also readily accomplished by this method; however, it is often associated with rapid changes in central and systemic pressures resulting in increased myocardial oxygen demand. Use of bicarbonate dialysate and a more biocompatible dialysis membrane such as polyacrylonitrile may lessen such problems. It is our practice to perform "heparin free" hemodialysis in the postoperative setting. Frequent saline flushes of the dialyzer or use of citrate have been very successful.

Continuous arteriovenous hemofiltration (CAVH) is a

Table 5-7 Advantages and Disadvantages of Renal Replacement Therapies

	HD	PD	CAVH
Volume removal	++	+	++++
Hyperkalemia and hypercatabolism	++++	++	+
Myocardial stress	− −	0	0
Hypotension	− − −	0	−
Anticoagulation requirement	0 or −	0	− − −
Access placement	−	− − −	− −
Potential infection	0 or −	− − −	−

HD, hemodialysis; PD, peritoneal dialysis; CAVH, continuous arteriovenous hemofiltration; +, advantage; −, disadvantage.

relatively new technique in which the arterial and venous pressure difference is used by connecting arterial and venous catheters to a hemofilter. The resulting transmembrane pressure creates a significant volume of ultrafiltrate which can be augmented to 1.0–1.5 L/h by connection of the ultrafiltration port to wall suction. A replacement fluid such as Ringer's acetate is infused, thereby achieving urea clearances of 5–20 mL/min which may not be sufficient in the severely hypercatabolic patient. Unlike acute hemodialysis, two catheters (or a Scribner shunt) are required. Frequent clotting of the hemofilter is mitigated by a constant heparin infusion, which may have adverse consequences in the postcardiac surgery patient. For the most part, CAVH in the postcardiac surgery patient should be reserved for individuals whose wounds are well healed and who sustain an adverse event like prolonged sepsis (the most frequent cause of death in these patients) requiring infusion of large, continuous volumes of fluid for administration of pressors, antimicrobials, and nutrition. A recent refinement of this technique (CAVHD) can enhance clearances over conventional CAVH. In most centers, frequent and often daily hemodialysis is usually the more viable option. The utility of peritoneal dialysis varies from center to center. Reasonable clearances which achieve daily volume reduction of several liters a day can be obtained, although hemodialysis remains the treatment of choice for severe hyperkalemia. Acute and chronic peritoneal dialysis catheters may be used in the perioperative setting although the former has been associated with very high rates of infection.

Cardiovascular surgery and the chronic dialysis patient

We have previously noted that CRF per se is not a major risk factor for cardiovascular surgery. Many of the points discussed in ARF are applicable to chronic dialysis patients. These individuals are usually managed in concert with the nephrology group. It is our practice to have the patient well dialyzed and volume optimized, with the last treatment completed the day before surgery. In specific instances, dialysis may be required immediately before surgery. In the hemodialyzed individual no systemic anticoagulant is used and frequent saline flushing (every 15–20 minutes) of the dialyzer usually limits the need to change the dialyzer because of clotting. Blood products should be infused at separate sites if this technique is used. Intraoperatively, attention to the volume status and electrolyte disorders usually prevents the need for immediate dialysis following surgery. Most patients can be subsequently managed on their routine schedule. In the case of the patient with hemodialysis, the arteriovenous access should be monitored closely for evidence of clotting that may result from perioperative hypotension. Blood pressure determinations, arterial-venous blood drawing, or fluid administration should be avoided on the access extremity except in an emergency. The access site is especially prone to infection in the setting of perioperative sepsis, often resulting from infected intravenous sites or pneumonia and should be examined closely in the febrile patient. The limited clearances of aminoglycosides and vancomycin in the patient with advanced CRF may be advantageous in treating life-threatening infection. Vancomycin may be administered every 5–10 days (follow levels) and the loading dose of gentamycin given after each dialysis. The clearances of other antibiotics are listed in multiple references.

A variety of medications employed in the perioperative setting require dosage modifications which may vary depending on the dialytic modality used (see Maher, JF). It should additionally be noted that the effects of analgesics or sedatives in these patients may be prolonged and very small, frequent dosing is preferable.

Nutritional guidelines for the CRF patients are similar to those noted for ARF. Although protein requirements are higher in the patient with minimal renal function, the protein catabolic rate is easily estimated, thus simplifying the task of devising an appropriate nutritional regimen and dialysis schedule. However, 10–13 g amino acid is lost in each treatment by conventional hemodialysis. Peritoneal dialysis promotes 12–20 g protein loss daily in addition to amino acid depletion. Thus, the minimum protein requirement for CRF patients in the perioperative period is about 1 g/kg/d and this may need to be augmented if the dialysis treatment period is increased.

SUGGESTED READING

Bevan DR. Renal function in anaesthesia and surgery. London: Academic Press, 1979.

Brenner BM, Lazarus MJ. Acute renal failure. New York: Churchill Livingstone, 1988.

Maher JF. Replacement of renal function by dialysis. Dordrecht, Netherlands: Kluwer Academic Publishers, 1989.

O'Rourke RA, Brenner BM, Stein JH. The heart and renal disease. New York: Churchill Livingstone, 1984.

Ream AK, Fogdall RP. Acute cardiovascular management. Philadelphia: J.B. Lippincott Company, 1982.

Roe BB. Perioperative management in cardiothoracic surgery. Boston: Little, Brown and Company, 1981.

Rose BD. Clinical physiology of acid-base and electrolyte disorders. New York: McGraw Hill, 1989.

Tilney NL, Lazarus JM. Surgical care of the patient with renal failure. Philadelphia: Saunders, 1982.

Endocrine and Metabolic Diseases

Andrew J. Green, M.D.

6

DIABETES MELLITUS

Diabetes mellitus is a disorder of fuel metabolism characterized by hyperglycemia due to an absolute or relative deficiency of insulin. It is diagnosed by a fasting blood sugar level of greater than 140 mg/dL in a nonstressed, nonpregnant adult on two occasions by two random blood glucose measurements in excess of 200 mg/dL or by an abnormal response to an oral glucose load (Table 6-1). There are three general diabetic syndromes.

Type I diabetes mellitus

This disorder is characterized by *absolute insulin deficiency* due to destruction of pancreatic B cells, usually by an autoimmune process. These patients comprise about 15% of the diabetic population. It generally presents in the young (under age 40), and patients are usually of normal body weight. Occasionally it presents in the elderly. Family history is frequently negative for diabetes. Because of the absolute insulin deficiency, these patients are prone to diabetic ketoacidosis (DKA) and depend on exogenous insulin for survival. For this reason, they are sometimes called insulin–dependent diabetics. Prior to the insulin era, these patients inevitably died. *Insulin must never be denied a type I diabetic,* even for a brief period.

Type II diabetes mellitus

This disorder is characterized by *insulin resistance* and comprises 80% to 85% of the diabetic population. Circulating insulin levels are normal or even elevated but are inappropriately low for

---

Table 6-1 Criteria and Technique for Screening and Diagnosis of Diabetes Mellitus

---

Screening Indications

Screening tests for diabetes mellitus (DM) are indicated when the patient
- has a strong family history of diabetes mellitus
- is markedly obese
- has a history of giving birth to infants > 9 lbs (4000 grams)

Screening Criteria

In adults (except pregnant women) a fasting plasma (or serum) glucose is the preferred screening test. A fasting plasma glucose > 140 mg/dL suggests diabetes (see below), while a fasting plasma glucose < 140 mg/dL but ≥ 115 mg/dL is an indication for glucose tolerance testing. A fasting plasma glucose < 115 mg/dL indicates normal glucose tolerance.

Diagnostic Criteria for DM and Impaired Glucose Tolerance in Nonpregnant Adults

The diagnosis of DM is restricted to individuals with any one of the following:
- Random plasma glucose of ≥ 200 mg/dL, plus classic signs and symptoms
- Fasting plasma glucose ≥ 140 mg/dL on two occasions
- Fasting plasma glucose < 140 mg/dL, but at least two abnormal glucose tolerance tests
- Abnormal glucose tolerance test is defined as a two hour sample ≥ 200 mg/dL and at least one intervening sample ≥ 200 mg/dL

The diagnosis of impaired glucose tolerance is restricted to individuals with *all* of the following:
- Fasting plasma glucose <140 mg/dL
- A 2 hr oral glucose tolerance test level between 140 and 200 mg/dL
- An intervening oral glucose tolerance test level ≥ 200 mg/dL

Technique for Oral Glucose Tolerance Testing of Nonpregnant Adults

Subject selection:

Individuals tested should be in an unstressed condition. This test should not be done in persons who are malnourished, or who have restricted their carbohydrate intake to less than 150 g/day for 3 or more days. Patients experiencing acute medical or surgical stress, or who have been confined to bed for more than 3 days should not be tested as these conditions also affect glucose tolerance. It is preferable that all medications be stopped 3 days prior to testing whenever possible.

Test technique:

The test should be scheduled in the morning after an overnight fast. The subject must remain quietly seated, NPO, and refrain from smoking. A baseline blood sample is drawn for determination of the plasma glucose, and 75 g glucose administered in a standard solution (1 g glucose/cc). Begin timing as the subject begins to drink. Obtain blood samples at 30, 60, 90, and 120 minutes.

Modifed from: Rifkin, H. (ed) The physician's guide to Type II Diabetes (NIDDM): diagnosis and treatment, American Diabetes Association, 1984.

the degree of hyperglycemia present, indicating a component of pancreatic β-cell dysfunction. Type II diabetes usually presents after the age of 40, and about 85% of patients are obese. Family history is usually positive. A small proportion of type II diabetics present at a young age and have an autosomal dominant form of transmission. This syndrome is (clumsily) called maturity-onset diabetes of the young, or MODY. Because type II diabetics produce insulin, they do not depend on exogenous insulin for survival (although they may need it to control hyperglycemia) and are sometimes called non–insulin-dependent diabetics. Most type II diabetics are managed without insulin, and with diet alone or diet and an oral hypoglycemic agent, which enhances insulin secretion.

Type other or secondary diabetes

A small minority of diabetic patients (1% to 2%) develop hyperglycemia due to another condition that causes insulin deficiency or insulin resistance. Examples include end-stage pancreatitis or pancreatectomy, hypercortisolism, either exogenous or endogenous (Cushing's syndrome), acromegaly, and rare heritable syndromes of insulin resistance or secretion of abnormal insulins. These patients are managed in a way similar to type I or type II diabetic patients, depending on whether their syndrome is characterized by insulin deficiency or resistance, respectively. Gestational diabetes, or diabetes due to pregnancy, is also a part of this subset. The management issues raised by the gestational diabetic are beyond the scope of this chapter.

Management of the hospitalized diabetic patient

Diet: The diabetic diet should promote good nutrition and maintenance of optimal weight. A proper diet consists of approximately 50% to 60% carbohydrate, 20% protein, and 20% to 30% fat, divided between three meals, and often a bedtime snack in patients receiving insulin. The house officer is responsible primarily for determining the number of calories prescribed. Consultation with a nutritionist is always desirable.

Caloric prescription is based on ideal body weight and activity. Hospitalized patients are generally sedentary, but allowance for calories equal to moderate activity should be provided to postoperative patients to promote tissue repair.

Ideal body weight is estimated on the basis of height, gender, and frame size. For women of medium frame, ideal body weight approximates 100 lb for 5 ft of height, plus or minus 5 lb/inch above or below 5 ft. Add or subtract 10% for large or small frame. For men of medium frame, ideal body weight approximates 106 lb for 5 ft, ±6 lb/inch, with the same 10% correction for large or small frames.

Caloric prescription is based on basal requirements plus activity (or stress) requirements. Basal requirements are estimated by ideal weight multiplied by 10. Activity requirements are three times ideal weight for sedentary activity, five times for moderate activity or usual postoperative stress, and ten times for heavy activity or severe stress (e.g., high fever, sepsis). Thus, a 5 ft 9 inch man of medium frame should receive $[106 + (9 \times 6)] \times 10$ plus $[106 + (9 \times 6)] \times 3$, or 2080 calories preoperatively. It would make sense to round off to the nearest hundred and prescribe 2100 calories.

Blood glucose monitoring: Monitoring of the blood glucose level is essential in the management of hospitalized diabetic patients. Estimation of venous plasma blood glucose can be obtained rapidly and painlessly via a drop of capillary blood obtained by finger stick with a lancet. Automatic lancing devices are less traumatic than a manual stick and should always be used. Pricking the side of the distal phalanx, rather than the sensitive pulp of the finger is recommended. The drop of capillary blood is placed on a glucose–oxidase-treated strip, which undergoes a color change proportional to the blood glucose concentration. A digital readout is provided by a reflectance meter and is accurate to within 10% to 15%. The quality of results depends on the quality of the technique. Care must be taken that the drop of blood obtained covers the reagent pad completely and that the timing of blotting the specimen is precise.

Blood glucose monitoring has replaced urine glucose monitoring for several reasons. First, it is direct and provides instantaneous data. Even under the best of circumstances, urine glucose determinations can only reflect the blood glucose concentration at the time the urine was being filtered. Second, renal thresholds for glucose vary even in patients with apparently healthy kidneys. If renal disease is present, as is common in hospitalized diabetic patients, all bets are off: renal threshold can be high or low. Thus, the urinary glucose value may be misleading. Third, urine glucose should be negative when blood sugars are in the normal or near-normal range. This is the target range for most patients, so urine glucose values are not helpful here. It also follows that urine glucose levels are useless for the diagnosis of hypoglycemia.

While urine testing for glucose cannot be recommended in hospital, it remains valuable for testing for the presence of ketones. A good guideline for testing for urinary ketones is any time the blood sugar level is greater than 350–400 mg/dL.

The frequency of blood glucose monitoring is tailored to the individual patient. Patients whose diabetes is controlled by diet alone, or by diet and an oral hypoglycemic, may be checked once or twice daily. Patients requiring insulin will need more frequent monitoring, usually before meals and at bedtime. *The timing of blood glucose monitoring is critical for interpretation of results.* Specimens should be obtained preprandially; otherwise the glycemic peak that normally follows eating could be misinterpreted as hyperglycemia. Orders should be written to reflect this; i.e., they should be written as before meals and at bedtime rather than four times daily, every 6 hours, or according to clock time. This recognizes the reality that patients are served meals at different times on different days. Obviously, a blood sugar level obtained at noon before lunch has a different meaning than a blood sugar level obtained at noon after lunch.

Goals of blood glucose management: If following a prescribed diet does not control hyperglycemia, medications are used. Before considering these, it is important to establish the goals of therapy. Clearly, extremes of hyperglycemia must be avoided, as these predispose to metabolic decompensation. Normalization or near-normalization of blood glucose is believed to promote wound healing and tissue repair by preventing fluid and electrolyte imbalance, optimizing neutrophil function, and promoting tissue oxygenation. Over the long term, the risk of developing the complications of diabetes is related to the adequacy of glycemic control. However, the benefits of "tight" control of blood sugar must be weighed against the risk of induction of hypoglycemia. In the relatively young and healthy patient, the cost:benefit ratio weighs on the side of tight control. In practical terms, this means striving for a fasting blood glucose level of 60–120 mg/dL and preprandial blood glucose levels of less than 150 mg/dL. In the older patient, and particularly those with cardiovascular disease, more caution is in order, because the catecholamine surge that is part of hypoglycemic counterregulation places a large oxygen demand on the myocardium. In patients with whom it is desirable to avoid hypoglycemia, appropriate goals are fasting glucose levels of 100–150 mg/dL and preprandial glucose values of less than 200–250 mg/dL. In the perioperative period, while a patient is unable to communicate symptoms of hypoglycemia, it is appropriate to maintain blood glucose levels at 150–250 mg/dL to decrease the risk of inducing hypoglycemia.

Oral hypoglycemic agents: These medications are described in Table 6-2. All work the same way—by augmenting the β-cell secretory capacity. Selection of an agent is therefore largely arbitrary. Many endocrinologists prefer the second generation oral hypoglycemics, glipizide and glyburide, because they permit convenient once or twice daily dosing, have dual routes of hepatic and renal metabolism, and generally lack side effects.

The author's opinion is that all currently available agents are acceptable with the exception of chlorpropamide. Chlorpropamide has a very long half-life (36 hours in people with normal renal function) which puts patients at risk for late and prolonged hypoglycemia. In addition, it causes a disulfuram-like reaction in many patients and frequently causes hyponatremia due to syndrome of inappropriate antidiuretic hormone (SIADH). Since a number of equally effective agents are available that do not carry this burden of side effects, it seems reasonable to consider this drug obsolete. Of the remaining drugs, hypoglycemia may be most frequent with glyburide, the most potent agent, particularly in elderly patients.

Table 6-2 Sulfonylureas Available in the United States

Generic name	Brand name	Dosage range (mg/day)	Duration (h)	Comments
First Generation				
Acetohexamide	Dymelor	250–1500	12–18	Hepatic metabolism to an active metabolite; given 2–3 times daily
Chlorpropamide	Diabinase	100–750	60	~70% hepatic metabolism to less active metabolites, ~30% excreted intact by kidneys; can cause nephrogenic SIADH and disulfiram-type reaction; given once daily.
Tolazamide	Tolinase	100–1000	12–24	Hepatic metabolism to active and inactive products. Given 1–2 times daily
Tolbutamide	Orinase	500–3000	6–12	Hepatic metabolism to an inactive product; given 2–3 times daily
Second Generation				
Glipizide	Glucotrol	2.5–40	8–24	Hepatic metabolism to inactive products; given 1–2 times daily
Glyburide	Diabeta Micronase	1.25–20	12–24	Hepatic metabolism to inactive products; given 1–2 times daily

Insulin: The commonly used insulins are referred to as rapid-acting (regular and semilente) and intermediate-acting (NPH and lente) (Table 6-3). Each insulin preparation is available from several sources: mixed beef/pork, purified pork or beef, and biosynthetic (recombinant DNA) or semisynthetic human insulin. Pork insulin differs from human at only one amino acid residue, and so purified pork insulin is no more immunogenic than human insulin. Beef insulin differs at three amino acid residues, and so is relatively immunogenic. The less highly purified mixed beef/pork insulin also contains small amounts of contaminants, such as proinsulin and other pancreatic peptides. Each brand of insulin has a slightly different pharmacokinetic profile (in other words, all NPH is not alike) and so it is advisable to maintain patients on their usual brand. The available insulins and their pharmacokinetics are listed in Table 6-3. When starting a patient on insulin for the first time, use human or purified pork insulin.

Numerous successful insulin regimens are available. Nothing succeeds like success, and any regimen that meets the goal of around-the-clock euglycemia or near-euglycemia is satisfactory. To accomplish this in nearly all type I diabetics and many type II diabetics, it is necessary to mimic normal physiology, i.e., provide an insulin peak after each meal. A convenient way of doing this is the time-honored "mixed-split" regimen, i.e., *mixing* rapid- and intermediate-acting insulins and *splitting* the dose into two injections, before breakfast and before dinner. Thus, the rapid-acting insulin injected before breakfast peaks around the time breakfast calories are absorbed, and the intermediate-acting insulin injected before breakfast peaks around lunchtime. Similarly, rapid-acting insulin injected before dinner covers

Table 6-3   Pharmacokinetics of Commercial Insulin Preparations

Preparation	Onset of Action (hours)	Peak Action (hours)	Duration of action (hours)
Regular	0.5–1	2–4	4–6
Semilente	1–2	3–6	8–12
NPH	2–4	6–14	14–20
Lente	2–4	6–14	16–20
Ultralente	6–14	minimal	18–36

* Actions given are approximate. There is significant inter- *and* intra-individual variations based on injection site, temperature, exercise of the injected area, etc.

dinnertime calories, and the intermediate-acting insulin covers the bedtime snack and provides a good level of insulinemia overnight. Accordingly, on a split-mixed regimen, insulin dosages are titrated as follows: to raise or lower the fasting blood sugar, lower or raise the evening NPH (or Lente); to change the prelunch blood sugar, titrate the morning regular (or semilente); to change the predinner blood sugar, titrate the morning NPH; to change the bedtime blood sugar, titrate the evening regular. This concept is illustrated in Figure 6-1. The practice of "covering" an elevated blood sugar with additional doses of regular insulin in the metabolically stable patient is to be strongly discouraged because additional insulin peaks at odd times inevitably yield confusing results. Dosage adjustments should be made as above on the next day. If hyperglycemia is severe (greater than 300 mg/dL), it is appropriate to add 2–6 U regular insulin to the next scheduled dosage on a one-time basis.

Managing the short procedure: For the purposes of this discussion, a short procedure is one lasting no more than an hour or two and not requiring general anesthesia, such as angiography, gastrointestinal endoscopy, or minor surgery. Generally patients are NPO after midnight. Efforts should be made to schedule the patient as early in the day as possible; ideally the diabetic patient should be "first case."

The type I diabetic patient: Since the type I diabetic is wholly dependent on exogenous insulin, it is important to *never hold the insulin dose.* An unexpected delay in the procedure or in transport could allow the insulin level to drop to the point that DKA might develop, and this can happen rapidly. The goal of management, therefore, is to ensure a sufficient insulinemia to prevent ketosis and at the same time avoid hypo- or severe hyperglycemia (a range of blood glucose of 150–250 mg/dL is appropriate). There are several fairly simple ways of achieving this. If the efforts of scheduling the patient early have been successful, and it is anticipated that the procedure will be completed by around lunchtime, it is acceptable to begin an infusion of 5% dextrose at 100–150 mL/h and administer half the usual insulin dose subcutaneously at breakfast time. Blood glucose concentrations should be monitored every 1–2 hours until the patient leaves the floor and on return. If the blood glucose level drops below 100, either increase the rate of the D_5 infusion or give 10–25 mL D_{50} intravenously. If the patient is able to eat lunch on return from

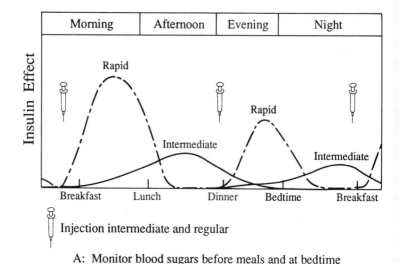

Injection intermediate and regular

A: Monitor blood sugars before meals and at bedtime

B: To adjust: titrate:
   Fasting blood glucose   evening intermediate
   pre-lunch   morning regular
   pre-dinner   morning intermediate
   bedtime   evening regular

C: Typical adjustment regimen:

blood sugar	adjustment
less than 70	decrease 2 units
71 - 140	no change
141 - 200	increase 2 units
201 - 250	increase 4 units
251 - 300	increase 4 - 6 units
more than 300	increase 4 - 8 units

Figure 6-1 Pharmacokinetics and titration of the split-mixed regimen.

the procedure, administer approximately 25% of the total morning insulin dose as regular insulin. (For example, if the patient normally receives 15R + 25N before breakfast, give 7R + 12N along with the dextrose infusion before the procedure, and 10R before lunch). Once it is clear the patient is tolerating food, stop the dextrose infusion.

If the procedure is to be performed later in the day and the patient maintained NPO for a long period or if it is anticipated that the patient will not tolerate food after the procedure, a better alternative is to administer 10% dextrose at 100–150 mL/h along with an insulin infusion. The details of how to prepare and titrate the insulin infusion are given below (see Diabetic emergencies).

Other alternatives are also acceptable. As long as insulin is not withheld entirely and patients' blood glucose levels are monitored frequently, they should do well.

The type II diabetic: Since these patients do produce endogenous insulin, they are inherently more metabolically stable than the type I diabetic. Type II diabetic patients rarely become severely hyperglycemic when they are fasted, so long as good hydration is maintained. If the patient is controlled with diet or an oral hypoglycemic, it is safe to hydrate gently with normal saline and hold medication. Blood glucose levels should be monitored every 2–4 hours. Extra caution must be exercised when dealing with patients who are taking chlorpropamide (Diabinase), because its long half-life may produce late hypoglycemia in a fasted patient. It is also safe to treat insulin-requiring type II diabetics in this fashion (i.e., hold medication, hydrate, and observe) but *only if certainty exists that they are, in fact, type II.* If uncertainty exists as to the type of diabetes in patients using insulin, they should be treated as type I (see preceding section). If the blood glucose level goes above 300 mg/dL, 5–10 U regular human insulin should be administered subcutaneously or intravenously. Patients returning in time for lunch should receive half their usual dose of oral medication at that time.

Perioperative management of the diabetic patient: The management of the diabetic patient who is to undergo a major surgical procedure differs from that of the patient who undergoes a short procedure. First, it can be anticipated that patients will often be NPO for more than 48 hours. Nutrition is frequently neglected under these circumstances in favor of more pressing issues, but it is difficult to see this as advantageous. A minimal level of short-term nutrition should be provided. Second, the stresses of surgery and anesthesia in the perioperative period tend to cause hyperglycemia and increase the risk of DKA. A system providing flexibility and ease of titration is desirable.

The best way to accomplish these goals is administration

of an intravenous insulin infusion in conjunction with an infusion of 10% dextrose at 75–150 mL/h with frequent blood glucose monitoring of all diabetic patients. The details of how to prepare and titrate the insulin infusion are given below. Ten percent dextrose given at a rate of 100 mL/h provides 240 g glucose in 24 hours, or 960 calories. This is not adequate nutrition, but it is enough to minimize protein wasting over the short term. An ampule of multivitamins should be added to the first liter of D_{10} each day. The insulin-dextrose infusion should be started preoperatively and can be maintained by the anesthesiologist in the operating room and recovery room, and in the SICU or hospital floor until the patient is able to eat.

An alternative to the continuous infusion of intravenous insulin is the hourly bolus of intravenous insulin. An infusion of 5% or 10% dextrose is started at 75–150 mL/h, and approximately 1/20 of the usual total daily insulin dose is given as an intravenous bolus, with hourly blood sugar monitoring, and repetition and adjustment of the bolus dose accordingly. The disadvantage of this technique is that it requires close attention to the clock time and great care to ensure that doses of insulin are not missed.

The third alternative for perioperative management of the diabetic patient is administration of subcutaneous regular insulin. Ten percent dextrose is given at 75–150 mL/h as with the other regimens. One-fourth of the total daily insulin dose is given as regular subcutaneous at 7:00 to 8:00 AM and repeated every 6 hours. Blood glucose is monitored every 2–4 hours (hourly intraoperatively). Small doses of intravenous insulin can be given if hyperglycemia develops before the next scheduled dose, and the rate of the dextrose infusion increased if the blood glucose level dips below 125 mg/dL. This approach is acceptable for all types of surgery *except cardiac surgery,* because hypothermia prevents perfusion of the subcutaneous tissue, rendering absorption unreliable. An *intravenous insulin regimen must be used for cardiac surgery or any procedure utilizing hypothermia*. This approach lacks the flexibility of dose titration of the intravenous insulin infusion but is the simplest and is often very satisfactory.

Diabetic complications

Since the advent of the insulin era, the most important cause of morbidity and mortality among diabetic patients has been the long-term complications of diabetes, which appear after about 10 years of disease. All diabetics, regardless of type, are prone to the same complications, which is one of the reasons why it is thought that hyperglycemia or other metabolic complications of the diabetic milieu is responsible. The complications of diabetes involve the microvasculature and macrovasculature, leading to the high prevalence of diabetes among patients requiring cardiovascular and peripheral vascular surgery. Usually other complications coexist.

Retinopathy: Microaneurysms are the first lesions of early, or background, diabetic retinopathy. The walls of microvessels weaken, form outpouchings, and hemorrhage, leading to the characteristic dot and blot hemorrhages. Transudation of plasma proteins leads to the development of refractile-appearing hard exudates. Capillary closure leads to ischemia. Background retinopathy rarely impairs vision, unless it causes macular edema. In some patients proliferative retinopathy develops in response to ischemia. Fragile new vessels grow, unsupported by the retinal stroma, and project anteriorly into the vitreous. If these vessels break, vitreous hemorrhage results, which immediately obscures vision. If the clot organizes into a scar, it may place traction on the retina, leading to detachment and permanent blindness.

Nephropathy: Proteinuria is usually the first sign of diabetic nephropathy. Once azotemia develops, progression to complete renal failure is the rule in less than 5 years. Urinary tract infections are also common among diabetics, due to relative immunocompromise and the high prevalence of atonic bladder. Great care must be taken to avoid or minimize nephrotoxic insults, because acute renal failure commonly results. This includes vigorously hydrating the patient before any procedure using iodinated contrast material (including computed tomography scans and intravenous pyelograms), avoiding aminoglycoside antibiotics when possible, and meticulously following drug levels when not possible, avoiding hypotension, and carefully screening for urinary tract infections. Indwelling bladder catheters should be avoided when possible and removed promptly when not avoidable. Careful control of hypertension is important and has been shown to decrease the rate of decline of renal function.

Neuropathy: There are three general neuropathic syndromes: peripheral sensorimotor neuropathy, mononeuropathy, and autonomic neuropathy. Sensorimotor neuropathy is the most common and typically presents in the feet with loss of sensation or tingling or painful paresthsias, which progress from distal to proximal. The intrinsic muscles of the hands and feet are typically involved early. Loss of sensation is subtle initially but may progress to complete anethesia. As the disease progresses, larger muscles of the leg become atrophic. Mononeuropathies and radiculopathies are lesions of a single nerve, probably due to infarction. Any nerve may be involved. Cranial neuropathies may lead to unilateral oculomotor palsy or Bell's palsy. Peroneal involvement may lead to inability to dorsiflex the foot (foot drop). Truncal radiculopathy may imitate the pain of shingles or even an intra–abdominal crisis. Autonomic neuropathy is common. As mentioned above, it may cause an asymptomatic atonic bladder, predisposing to urinary tract infection. Other autonomic syndromes include gastroparesis, diarrhea alternating with constipation, sexual dysfunction, orthostatic dizziness, night sweats, and hypoglycemic unawareness.

Vascular disease: The histopathology and the consequences of the atherosclerosis associated with diabetes are identical to atherosclerosis occurring in the general population, although it is more common, occurs at an earlier age, and frequently is more severe. It is not clear if hyperglycemia plays a major role directly, or if the obesity, hypercholesterolemia, and hyperlipidemia commonly associated with poorly controlled diabetes are responsible. Myocardial infarction and stroke account for most (early) mortality among diabetics, and gangrene of the lower extremity is fifty times more common among the diabetic population. Smoking is a synergistic risk factor.

The diabetic foot: Since the foot may be considered a vascularized neuromuscular unit, it is not surprising that it is often involved in patients with long-standing diabetes. Sensorimotor neuropathy is a prerequisite. Toe flexors are involved earlier and more severely than toe extensors. This causes muscle imbalance, leading to abnormal weight-bearing under the metatarsal heads. Pressure leads to ulceration in this area. Lack of pain sensation prevents the usual protective mechanisms from coming into play. Poor vascular supply causes poor wound healing and leaves the foot susceptible to infection. Nonhealing ulcers, gangrene, and amputation often result. The feet of diabetic patients must be inspected regularly and carefully and any signs of skin breakdown or infection treated vigorously.

Diabetic emergencies

Hypoglycemia: Hypoglycemia is the most common diabetic emergency. Symptoms of mild hypoglycemia are mediated by epinephrine secreted as part of the counterregulatory response and resemble those of anxiety: diaphoresis, tachycardia or palpitations, tremulousness. Symptoms of slightly more severe hypoglycemia include weakness, hunger, and dizziness. Severe hypoglycemia causes symptoms of brain dysfunction (neuroglycopenia): feeling "out of it," confusion, disorientation, slurred speech, combativeness. Patients with autonomic neuropathy may lack adrenergic symptoms, and so the first indication of hypoglycemia may be symptoms of neuroglycopenia. The end stage of severe, prolonged hypoglycemia is brain damage, coma, and death. In the unconscious, obtunded, or anesthetized patient, careful monitoring is indicated to detect (or better yet, prevent) hypoglycemia.

The treatment of hypoglycemia depends on its severity. Mild hypoglycemia (blood sugar level over 50, patient alert and oriented) should be treated orally. Most people have a tendency to overtreat, with resultant late hyperglycemia. Liquids are preferred, because they are absorbed more quickly, but any food containing carbohydrate will be effective. Adequate carbohydrate for mild hypoglycemia is present in 4–8 oz milk, fruit juice, or regular (not diet!) soda pop, four to six small hard candies or saltines, or two to three small cookies. Remember that 10–20 minutes is required for absorption from the gastrointestinal tract, and so a lag exists between ingesting carbohydrate and symptomatic relief. Blood glucose should be tested about an hour later to ensure an adequate glycemic response to treatment.

Severe hypoglycemia (defined by signs of neuroglycopenia) should be treated parenterally. Intravenous dextrose in any concentration is acceptable; about 25–50 grams of glucose is generally required. This can be accomplished most rapidly by intravenous push of 50% dextrose, provided a large-bore intravenous line is available. Again, overtreatment is to be avoided. D_{50} comes in 100-mL ampules; administer 0.5 to 1 ampule, and recheck blood sugar level. Usually neurologic recovery is rapid, but occasionally is not, especially if the patient has been unconscious for a long period. There is no advantage to raising the blood glucose level to over 150 mg/dL, but blood glucose value should be monitored every 30-60 minutes until the patient has recovered. If intravenous access is not available or difficult, give 1.0 mg glucagon subcutaneously. Glucagon raises the blood glucose concentration by stimulating hepatic glycogenolysis and is effective in 10–20 minutes. If venous access is a problem, it often makes more sense to administer glucagon subcutaneously immediately than to waste valuable minutes attempting to establish a secure line. The line remains necessary, but after administration of glucagon work can proceed with greater leisure.

Diabetic ketoacidosis: DKA is an emergency requiring urgent therapy. It results from severe insulin deficiency as a result of failure to receive insulin in a type I diabetic or marked peripheral insulin antagonism due to stress (commonly infection or infarction). Severe insulin deficiency results in peripheral lipolysis, which provides the substrate for hepatic ketoacid generation. Patients present with nausea, vomiting, abdominal pain, thirst, and variable degrees of stupor or coma. Severe hyperglycemia results in an osmotic diuresis, which causes fluid and electrolyte depletion. Hypotension may result, with tissue hypoperfusion leading to a superimposed lactic acidosis. The general strategy for treating DKA is three-pronged: diagnosis and treatment of precipitating cause, fluid and electrolyte repletion, and insulin administration. Careful monitoring is crucial.

Diagnosis and correction of the precipitating cause of DKA is a requisite for successful therapy. Careful history and physical examination are needed with particular attention to skin, oral cavity, and feet for signs of infection. Basic laboratory studies include chest x-ray, electrocardiogram (ECG), urinalysis, and cultures of blood and urine. In addition, obtain a complete blood count (CBC) with differential, electrolytes, magnesium, phosphorus, blood urea nitrogen (BUN), creatinine, and arterial blood gases.

Fluid: A large-bore intravenous line should be rapidly established to administer fluid. Since essentially all patients in DKA have a total body depletion of water and sodium, administer a liter of isotonic saline rapidly while awaiting initial laboratory results. If the patient is elderly, is suspected of having a myocardial infarction, or has a compromised cardiac status, monitoring of central venous or pulmonary capillary wedge pressure is necessary, and fluid is administered as rapidly as tolerated. A second liter of fluid should be given over the next hour. After 1–2 L normal saline has been administered, give 0.45 normal saline at 150–500 mL/h, adjusting the rate according to clinical response and urine output. Once the blood glucose level has fallen to 250–300 mg/dL, change to 5% dextrose half normal saline.

Electrolytes: *Potassium.* All patients in DKA are total body potassium depleted due to the osmotic diuresis. Acidosis causes H^+ to be exchanged for K^+ across cell membranes, and so the plasma concentration of K^+ may be high, normal, or low at presentation. Accordingly, K^+ should be administered once the plasma concentration is less than 5.0 mEq at 20–40 mEq/h. If the initial K^+ is low, more rapid administration may be needed, with ECGs every 2 hours. If renal impairment exists, K^+ repletion should be less aggressive.

Bicarbonate. There are several good reasons to avoid bicarbonate therapy in patients with DKA. Acute alkalinization of the peripheral circulation generates CO_2, which crosses cell membranes easily and may lead to a paradoxical acute *worsening* of acidosis intracellularly and in the central nervous system. Secondly, it shifts the oxyhemoglobin dissociation curve to the left, worsening oxygen delivery to the tissues. Finally, a retrospective analysis of patients treated for severe DKA showed no difference in outcome in patients receiving and not receiving bicarbonate. The other side of the coin is that severe acidosis depresses myocardial contractility and vascular tone, so most experts recommend administering bicarbonate if the arterial pH is less than 7.0–7.1, or the bicarbonate level is less than 5 mEq/dL. In this situation 88 mEq (2 ampules) of sodium bicarbonate should be added to the first liter of fluid, which is given as 0.45 normal saline, to avoid administering a hypertonic solution. One to 2 ampules of bicarbonate per liter can be given until the pH is 7.1–7.2. Bicarbonate should not be given when the pH is above 7.2, as overshoot alkalosis commonly results.

Insulin: Insulin is necessary to stop lipolysis and ketogenesis. Although in the past large doses of insulin (50–100 U every 2–4 hours) were used, most authorities currently prefer the "low-dose" approach because it leads to a lower incidence of hypoglycemia and hypokalemia. Either the intravenous route or intramuscular route is effective, though the former seems more humane. If intravenous access is difficult, an initial intramuscular dose of insulin is a good idea, so it can begin to act while a line is being established. Begin therapy with a bolus of 10 U regular insulin intramuscularly or intravenously, followed by an insulin infusion at 6–10 U/h (or about 0.1 U/kg/h). If the hyperglycemia or acidosis does not respond within 2 hours, double the dose of insulin every 2 hours until a response is seen.

Preparing and managing an insulin drip. There is no need to rely on the pharmacy. Simply add 10 U regular insulin to 100 mL normal saline, or 50 U regular insulin to 500 mL normal saline, to give a dilution of 1 U/10 mL, which is easy to titrate. Since insulin adsorbs to plastic, add 5 mL 25% albumin or flush the line with 30–50 mL solution before infusing into the patient. It is also acceptable to add a few milliliters of the patient's blood to the bag of saline, as long as strict attention to sterile technique is maintained. This results in a cloudy infusion bag, which has been known to precipitate concern among nurses and patients, and so may be less desirable on an aesthetic basis.

Continue the insulin infusion at the initial rate until the blood sugar level is 250–300 mg/dL. At that point, begin D_5 normal saline at 100–150 mL/h, and titrate the insulin infusion according to blood glucose every 1–2 hours, with a goal of maintaining the blood glucose level at 100–250 mg/dL. *Never stop the insulin drip!* This bears repeating. **Never stop the insulin drip!** The half-life of intravenous insulin is only minutes, and if the drip is turned off, DKA may rapidly recur. The drip may be titrated as low as 1–2 U/h. If at this point the patient's blood glucose level drops below 100 mg/dL, increase the rate of the D_5 infusion or switch to 10% dextrose at whatever rate necessary to maintain blood glucose in the target range.

Changing to subcutaneous insulin. The time to change from an intravenous to a subcutaneous regimen is when the patient is alert, feeling well, and able to resume a normal diet. It is advisable to give a trial of one or two clear liquid meals, maintaining the intravenous dextrose and insulin, to ensure that the patient tolerates food. At this point, give subcutaneous insulin about 30 minutes before mealtime, decrease the rate of the dextrose infusion at mealtime, and stop the insulin infusion 60–90 minutes *after* the subcutaneous dose of insulin. This is to allow sufficient time to permit absorption of insulin from the subcutaneous depot.

The dose of subcutaneous insulin may be estimated from the patient's previous subcutaneous regimen, or from the intravenous insulin requirement over the prior 24 hours. If the previous subcutaneous regimen had been effective, resume it at a 10% to 20% lower dose, anticipating that the patient may not eat as well as usual in the immediate recovery period. If the patient had not been well controlled, an increase in dose may be necessary.

If the patient has not received insulin previously or a new and improved regimen is deemed necessary, it can be estimated from the total amount of insulin infused the day prior. Give two-thirds the total dose before breakfast, with two-thirds of this as NPH or Lente and one-third as regular. Give one-third the total dose before dinner, with half as intermediate-acting and half as regular insulin. Alternatively, some endocrinologists prefer to give approximately 25% of the total dose as regular before meals and approximately 25% at bedtime as intermediate-acting insulin. This latter approach allows for observation of the glycemic response to each meal, with more precise titration of the insulin dose. Patients can continue on a regimen of four injections a day, or it can be modified to a traditional split-mixed regimen according to the rules given above.

Maintaining an insulin infusion. If a patient is stabilized after treatment for DKA, but not able to tolerate oral feedings, it is desirable to maintain a minimal level of nutrition by infusing 10% dextrose and insulin (see the discussion of the perioperative management of the diabetic patient). Infuse D_{10} at 75–150 mL/h and titrate the insulin drip to maintain the blood glucose level at 100-250 mg/dL. Initially this can be done by monitoring finger stick blood glucose every 2 hours and adjusting as follows:

Blood glucose	Insulin infusion
± 0–50 mg/dL	No change
± 51–100	± 0.5 U
± 101–150	± 1.0 U
± 151–200	± 2.0 U
+ >200	Bolus 4 U IV, +2.5 U
− >200	Increase D_{10} 50 mL/h −2.0 U

If blood glucose content drops below 100 mg/dL, give 25 mL 50% dextrose and decrease insulin infusion according to algorithm.

Clearly, this algorithm is meant as a guideline, and attention must be paid to long-term trends. For example, if the blood glucose level drops 30–40 mg/dL at each measurement, although the algorithm does not call for any changes, the patient is headed for trouble. Respond by decreasing the insulin infusion by half a unit or increasing the rate of dextrose infusion.

Table 6-4   Treatment of Diabetic Ketoacidosis

Evaluation	History and physical exam with attention to signs of infection/infarction, arterial blood gases, glucose, electrolytes, BUN/creatinine, CBC with differential, Mg, PO_4, ECG, Chest X-ray, urinalysis, blood and urine cultures
Fluid	1–2 L normal saline rapidly
	1–2 L normal saline at 500 mL/h
	1/2 normal saline at 150–500 mL/h
	D_5 1/2 N saline once blood sugar is 250–300 mg/dL
Electrolytes	K^+ at 20–40 mEq/h once plasma K^+ is < 5.0
	K^+ at 40–80 mEq/h into central vein if presenting K^+ is < 3.0 mEq/dL
	HCO_3 only if pH is < 7.1
	If pH is < 7.1, give 1–2 ampules HCO_3 in the first liter of saline, which should be 1/2 N. Continue with 1 ampule/L until pH is > 7.1.
Insulin	Immediate bolus of 10 U IM or IV
	Insulin infusion at 6–10 U/h (about 0.1 U/kg)
	To prepare an insulin drip:
	50 U regular insulin in 500 mL normal saline to give a concentration of 1 U/10 mL. Add 5 mL 25% albumin or flush line.

NEVER STOP THE INSULIN DRIP!

Monitoring	
Vital signs, urine output	hourly
Finger stick glucose	hourly
Arterial blood gases	q2–4h
Plasma Na, K, Cl, HCO_3, glucose	q2–4h
CBC, BUN, creatinine	q8–12h
Mg, PO_4	daily

Once the patient has clearly stabilized in the target range, it is acceptable to decrease the frequency of finger stick monitoring to every 4 hours.

Monitoring the patient in DKA: Initially, the patient should be evaluated with arterial blood gases, electrolytes, BUN/creatinine, magnesium, and phosphorus to assess the metabolic state, as well as ECG, CBC with differential, urinalysis, and cultures to seek a precipitating cause. Close monitoring of the patient is essential to a positive outcome and avoiding complications of therapy. This usually requires an intensive care setting. Patients should have hourly vital signs or continuous blood pressure monitoring if hemodynamically unstable. Urine output should be followed hourly. For the first 8–12 hours, follow hourly finger stick glucose values. Sodium, potassium, chloride, and bicarbonate should be followed every 2–4 hours (potassium more frequently if the patient is hyper- or hypokalemic). The BUN, creatinine, and CBC should be followed every 8–12 hours and magnesium and phosphorus daily. A flow sheet which clearly displays vital signs, blood glucose and other laboratory results, rate of insulin infusion, fluid input and output, and other medications administered is essential.

Table 6-4 summarizes the treatment of DKA.

THYROID DISEASE

Hyperthyroidism

Hyperthyroidism is defined as an excess of biologically active thyroid hormones in the circulation. There are many causes of hyperthyroidism; Graves' disease, toxic multinodular goiter, and overdose of exogenous thyroid hormone are the most common. Classic signs and symptoms of hyperthyroidism are generally fairly obvious and include goiter, resting tachycardia, tremor, diaphoresis, diarrhea, weight loss, and emotional irritability. Apathetic hyperthyroidism presents in older patients or those with underlying illness and requires a high index of suspicion to detect. High output congestive heart failure occurs occasionally. Because hyperthyroidism can precipitate angina, myocardial infarction, and virtually any arrhythmia (classically atrial fibrillation resistant to digoxin), it should be considered in patients presenting with these problems. Patients with borderline thyroid hyperfunction due to Graves' disease or multinodular goiter may develop overt thyroid toxicosis acutely if given an iodine load, as occurs with administration of iodinated radiographic contrast material.

Hyperthyroidism is diagnosed by the demonstration of elevated levels of circulating thyroid hormone and suppression of thyrotropin (TSH) measured by a supersensitive assay. The best test is the free thyroxine index (FTI), a multiple of the total thyroxine (T_4) and the triiodothyronine (T_3) resin uptake (T_3RU). The T_3 level is also elevated. An isolated T_4 should not be ordered, because it may be altered by changes in levels of thyroid-binding proteins. The T_3RU corrects for binding-protein abnormalities. The combination of the total T_4 and T_3RU yields the reliable FTI. These tests may be rendered unreliable in postoperative patients or in those who have severe nonthyroidal illness, and so must be interpreted cautiously in this context (see Euthyroid sick syndrome, below).

The primary risks of hyperthyroid patients who undergo invasive procedures are precipitation of arrhythmias due to increased myocardial irritability and precipitation of thyroid storm. Thyrotoxic arrhythmias are difficult to control pharmacologically. Elective procedures or operations should be deferred until hyperthyroidism is controlled by antithyroid medication or radioactive iodine. Patients requiring surgery emergently require a more aggressive approach directed at reducing levels of thyroid hormone as rapidly as possible and antagonizing its effects peripherally.

Urgent treatment of hyperthyroidism requires the following:

1. β-Blockade with propranolol: 20–40 mg every 6 hours orally or 2–10 mg by slow intravenous infusion every 6 hours to reduce the heart rate to less than 90.
2. Antithyroid medication: either propylthiouracil (PTU), given as a loading dose of 1000 mg orally or via nasogastric tube, followed by 300 mg orally every 8 hours *or* methimazole 100 mg loading dose orally or by nasogastric tube, followed by 30 mg orally daily or bid. PTU is generally preferred because it inhibits peripheral conversion of T_4 to T_3.
3. Inorganic iodide: administered *1 hour after* antithyroid medication: either saturated solution of potassium iodide (SSKI)

5 drops orally tid, or sodium iodide 500 mg orally or intravenously every 8–12 hours.

4. Hydrocortisone 100 mg intravenously every 8 hours, to protect against the possibility of decreased adrenal reserve.

Thyroid storm is by definition acute, severe, life-threatening hyperthyroidism. The diagnosis is based on clinical impression, as there is no precise cutoff that distinguishes it from uncontrolled hyperthyroidism. It is characterized by hyperpyrexia, delirium, marked tachycardia and other arrhythmias, nausea, vomiting, heart failure, and vascular collapse. It is usually triggered in a patient with mild or undiagnosed hyperthyroidism by illness, surgery, trauma, or exposure to an iodine load, as when given iodinated contrast. Treatment is the same as for preparation of a thyrotoxic patient for urgent surgery, with additional supportive measures such as cooling blankets, volume expansion, electrolytes and aggressive treatment of underlying or coexisting illness. Aspirin should be avoided, because it displaces thyroid hormone from its plasma–binding proteins.

Hypothyroidism

Hypothyroidism is a lack of circulating thyroid hormone. Primary hypothyroidism is common, especially in women. It may be spontaneous, due to an autoimmune process, or the result of radioactive iodine treatment or thyroid surgery. Diagnosis is made by a low free thyroxine index (FTI) and an elevated TSH level. Clues on physical examination include bradycardia, pale dry skin, nonpitting edema of the face and extremities, "hung-up" reflexes, and a thyroidectomy scar—a valuable sign often missed. Frequently physical examination is normal, and the patient may have only nonspecific complaints such as fatigue, constipation, muscle cramps, or cold intolerance.

Laboratory evaluation is usually normal, except for the alterations in thyroid hormone and TSH. Mild anemia may be present. In more severe cases creatinine phosphokinase, lactic dehydrogenase, and aldolase levels are elevated, due to release from skeletal muscle and reduced clearance. Pericardial effusions may be present but are rarely hemodynamically significant. The ECG characteristically shows low voltage, intraventricular conduction delays, and nonspecific ST-T changes.

Hypothyroid patients have decreased myocardial contractility, increased peripheral resistance, and decreased myocardial and peripheral oxygen demand. Consequent to this, volume contraction and decreased cardiac output occurs, but end-diastolic pressures are normal. Because of the reduced myocardial oxygen demand of hypothyroidism, thyroid hormone replacement can precipitate angina.

Patients with mild hypothyroidism generally have an uncomplicated perioperative course. If an operation or procedure is elective, it may still be appropriate to delay for several months to allow for replacement therapy. The usual replacement dose is $75-150\,\mu g\,T_4$ daily. In elderly patients or patients with cardiovascular disease, it is prudent to start therapy with a dose of $25-50$ μg and advance the dose by $25\,\mu g$ every 2–4 weeks, until the TSH normalizes. If a patient has severe coronary artery disease, however, it may be wiser to perform bypass surgery, if indicated, before instituting therapy with thyroid hormone. It has been shown that coronary revascularization can be safely performed in hypothyroid patients. Judicious volume expansion is necessary.

Euthyroid sick syndrome

All patients who experience severe illness or major surgery have changes in thyroid hormone metabolism. These include a decrease in peripheral conversion of T_4 to T_3, and changes in thyroid hormone binding to plasma proteins. The total level of circulating T_4 and T_3 is depressed. Although some controversy exists, most authorities believe that the level of free thyroid hormone—a tiny fraction of the total but the biologically significant one—is normal. TSH levels are normal, as is TSH responsiveness to hypothalamic thyrotropin-releasing hormone. An exception to this situation is the severely ill patient receiving high-dose glucocorticoids or dopamine, which inhibit pituitary secretion of TSH, and so may induce mild secondary hypothyroidism. In general, the levels of total T_4 and T_3 roughly correlate with the severity of illness. Mortality has been shown to be significantly greater in patients with total T_4 levels under 3 μg/dL. This is thought *not* to be due to hypothyroidism, but merely to correlate with these patients' moribund state.

The question sometimes arises in a severely ill patient as to whether hypothyroidism is contributing to a poor response to therapy. Remember that depression of thyroid hormone levels is expected in such patients. Hypothyroidism can be reliably diagnosed if the TSH level is elevated. Otherwise, thyroid function tests are not reliable. Unless there is strong suspicion based on clinical evidence, such as obvious nonpitting edema and hung-up reflexes in a patient with a thyroidectomy scar, it is generally presumed that the patient has normal thyroid function. The situation becomes even more problematic in patients receiving dopamine or high-dose glucocorticoids, because these agents are known to cause secondary hypothyroidism. No evidence indicates that thyroid hormone replacement is of value in such patients. When patients recover, levels of thyroid hormone return to normal. Thus, final diagnosis may be retrospective.

ADRENAL DISEASE
Cushing's syndrome

Cushing's syndrome results from glucocorticoid excess, whether exogenous or endogenous. A full discussion of Cushing's syndrome is beyond the scope of this chapter. Metabolic consequences of Cushing's syndrome include hyperglycemia and hypokalemia if due to excess of cortisol, which has a mineralocorticoid effect and so promotes kaliuresis. Treatment is the same as for other patients with these metabolic disturbances, as well as the attempts to minimize the glucocorticoid excess. Since glucocoticoids are catabolic hormones, protein wasting results, with thin skin and atrophic musculature. These patients are particularly prone to poor wound healing, skin breakdown, and poor defense against infection, so meticulous care must be directed toward preventing these complications.

Adrenal insufficiency

Primary adrenal insufficiency is relatively rare and may occur due to metastatic, autoimmune, or tuberculous destruction of the adrenals. Such patients have combined glucocorticoid and mineralocorticoid deficiency. Much more common is suppression of the hypothalamic-pituitary-adrenal axis due to treatment with exogenous corticosteroids, with endogenous glucocorticoid insufficiency resulting when the exogenous steroids are withdrawn, or when a lack of adrenal reserve causes an inadequate stress response. Mineralocorticoid deficiency usually does not result, because the aldosterone-producing zona glomerulosa is not dependent on corticotropin (ACTH). Recovery from long-term suppression with exogenous glucocorticoid may take a year.

Table 6-5 Commercially Available Systemic* Glucocorticoids and Their Relative Potencies

Generic name	Brand name	Relative potency (cortisol = 1)
Oral preparations		
Cortisone	Cortogen, Cortone	0.8
Hydrocortisone	Cortef, Cortril, Hydrocort, Hydrocortone	1.0
Prednisone	Deltasone, Deltra, Meticorten, Paracort	4.0
Methylprednisolone	Medrol	5.0
Triamcinolone	Aristocort, Kenacort	5.0
Betamethasone	Celestone	30.0
Dexamethasone	Decadron, Dexasone, Hexadrol	30.0
Intravenous preparations		
Hydrocortisone hemisuccinate	Solu-Cortef	1.0
Hydrocortisone phosphate	Hydrocortone phosphate	1.0
Methylprednisolone hemisuccinate	Solu-Medrol	5.0
Dexamethasone phosphate	Decadron Phosphate	30.0

*In addition to systemic preparations, many glucocorticoids are provided in topical creams, ointments, aerosols, suppositories, eyedrops, etc. for their anti-inflammatory properties. These can have systemic effects if used in sufficient dosage/duration.

Adrenal suppression should be suspected in any patient who has received the corticosteroid equivalent of 20 mg or more of prednisone for longer than 3–4 weeks. Table 6-5 gives commonly used glucocorticoids and their dose equivalents.

Diagnosis of adrenal insufficiency or suppression is most conveniently made by the cosyntropin stimulation test. Cosyntropin is a synthetic analogue of ACTH. Exogenous steroids are withheld for 12–24 hours. Baseline cortisol is drawn at 8:00 AM the following day, followed by injection of 0.25 mg cosyntropin (1 ampule). Plasma cortisol determination is repeated 60 minutes later. A normal response is an increase over baseline of 7 μg/dL, usually to greater than 18 μg/dL. No significant side effects are associated with injection of cosyntropin.

Clinically, patients with adrenal insufficiency present with anorexia, nausea, weight loss, fatigability, and orthostatic hypotension. Patients with primary adrenal insufficiency become hyperpigmented due to high levels of ACTH. Electrolyte abnormalities are common. Glucocorticoids stimulate the distal tubular Na–K adenosine triphosphatase, whereas mineralocorticoid acts even more potently in the collecting ducts. Glucocorticoid deficiency commonly results in hyponatremia; mineralocorticoid deficiency results in hyponatremia and hypokalemia. Spontaneous hypoglycemia occurs in about half the patients with adrenal insufficiency.

Adrenal crisis: Acute adrenal crisis, or addisonian crisis, is a life-threatening emergency. It most often occurs when a patient with compromised adrenal reserve due to primary insufficiency or exogenous suppression is stressed by illness or surgery. The precipitating stress may be fairly trivial, such as a common cold. Patients present with anorexia progressing rapidly to nausea, vomiting, and abdominal pain. Patients are volume depleted and hypotensive. Typical laboratory abnormalities include hyponatremia, hyperkalemia (rarely greater than 7 mEq/dL), moderate metabolic acidosis, increased BUN, hypoglycemia, and, of course, a low plasma cortisol level.

If adrenal crisis is suspected, treatment must be immediate to prevent vascular collapse. If the diagnosis is in question, it is possible to do a rapid cosyntropin stimulation test without delaying therapy. Draw plasma for a baseline cortisol determination, followed by 0.25 mg cosyntropin intravenously. Immediately thereafter, give 10 mg dexamethasone phosphate (Decadron) or 20 mg methylpredisolone (Solu-Medrol) intravenously. Plasma is drawn at 60 minutes for cortisol determination. Hypotensive patients with normal adrenal function have baseline cortisol level of 10 μg/dL or greater, and increase by a least 7 μg/dL after cosyntropin. Addisonian patients have a baseline cortisol level less than 10 μg/dL and do not respond to cosyntropin. Fluid resuscitation and other treatment is given as in Table 6-6.

SUGGESTED READING

All topics are covered in detail in Felig P, Baxter JD, Broadhus AE, Frohmen LA, (eds)., *Endocrinology and metabolism. 2nd ed.,* New York: McGraw Hill; 1987, as well as other endocrinology

Table 6-6 Treatment of Adrenal Crisis

1. Insert large-bore IV, draw blood for glucose, electrolytes, BUN, cortisol, and culture.
2. If diagnosis is in question, administer cosyntropin stimulation test with dexamethasone or methylprednisolone, as described in text.
3. Infuse normal saline or D_5 normal saline aggressively: 1 L/h or as fast as tolerated for 3 L. Once blood pressure is stable, hydrate according to clinical response. Do not use hypotonic saline.
4. Simultaneously with step 3, give 200 mg hydrocortisone IV (phosphate or succinate), followed by 100 mg q6h.
5. Seek and treat precipitating factors: cultures of blood, urine, sputum; signs of meningitis; infarction; trauma.

texts. The references below provide additional details on selected topics.

Chopra IJ, Hershman JM, Pardridge WM and Nicoloff JT. Thyroid function in nonthyroidal illnesses. *Ann Intern Med*. 1983; 98:946–957.

Faber J, Kirkegaard C, Rasmussen B, et al. Pituitary-thyroid axis in critical illness. *J Clin Endocrinal Metab*. 1980; 65:315–320.

Flier JS, Moore MJ. The metabolic derangements and treatment of diabetic ketoacidosis. *N Engl J Med*. 1983; 309:159–169.

Galloway JA, Bressler R. Insulin treatment in diabetes. *Med Clin North Am*. 1978; 62:663.

Goldman DR. Surgery in patients with endocrine dysfunction. *Med Clin North Am*. 1987; 71:499–509.

Hay ID, Duick DS, Vlietstra RE, et al. Thyroxine therapy in hypothyroid patients undergoing coronary revascularization: a retrospective analysis. *Ann Intern Med*. 1984; 95:456.

Lebovitz HE, Feinglos MN. Sulfonylurea drugs: mechanism of antidiabetic action and therapeutic usefulness. *Diabetes Care*. 1979; 1:189–199.

Lever E, Jaspan JB. Sodium bicarbonate therapy in severe diabetic ketoacidosis. *Am J Med*. 1983; 75:263.

Molitel ME, Reichlin S. The care of the diabetic patient during emergency surgery and postoperatively. *Orthop Clin North Am*. 1978; 9:811.

Peripheral Vascular Disease

Robert A. Mason, M.D.

7

Vascular occlusive disease of the coronary arteries is the most common, and one of the most lethal, manifestations of atherosclerosis. At the same time, atherosclerosis is not isolated to a single vascular bed, but rather is a systemic process influenced by genetic, local, and systemic factors.

Atherosclerosis is a disease process initially involving the arterial intima and consisting of a spectrum of cellular proliferation with the accumulation of intra- and extracellular lipids. With the subsequent inflammatory changes, varing degrees of necrosis and scarring involve the full thickness of the arterial wall. An enlarging plaque encroaches on the lumen, resulting in stenosis or occlusion. Ulceration of the atheroma can result in platelet, thrombotic, and atheromatous emboli.

Intimal thickening with proliferating cellular elements consistent with the initial stages of atheroma development can be found in childhood and is progressive throughout life. The initial stages of atheroma development may represent adaptation of the arterial wall to hemodynamic stress and the aging process. The rate of development, however, is influenced by a multitude of local, mechanical, and systemic factors against a background of genetic predisposition. Well-defined systemic risk factors appear to influence the atherosclerotic process in the coronary, as well as the noncoronary, arterial tree (Table 7-1).

Although local and mechanical factors may differ with different vascular beds, the genetic and systemic risk factors are shared by both coronary and noncoronary arteries. It is, therefore, not surprising that patients with peripheral or cerebral vascular disease will have a high incidence of coronary artery

---

Table 7-1   Systemic Risk Factors for Atherosclerotic Vascular Occlusive Disease

---

Advanced age
Smoking history
Hyperlipidemia
Hypertension
Diabetes mellitus
? Family history
? Sedentary life-style

---

disease. Likewise, those patients with symptomatic coronary artery disease are a select population in which significant occlusive disease is more likely to be found in other parts of the arterial tree. Concomitant vascular disease not only complicates the performance of cardiac surgery and the postoperative recovery, but can also affect the longevity and the quality of the patient's remaining life.

EVALUATION OF NONCARDIAC VASCULAR DISEASE

The initial preoperative evaluation of the cardiac patient necessitates the careful evaluation of the remainder of the vascular tree. Fortunately, the diagnosis of vascular disease lends itself very well to a thoughtful history and careful physical examination.

Identification of the known risk factors such as a smoking history, advanced age, and other concomitant medical illnesses, such as hypertension and diabetes, should suggest the likelihood of vascular disease. Specific questioning regarding a previous stroke or transient ischemic attacks can alert the physician to significant cerebral vascular disease and the increased incidence of neurologic complications following coronary artery bypass grafting (CABG). A history of previous vascular surgery or calf and thigh claudication is indicative of peripheral vascular disease, and difficulty may be encountered in procedures which require arterial access through the groin, such as cardiac catheterization or insertion of intra-aortic balloon pump (IABP). In addition, it makes little sense to subject a patient to open heart surgery to improve exercise-induced angina, only to find that severe claudication continues to limit ambulation (Table 7-2).

Thrombophlebitis in the past or a history of varicose veins may affect the availability of the saphenous vein for a bypass

Table 7-2   Signs and Symptoms of Vascular Disease and the Potential Complications of Bypass Surgery

Symptom	Physical sign	Vascular abnormality	Potential complication
Claudication	Absent pulses	Vascular occlusion	Difficulty with vascular access, catheterization, IABP
Asymptomatic	Pulsatile abdominal mass	Aortic aneurysm	Difficulty with vascular access Arterial embolism Rupture
Transient ischemic attack, cerebrovascular accident	Cervical bruit, neurologic deficit	Ulcer/stenotic carotid artery	Perioperative stroke
History of hypertension	Hypertension Renal dysfunction	Renal artery stenosis	Renal failure Difficult to control blood pressure
Phlebitis	Leg edema Venous insufficiency	Deep venous occlusion	Recurrent phlebitis Lower extremity wound problems Pulmonary embolus

graft. The risk of recurrent thrombophlebitis or pulmonary embolism complicating the postoperative recovery are also increased in patients with chronic venous insufficiency. The onset of significant hypertension at an early age or hypertension with concomitant renal dysfunction in the more elderly patient should raise the suspicion of renal vascular disease. If renal artery disease is bilateral, there is an increased risk of acute renal failure complicating the use of cardiopulmonary bypass.

The physical examination should include a thorough investigation of all peripheral pulses. The absence of a palpable pulse indicates proximal stenosis/occlusion. The presence of a bruit in the neck, supraclavicular region, abdomen, or groin suggests underlying arterial disease. Aneurysmal disease may present as a pulsatile mass in the epigastrium, groin, or popliteal region. Unilateral leg edema, venous stasis ulceration, increased ankle pigmentation, or skin changes of a postphlebitic syndrome suggests chronic venous disease. Whether the diagnosis of concomitant vascular disease is clear or suspected, the noninvasive vascular laboratory can be used to confirm, localize and document the degree of vascular impairment.

Noninvasive arterial evaluation

Doppler velocity detector: The Doppler effect is based on the physical principle that an observed change of frequency is caused by relative motion, as first described by Christian Doppler in 1842, and so named after him. With the aid of a piezoelectric crystal* an ultrasonic sound wave is generated in the range of 2 to 10 MHz and transmitted to the skin through an acoustic gel that serves as a coupling agent. The sound wave is reflected back from the underlying structures, including red blood cells and detected by a receiving piezoelectric crystal. The erythrocytes flowing within larger vessels are moving with each cardiac cycle and, therefore, the frequency of the reflected wave from the moving red cells will be shifted in a manner proportional to their velocity. The change in frequency (Δf) between the transmitted and the reflected sound wave is described by the formula:

$$\Delta f = \frac{2fV\cos}{C}$$

in which f is frequency of transmitted sound wave, V is velocity of erythrocytes, cos is angle of incidence between the sound beam and the longitudinal axis of the artery, and C is velocity of sound in tissue. By maintaining the transmitting frequency, the angle of incidence, and the velocity of sound in tissue constant, the shift of frequency is proportional to the velocity of the erythrocytes. This signal is amplified and can be presented as an audible signal or recorded as a waveform. By varying the frequency of the transmitted sound wave the depth of tissue penetration can be varied. In general, a low frequency (2–5 MHz) is most useful for investigating deeper structures such as

*A ceramic crystal capable of vibrating at high frequency when an electric current is applied and thus producing an ultrasonic sound wave, the frequency of which is related to the electric current applied. If a receiving piezoelectric crystal is vibrated by an ultrasonic sound wave, it will emit an electric current the magnitude of which is determined by the frequency of the sound wave.

mesenteric vessels, while a high frequency (8–10 MHz) gives a shallow penetration with a sharp focus and is most useful for determining blood flow velocity in carotid arteries or the arteries and veins of the limbs.

Valuable information can be obtained from both the audible and the recorded signals by pattern recognition. In addition, the Doppler shift signal can be subjected to a real-time, fast fourier transformation system that allows the display of a computer-generated real-time velocity spectrum. Waveform patterns consistent with reduced flow, turbulent flow, or the "jet effect" of a high-grade stenosis can be recognized.

A pulsed Doppler flow detector transmits short bursts of ultrasound. Because sound travels through the tissue at a fixed rate, the time required for the sound wave to reach a particular point and return to the receiving crystal depends on the distance from the crystal. By time-gating the receiving crystal the Doppler shift at a defined point along the path of the ultrasound beam can be obtained (Figure 7-1). By combining a pulse Doppler with gray scale ultrasonography (duplex scan)

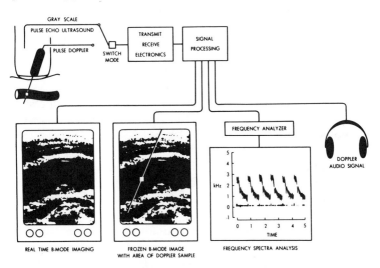

Figure 7-1   Duplex system: A pulse echo ultrasound probe is used to obtain a gray scale or B-mode image of the underlying vessel. With the scanning head held in place and steady, the pulsed Doppler within the scanning head is switched on. By time-gating the area of Doppler, sample can be adjusted on the frozen B-mode image. Once the area of interest is selected, the Doppler signal is then subjected to frequency analysis.

precise sampling of the Doppler signal at different points across the lumen of a vessel can be obtained. This technique has quietly revolutionized the detection of extracranial carotid artery disease (Figure 7-2).

Although the use of Doppler ultrasound devices have become increasingly sophisticated and expensive, a great deal of information can be obtained with a simple hand-held Doppler flow detector.

By placing on the patient a blood pressure cuff attached to a manometer, and using the Doppler flow probe to detect the first return of blood flow, the systolic blood pressure can be determined at different segmental levels of the extremities. Because the large arteries represent a low-resistant conduit, a drop in the systolic blood pressure between two levels indicates an impediment to blood flow. This technique is not only useful to demonstrate the level of obstructing arterial lesion, but can help to quantify the degree of impairment of blood flow by a particular stenosis or series of stenoses.

Occlusive disease of the arm is unusual; therefore, the systolic blood pressure measured in the upper extremity can, in general, be equated to the central aortic pressure. By comparing the ankle systolic pressure with that of the arm, an ankle-brachial index can be calculated that normally will be a value of one. A low ankle-brachial index indicates a limited blood flow to the foot. This index can be used to confirm the clinical diagnosis and serves as a means to follow the progression of vascular disease and predict the degree of ischemia of the involved extremity.

Pulse volume recording: There is, however, a group of patients, particularly those with diabetes, in whom the measurement of blood pressure with an occluding cuff technique is inaccurate because of calcific noncompressible vessels. Plethysmographic techniques, based on the measurement of changes in volume, have been perfected and have become a useful adjunct in the noninvasive vascular laboratory. The blood volume within an extremity varies over the cardiac cycle. Because the other tissues within the extremity are stable, measurement of relative changes in the volume of a segmental portion of the extremity can be equated to the blood volume within that segment. These volume changes are measured with a specifically

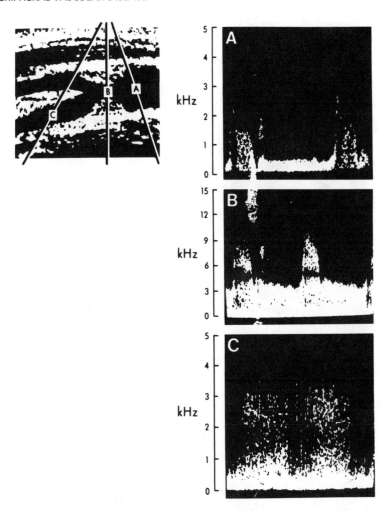

Figure 7-2. The Doppler signal is sampled and analyzed at numerous points within the arterial lumen in this example of a carotid bifurcation stenosis (flow is from left to right). *A.* Prior to the stenosis there is a pulsed waveform, but there is a broadening of the spectrum indicating there are multiple different velocities within the Doppler sample or turbulent flow. *B.* Sampling at the point of maximal stenosis, there is a rapid velocity (peak velocity at this point is 9.2 KHz, the higher the frequency shift indicates a higher blood velocity) or jet effect. *C.* Sampling beyond the stenosis, there is considerable spectral broadening indicative of a very turbulent flow with loss of pulse wave pattern.

designed circumferential air bladder cuff and are amplified and recorded on a strip chart as a waveform. The degree of impairment of blood flow can be assessed by pattern recognition of the waveform measured at different segmental levels of the extremity. The plethysmographic waveform is less affected by rigidity of the vessel wall and, therefore, when combined with Doppler systolic segmental pressure measurements, becomes an effective diagnostic tool in the vascular laboratory.

Noninvasive venous evaluation

Clinical examination can identify changes caused by chronic venous insufficiency, but it is notoriously inaccurate in defining acute venous disease, especially acute deep vein thrombosis (DVT). The association of lethal pulmonary embolism with DVT makes its diagnosis in the perioperative period an important function of the vascular laboratory. Both the Doppler and plethysmographic techniques have proven useful in the diagnosis of deep venous obstructive disease.

A characteristic audible Doppler signal is used to detect blood flow in the deep veins of the extremities. By assessing the changes in the Doppler signal with various maneuvers, such as a Valsalva maneuver, that alter venous blood flow, obstruction of deep veins can be identified. The Doppler venous examination can identify acute occlusion of the deep veins, especially in the thigh and ileofemoral regions, with a moderate degree of accuracy. The accuracy of the venous evaluation for DVT in the vascular laboratory is further increased with plethysmography. In brief, a venous occluding cuff is placed on the thigh and a plethysmographic monitor placed on the calf to detect changes in volume. Most commonly used is impedance plethysmography, in which changes in volume are detected by the change in the impedance to an electric current passing between two electrodes placed on the calf. The venous occluding cuff is inflated, creating an increase in blood volume within the distal leg. Because the venous system has a relatively high compliance, a moderate volume expansion will follow until an equilibration is reached (Figure 7-3). If thrombus obstructs the large deep veins, then their capacity to expand will be limited and the total ability of the leg to increase in volume will be limited. At the point of equilibrium, the venous occluding cuff is deflated, allowing the expanded venous volume to return to normal. If there is free outflow through

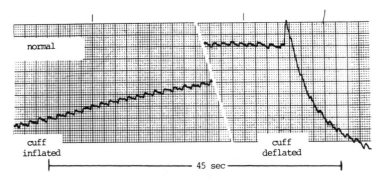

Figure 7-3. A normal impedance plethysmographic tracing notes when the venous occlusion cuff is up. *A.* There is a moderate volume expansion representing venous capacitance, when the cuff is deflated. *B.* There is a rapid return to baseline indicated on an obstructed venous outflow.

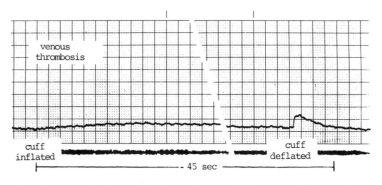

Figure 7-4. An abnormal impedance plethysmographic tracing: note a very small increase in volume after the occluding cuff is inflated. *A.* Indicating a limited venous capacitance, when occluding cuff is deflated. *B.* There is a slow return to baseline, indicating an impediment to venous outflow.

the major deep vein channels, the rate of fall in expanded volume is rapid (see Figure 7-2). However, if the major venous channels are obstructed, then this rate will be abnormally slow (Figure 7-4).

The combination of impedance plethysmography and Doppler examination of the deep venous system has a high degree of accuracy (over 90%) in identifying obstructive lesions in its deep veins of the lower extremities. Recently the technology of pulse Doppler combined with B-scale ultrasound (duplex scan) has proven increasing accurate in diagnosis of deep venous disease. With the duplex scan an ultrasound picture and a Doppler velocity profile can be determined along the length of vein in a noninvasive way.

Other minimal invasive techniques such as plain radiography, computed tomography (CT) and magnetic resonance imaging (MRI) are useful in defining specific vascular problems.

Invasive techniques

Contrast angiography has been one of the main diagnostic procedures used to evaluate both the arterial and the venous circulation. Improved technology of imaging equipment, less toxic contrast media and the development of guidewire directed percutaneous catheter placement (Seldinger technique) have improved the quality and safety of angiography. Nonetheless, angiography is still an invasive procedure with a small, but very real, incidence of complications. Its use in the diagnosis of noncoronary vascular disease has been displaced by the newer noninvasive modalities discussed in the previous section. Using a combination of Doppler velocity detector, duplex scan, and CT imaging directed by a thoughtful and careful clinical examination, there is little need for angiography as a diagnostic aid. On the other hand, angiography remains a critically important part of directing therapeutic intervention. The information provided by angiography provides the vascular surgeon with a "road map" in planning a surgical approach to correction of a particular vascular problem. The degree of involvement of a specific arterial segment can be seen as well as the anatomy and quality of the distal vessels, which remains an important consideration in planning a revascularization procedure. Angiography remains critical in directing the newer percutaneous balloon and laser angioplasty and atherectomy techniques.

Intravenous digital subtraction angiography (DSA) has recently become available and has allowed arterial imaging with an intravenous bolus injection of contrast. Although this technique eliminates the need for an arterial puncture, the large dose of contrast and the quality of images prevent it from replacing conventional intra-arterial angiography for directing interventional therapy. The noninvasive techniques such as duplex scan have eliminated the use of intravenous DSA as a screening procedure. Intra-arterial DSA has proven useful in imaging defined vascular beds with small doses of dilute contrast, especially when there is limited flow beyond a stenosis.

SPECIFIC PARTS OF THE VASCULAR TREE THAT MAY INFLUENCE CARDIAC SURGERY

Aortic disease

Degenerative or atheromatous involvement of the ascending aorta can have a direct complicating effect on coronary surgery, given the need to manipulate the aorta in cannulating and cross-clamping. Although disease of the aorta beyond the ascending portion has little direct effect on the performance of cardiac surgery, it can markedly complicate access to the arterial tree for diagnostic and therapeutic cardiac catheterization. In addition, the use of the IABP is far more hazardous. Aortic disease clearly has an effect on patient longevity and, therefore, long-term outcome.

Atheroma development in the ascending aorta typically consists of a thickened plaque with a soft grumous center and varying degrees of calcification, creating a potentially treacherous problem for the cardiac surgeon. There is an associated risk in cross-clamping and cannulating of producing an aortic tear or embolization of the grumous content of cholesterol-laden particulate matter with devastating effects to the central nervous system (CNS), visceral vessels, and lower extremities (Figure 7-5).

A highly calcified aortic knob on chest x-ray in a patient with diffuse atheromatous disease should raise the suspicion. A CT scan of the upper chest can give the cardiac surgeon an idea of the "quality" of the ascending aorta, but frequently it is only the intraoperative assessment of the aorta that will define this "high-risk aorta."

Thoracic aorta: Cystic medial necrosis is a degenerative process common to the thoracic aorta in which there is destruction of the elastic and collagen elements of the aortic wall, resulting in a predisposition to intramural aortic dissection or aneurysmal dilatation. Congenital abnormalities as seen in Marfan syndrome and acquired infections such as syphilis are known to have a high incidence of cystic medial necrosis of the thoracic aorta. However, atherosclerosis remains the most common etiologic factor.

193

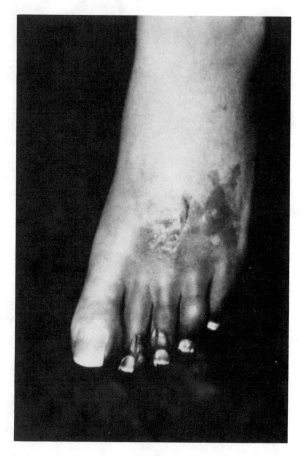

Figure 7-5 A. Necrosis of the forefoot in a patient suffering from embolization of atheromatous debris showered during aortic cross-clamping in a coronary artery bypass procedure.

The thoracic aorta is subjected to multiple stresses with each beat of the cardiac cycle. The sudden pulse pressure with left ventricular ejection with the 180° change in direction of the blood stream by the aortic arch, the longitudinal shear of the viscous blood along the luminal surface, and the flexion stresses created by the motion of the beating heart and a relatively fixed aorta are all factors in initiating an intimal tear. If there is medial necrosis weakening the aortic wall, blood can dissect both proximally and distally, creating an acute aortic dissection. Aortic dissection can affect the entire aorta or may be isolated to only

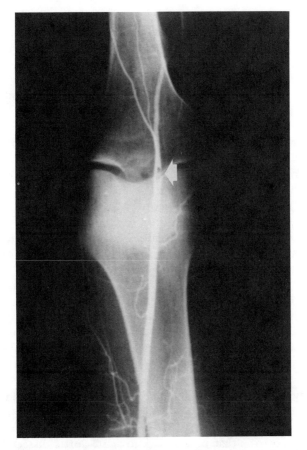

Figure 7-5 B. Angiogram of the same patient (7-5 A) showing embolic debris occluding popliteal artery.

the ascending or descending. With the destruction of the intima and part of the medial layers of the aorta, the blood stream is contained by the remaining medial remnants and the adventitia, thus forming a pseudo or false aneurysm.*

Acute aortic dissection usually presents as a catastrophic event with a high mortality and is associated with a multitude of complications including acute aortic valvular insufficiency, cardiac tamponade, coronary occlusion, CNS and visceral

*The wall of a false aneurysm does not have all layers of the arterial wall, whereas a true aneurysm is the dilatation of the entire wall of the vessel.

ischemia, and rupture of the aorta. The diagnosis of aortic dissection is suspected by the finding of a widened mediastinum in a patient presenting with acute onset of chest pain. A CT scan of the chest will also be useful in diagnosing and defining the size and limits of the accompanying false aneurysm created by the expansion of hematoma and false lumen within the media of the aorta. Ultimately, aortography is used to define the intimal tear creating the entry point as well as the compromise of the orifices of branch arteries along the dissection.

The majority of dissections involving the ascending aorta come to surgical repair early. However, a small group of patients will survive to have a chronic aortic dissection. If a patient with a chronic ascending aortic dissection requires CABG, the complicating dissection can rarely be ignored. The aorta, and perhaps the valve, will require repair, thus increasing the risk and magnitude of the surgery. The surgical mortality of repair of the ascending aorta is in the range of 10% to 20%.

Coronary surgery can be carried out in a patient with a chronic stable dissection of the descending aorta, but it must be remembered that the thoracic aorta is diseased and a higher incidence of embolization, tear, and technical difficulties must be anticipated. A chronic aortic dissection would, in most incidences, prohibit the use of the IABP.

Aneurysmal aortic disease: The incidence of true thoracic aneurysms increases with age; most are found after the fifth decade. The same destruction of the elastic and collagen fibers in medial necrosis that predisposes to acute aortic dissection is also an important factor in the etiology of thoracic aneurysm.

Most thoracic aneurysms are asymptomatic, causing symptoms only when they become moderately large, and then are symptomatic only as a result of compression on adjacent structures. Dilatation of the aortic valve annulus associated with ascending aortic aneurysm can present with aortic valve insufficiency. All thoracic aneurysms do, however, have the potential for catastrophic rupture carrying a near 100% mortality and therefore their presence represents a risk to the patient. The greater the diameter of the aneurysm, the greater the risk of rupture. The physical principle underlying LaPlace's law which states that for a tube at a given pressure the wall tension is directly related to the radius of the tube ($T = P \times R$). Therefore, as an aneurysm enlarges in diameter, the wall tension

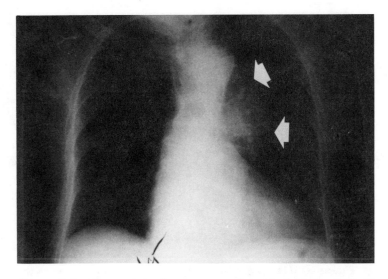

Figure 7-6. Large thoracic aneurysm in elderly asymptomatic woman; aneurysm was found on a routine chest film.

greatly increases, promoting a more rapid dilatation. In general, the greater the diameter, the more rapidly it expands. Thoracic aneurysms are frequently found on routine chest film (Figure 7-6). Their presence can be confirmed and their size best assessed with a CT scan. Angiography is not required for diagnosis and is needed only when surgical repair is contemplated. The presence of a thoracic aneurysm, unless affecting the ascending aorta, does not affect the procedure or recovery from CABG. It is, however, a factor in assessing the patient's overall longevity. The repair of a thoracic aneurysm can be a significant surgical undertaking, with the risk depending on the size and location. In general, if the aneursym involves the arch and has a diameter of less than 7 cm, it can be followed. A rapid growth (more than 1 cm/y), a diameter greater than 7 cm, or significant symptoms from compression are indications to consider elective surgical repair. Aneurysms involving the descending aorta, but remaining above the diaphragm, carry a lower risk of operative repair, though the risk of paraplegia complicating surgical repair remains in the range of 10%. Therefore, each patient must be considered individually and there are no absolute guidelines regarding a particular size that necessitates operative repair.

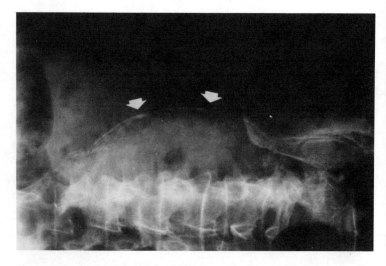

Figure 7-7. **Large abdominal aneurysm is demonstrated on the flat plate of the abdomen. The aneurysmal wall is denoted by the thin rim of calcium within the outer wall of the aneurysm.**

Abdominal aortic aneurysm: Like the thoracic aortic aneurysm, the abdominal aortic aneurysm is seen more frequently in the older patient population, most being in the sixth or seventh decade. Most are asymptomatic, found incidentally on physical examination or abdominal film (Figure 7-7). Similar to the thoracic aneurysm, the abdominal aortic aneurysm carries the same potential of catastrophic rupture with 100% mortality when untreated. The risk of rupture increases in an exponential fashion with increased size (diameter). The majority (95%) are in an infrarenal location and are amenable to surgical repair with a low operative risk when repaired electively. For this reason, surgical repair is undertaken for aneurysms of smaller diameter. An abdominal aortic aneurysm diameter greater than 4 cm should be considered for surgical repair if the patient is in good medical condition and the operative risks are low.

The diagnosis of abdominal aortic aneurysm is suspected by the finding of a pulsatile mass in the epigastrium on physical examination and the size established by ultrasound or CT scan. The CT scan can give valuable additional information regarding location, quality of the wall, and other associated abnormalities (Figure 7-8). Angiography studies are reserved for specific indications in patients being evaluated for surgical repair.

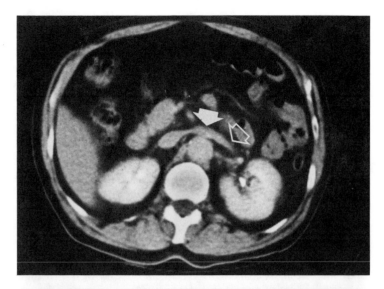

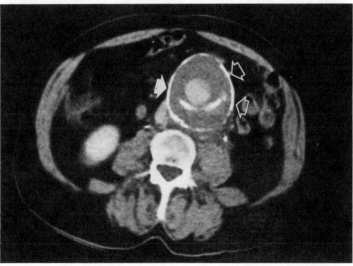

Figure 7-8.   A CT scan of the same patient in Figure 7-7. *A.* Note at the level of the left renal vein, the aorta is of normal caliber, indicating the infrarenal location of the aneurysm. *B.* Twenty millimeters lower, the aorta is clearly aneurysmal. Note calcium in the outer wall.

Aneurysmal disease of the aorta can render the aorta quite tortuous, increasing the difficulty of catheter passage during cardiac catheterization from the femoral approach. The risk of abdominal aortic aneurysmal disease is a relative contra-indication to the use of IABP. There is increased difficulty in positioning of the balloon because of the tortuosity of aorta and iliac vessels. In addition, there is a very real risk of em-bolization of thrombotic material lining the aneurysm, caus-ing limb-threatening ischemia. In using the IABP in a patient with an abdominal aneurysm, the benefit must be great to offset the inordinate risk of serious complications. In a patient with a thoracic aortic aneurysm, the IABP is contraindicated. The aneursymal dilatation of the aorta precludes effective counterpulsation and the risk of lethal embolization or aortic rupture is prohibitive.

Aortic iliac occlusive disease: Occlusive disease of the distal aorta and iliac vessels may limit the ability to catheterize the patient from a femoral approach. If passage of the catheter is accom-plished, there is an increased risk of iatrogenic dissection, plaque embolization, and acute thrombosis of the iliac and femoral vessels with subsequent limb-threatening ischemia. Ex-tensive aortic atherosclerotic disease may involve the orifices of the renal and mesenteric vessels, increasing the risk of acute renal failure or mesenteric ischemia following coronary sur-gery. Ischemia of the lower extremities can result in wound complications if the saphenous vein is harvested for a CABG.

The use of the IABP in stabilizing cardiac patients and as an adjunct to surgery has increased recently. Significant aortic occlusive disease may prohibit the introduction of the balloon through the femoral vessels. The risk of serious dissection of the iliac arteries, thrombosis, and embolization is significantly increased in aortoiliac occlusive disease (Figure 7-9).

Cerebral vascular disease

Cerebral vascular accident is one of the more devastating com-plications of CABG for patients, their families, and their physi-cians. While the incidence is relatively low (currently 1.7% to 3% reported in large series), more than half of them result in a permanent neurologic deficit. There are multiple different causes of perioperative stroke, including dislodgement of mu-ral thrombus from the ventricle, local or regional cerebral

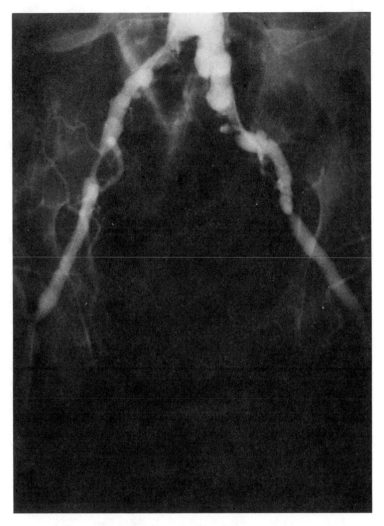

Figure 7-9. Angiogram of a patient with aortoiliac occlusive disease. The use of an IABP requiring passage of the balloon through these iliac arteries would carry a very high risk of complications.

hypoperfusion, emboli released from the ascending and arch aorta, and carotid bifurcation. However, a small group of patients undergoing CABG have preexisting cerebral vascular disease and are at a higher risk of developing perioperative stroke. The focus of this section will be on the identification, prediction of risk, and management of this select group of patients.

Atherosclerosis of the extracranial carotid and aortic arch is a risk factor for the development of ischemic cerebral vascular accident. Such strokes can arise from embolization of thrombus, platelet aggregations, or atheromatous debris from the ulcerated surface of an atheromatous plaque. A high-grade stenosis of the carotid bifurcation, especially if bilateral, can result in regional cerebral hypoperfusion during periods of hypotension. Thrombosis of a stenotic internal carotid artery carries a risk of embolization or extension of the thrombosis into intracerebral collateral pathways, precipitating a stroke. Patients presenting with lateralizing symptoms, such as transient ischemic attacks, are a higher risk group. Approximately one-third of these patients will suffer a sustained stroke over a period of 5 years with the highest risk occuring within the first 6 months after symptoms appear. The stroke risk of CABG in this group is not well defined; however, the opinion of most clinicians is that CABG surgery does carry an exaggerated risk of neurologic complications in the symptomatic patient. Certainly the risk of a perioperative neurologic complication is much higher in patients with ongoing lateralizing symptoms than in those without. It is, therefore, appropriate to question patients carefully regarding symptoms of transient ischemic attacks preoperatively and if these are elicited, further evaluation is indicated.

Those patients who have suffered a completed stroke, but have recovered, are also at a higher risk of a recurrent stroke (in the range of 6% to 11%/y). They too should have additional evaluation of the cerebral vascular circulation before proceeding with elective CABG surgery.

The evaluation of the symptomatic patient needs to include a CT scan of the head which will identify areas of previous infarcts, some of which may have been silent. A mass lesion, if present, is diagnosed with the aid of a CT scan. A noninvasive duplex scan of the carotids has a high degree of accuracy in identifying and quantifying atheromatous lesions involving the carotid bifurcation.

If these noninvasive studies suggest a significant carotid lesion that is appropriate for the patient's symptoms, cerebral angiography will characterize the atheromatous involvement of the aortic arch, carotid vessels, intracerebral vessels, and patterns of collateral circulation. With this information, a more rational judgment can then be made regarding possible carotid surgery and timing of coronary surgery. Cerebral angiography, however, is an invasive procedure and carries just under 1% risk of precipitating a stroke event in most centers. Therefore, if the CT and duplex scans do not suggest cerebral vascular disease, other sources of symptoms must be investigated prior to proceeding to angiography. These include emboli from a cardiac source, cardiac arrhythmias, vasospastic or hypertensive encephalopathy, seizure disorder, collagen vascular arteriopathies, and metabolic derangements. If the patient continues to have lateralizing neurologic symptoms without a defined etiology, then cerebral angiography before proceeding to elective CABG is indicated.

If the evaluation does identify a significant carotid bifurcation lesion as a source for the patient's symptoms, the treatment and its timing are the next questions to address. The therapeutic options include anticoagulation, antiplatelet drugs, or surgical intervention with carotid endarterectomy. The data regarding the effectiveness of anticoagulation as a means to prevent stroke in this group of symptomatic patients are mixed, although there is a definite increased risk of intracerebral hemorrhage with long-term anticoagulation. Antiplatelet medication in several large multicentered trials has shown, in patients with transient ischemic attacks, a reduction in the total number who suffered stroke or death. However, a scrutiny of these studies reveals that the effectiveness of antiplatelet therapy was in the reduction of death due to myocardial infarction, and indeed did not reduce the stroke rate.

Surgery in the form of carotid endarterectomy (CEA) on the appropriate lesion has been shown in numerous different studies to reduce the increased risk of completed stroke to that of an age-related general population (less than 2%/y). The risk of CEA varies, but for most large centers, it is now in the range of a 1% mortality and a 2% stroke risk. Therefore, surgical treatment offers the best reduction in stroke risk and remains the treatment of choice for the good risk patient with symptomatic extracranial carotid atheroma.

The major operative risk for patients undergoing CEA is that of myocardial infarction. Careful consideration must, then, be given to the status of the coronary disease in those patients with concomitant symptomatic carotid and coronary disease. If the coronary disease is moderate and does not preclude safe anesthetic induction, then elective endarterectomy of the symptomatic carotid artery should be done and the coronary procedure staged at a later date. On the other hand, if the coronary disease is life-threatening, as in patients with severe left main stenosis, three vessel disease with ventricular dysfunction or unstable angina, the operative risk for CEA becomes excessive (Figure 10, *A*). For these patients there has been a recent enthusiasm for a combined operative approach; that is, one in which the patient is anesthesized and a carotid operative team proceeds with CEA while the cardiac team prepares for cardiopulmonary bypass and harvests the saphenous vein or dissects the mammary artery for bypass grafting. Upon completing CEA, the patient is placed on cardiopulmonary bypass and the coronary surgery proceeds. The details of this simultaneous technique have been standardized and it can now be carried out with reported morbidity (stroke) and mortality rates of 3.2% and 4.6%, respectively. These rates are not much different from the additive morbidity and mortality of two separate procedures.

With the introduction of noninvasive, accurate Duplex screening, a group of patients representing 3% to 4% of patients undergoing elective CABG with asymptomatic, yet significant carotid disease, has been identified. Small as this group is, it represents a complex clinical problem without a clear consensus of opinion. There has been concern that a patient with an asymptomatic yet significant stenosis (85% cross-sectional area reduction) would be at a high risk of perioperative stroke in the face of cardiopulmonary bypass, blood loss, or hypotension during the operative procedure. Prospective randomized studies are underway to ascertain whether simultaneous CEA with CABG will reduce the perioperative neurologic morbidity of cardiac surgery in patients found on screening to have asymptomatic yet significant carotid occlusive disease. To date, simultaneous prophylactic CEA has not substantially reduced the incidence of neurologic complications of CABG. Other well-conducted studies have failed to define the suspected increase in perioperative stroke in patients with asymptomatic carotid disease. However, these patients are indeed at a higher risk (range of 2.5% to 7%/y) of developing stroke during their remaining lifetime than the general age-related population (stroke risk approximately 2%/y). Over half these patients will develop warning symptoms of transient ischemic attacks prior to the onset of a fixed stroke. Whether prophylactic CEA (staged following successful coronary revascularization) with an inherent 1% mortality and 2% stroke rate or nonoperative observation of the carotid disease in this group of patients is the best option remains a clinical judgment that varies from center to center. There is, however, a subgroup of these asymptomatic patients that has bilateral high-grade internal carotid stenosis or a high-grade stenosis with an occluded contralateral carotid. This group of patients is at an exaggerated risk of developing stroke without warning and, therefore, should be considered for prophylactic CEA. They may well represent a subgroup in whom the risk of perioperative stroke is high, and would benefit from CEA prior to, or simultaneously with, CABG (Figure 7-10, B).

Given that the incidence of asymptomatic, significant carotid disease is low (3% to 4%) overall in patients undergoing CABG, and the majority of patients will not require prophylactic CEA, who then should undergo noninvasive screening?

A cervical bruit in the past has been used as a marker for carotid artery disease; however, this is not very reliable. There is a poor correlation between a cervical bruit and significant occlusive carotid disease. In one study, only 37% of patients with cervical bruits had significant carotid disease, whereas of those patients with identified significant carotid stenosis only 27% had a detectable cervical bruit. Although the cervical bruit is not a good predictor of carotid disease, it does identify those patients with a more widespread atherosclerotic vascular disease. Therefore, those patients with an asymptomatic carotid bruit or other evidence of peripheral vascular disease, who are undergoing evaluation for CABG, should have noninvasive carotid screening by duplex scanning. There has been a positive correlation noted between left main coronary stenosis and carotid bifurcation disease, so these patients also should undergo Duplex evaluation. If screening indicates bilateral high-grade stenosis or unilateral stenosis greater than 60% cross-sectional area with contralateral occlusion, then carotid angiography should be done to confirm these findings. A decision can then be made regarding prophylactic carotid surgery.

Thus, all patients with lateralizing symptoms suggestive of carotid disease, including those recovered from a recent

INITIAL EVALUATION

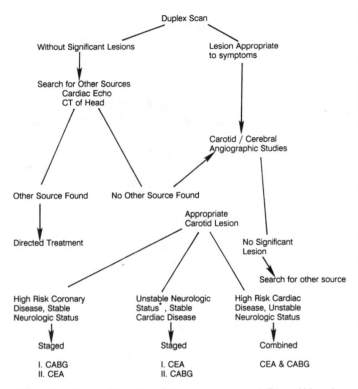

Lateralizing Neurologic Symptoms
Stroke in Past

Duplex Scan

Without Significant Lesions

Lesion Appropriate
to symptoms

Search for Other Sources
Cardiac Echo
CT of Head

Carotid / Cerebral
Angiographic Studies

Other Source Found   No Other Source Found

Appropriate
Carotid Lesion

Directed Treatment

No Significant
Lesion

Search for other source

High Risk Coronary
Disease, Stable
Neurologic Status

Unstable Neurologic
Status*, Stable
Cardiac Disease

High Risk Cardiac
Disease, Unstable
Neurologic Status

Staged

Staged

Combined

I. CABG
II. CEA

I. CEA
II. CABG

CEA & CABG

* Unstable Neurologic Status = Frequent lateralizing symptoms, crescendo TIAs, or high grade
stenosis (95 - 99%)n

Figure 7-10 A. Algorithms for patients with symptomatic cerebral vascular disease and coronary artery disease.

cerebrovascular accident, should undergo noninvasive screening. If significant disease involving the common or internal carotid is demonstrated, angiography should be done to confirm and define the lesion. If the cardiac disease is stable and nonthreatening, then staged prophylactic CEA followed by CABG is recommended. If the cardiac disease is of a more unstable or dangerous nature, then simultaneous CEA and CABG should be considered. Asymptomatic carotid disease appears to present less of a risk to the cardiac surgeon. Those patients with a cervical bruit, extracardiac manifestations of

INITIAL EVALUATION

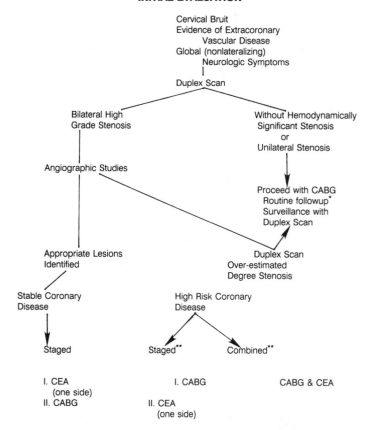

Cervical Bruit
Evidence of Extracoronary
Vascular Disease
Global (nonlateralizing)
Neurologic Symptoms
|
Duplex Scan

Bilateral High
Grade Stenosis

Without Hemodynamically
Significant Stenosis
or
Unilateral Stenosis

Angiographic Studies

Proceed with CABG
Routine followup*
Surveillance with
Duplex Scan

Appropriate Lesions
Identified

Duplex Scan
Over-estimated
Degree Stenosis

Stable Coronary
Disease

High Risk Coronary
Disease

Staged

Staged**

Combined**

I. CEA
  (one side)
II. CABG

I. CABG

II. CEA
  (one side)

CABG & CEA

* If lateralizing symptoms develop referable to stenotic lesion the workup with angiographic
    studies is indicated
** Decision regarding staged vs. combined should be made on individual patient basis.

**Figure 7-10 B. Algorithm for patients suspected of having asymp-
tomatic cerebral vascular disease and coronary artery disease.**

vascular disease or left main coronary disease, are at a higher
risk of having asymptomatic carotid disease, and should undergo Duplex screening. The treatment of a significant carotid
lesion then depends on the judgment and philosophy of the
managing physician and should be individualized to meet the
needs of the patient. The small group of patients with asymptomatic yet significant bilateral occlusive disease should be
treated in the same manner that patients with a symptomatic
carotid lesion are treated.

AVOIDING COMPLICATIONS ASSOCIATED WITH ARTERIAL ACCESS FOR DIAGNOSIS AND INTERVENTION

Utilization of intravascular access to the heart is increasing with the development of newer diagnostic and therapeutic techniques. While these developments have markedly improved our ability to treat ischemic heart disease, the vascular complications of their use are becoming more apparent.

The use of the Seldinger technique, together with recent advances in catheter design and materials and greater experience in catheterization laboratories, has served to reduce vascular-related complications of diagnostic catheterization to about 1%. Most of these complications are related to the local puncture site and include hematoma, false aneurysm, local thrombosis, plaque dissection, and arteriovenous fistula. The majority of these complications can be treated with local surgical procedures and rarely represent permanent or significant patient morbidity if recognized and treated promptly.

However, the increased use of the IABP is producing a large number of vascular-related complications. The larger size of the introducer, the rigidity and size of the balloon, the prolonged time it remains in place, and the direct trauma of the intra-arterial pumping action of the IABP itself are all factors that increase the risk of serious vascular morbidity. The incidence of major vascular complications related to the use of percutaneously placed IABP is in the range of 25% to 30% in several large, reported studies.

The complications can be divided into those created by the local arterial puncture and those induced by trauma to the arterial tree at a distance from the puncture site. The use of a larger-bore introducer increases the risk of a local dissection of an arterial plaque with resultant thrombosis and acute limb ischemia, the degree of which is related to the extent of the thrombotic process and the degree of collateral circulation. A low cardiac output in a failing heart will tend to aggravate the distal ischemia. Even without the lifting of an atherosclerotic plaque, the large diameter of the introducer and the balloon catheter may serve functionally to obstruct a narrow lumen artery, resulting in distal ischemia or thrombosis. Other local complications include thrombosis of the artery by clot and fibrin adhering to the balloon catheter and introducer that is sheared off upon its removal, infections secondary to a percutaneous indwelling foreign body, and hematoma or false aneurysm formation from the large puncture in the artery.

Minimizing the complications associated with use of the IABP requires a good evaluation of the circulation beyond the point of insertion, including palpation of distal pulses and assessment of signs of distal ischemia. A regular periodic assessment of distal circulation must, then, be carried out after insertion of the balloon to make possible the early recognition of developing ischemic complications. Close adherence to the recommended procedure for balloon removal, including allowing a brief, brisk bleed from the puncture site to flush adherent thrombus and an adequate period of compression at the puncture site, will serve to reduce the risk of hematoma and false aneurysm formation. If an ischemic complication develops during the use of the IABP, consultation with a vascular surgeon should be sought. Each situation must be assessed on an individual basis and, if necessary, a form of extra-anatomic bypass can be carried out to ensure salvage of the ischemic limb.

Another source of major morbidity associated with the use of the IABP is the precipitation of emboli either from dissection during the passage of the balloon catheter or from the trauma of the balloon's pumping a diseased artery. These emboli consist of small amounts of thrombus, platelet aggregates, and atheroma debris containing cholesterol crystals. The emboli can lodge in the mesenteric, renal, or extremity vascular beds, resulting in intestinal ischemia, renal failure, or ischemia of the limb. Spinal cord ischemia with resultant paraplegia has also been reported. The shower nature of these arterial-arterial emboli and their small size make successful surgical removal to restore blood flow to the involved vascular bed unlikely. Early recognition of this complication with expedient removal of the balloon catheter and treatment of the consequences of embolization, such as resection of infarcted gut, revascularization of an ischemic extremity, and supportive measures associated with renal ischemia, may reduce the ultimate patient morbidity and mortality. Aortic and iliac dissection or perforation by the balloon catheter can produce a significant morbidity and mortality. The use of a flexible guidewire over which the balloon catheter is passed and, in some instances, the surgical placement of a graft sheath beyond a segment of tortuous or diseased iliac artery, have reduced these complications. Aortoiliac dissection producing significant visceral ischemia or perforation with massive blood loss requires direct surgical intervention and is associated with a high mortality. Limb ischemia from iliac dissection can usually be managed with an extra-anatomic bypass.

Aneurysmal disease of the aorta and iliac vessels imposes an increased risk for any diagnostic or therapeutic intervention that requires passing a catheter through these arteries. The iliac arteries become quite tortuous as they are coiled by the expanding aneurysm. Forging such a tortuous lumen with a guidewire or catheter becomes difficult and is associated with increased trauma because the arterial wall is sheared by the catheter with each change in direction. The incidence of plaque disruption with dissection and emboli or perforation is thus increased. The aneurysmal cavity tends to fill with a friable proteinaceous laminated thrombus that can easily be dislodged by a catheter. The wall of an aneurysm also represents a weakened area of the artery and is more prone to perforation. For these reasons, the identification of an aortic or iliac aneurysm is a relative contraindication to intraluminal manipulation if an alternative route is available. The larger the size of the aneurysm, the higher the risk of associated complication. Certainly the use of the IABP in the face of a large aneurysm carries a high morbidity.

Aortoiliac occlusive disease increases the difficulty and risk of passing intraluminal catheters and is associated with a higher risk of local puncture site complications. The use of the smallest catheter and attempts to reduce the number of catheter manipulations will aid in reducing these complications. The use of heparin or low molecular weight dextran helps reduce the incidence of thrombotic complications.

Special care must be exercised in dealing with a patient who has had previous vascular surgery with the placement of an arterial graft. If a patient has a functioning femoral popliteal bypass and the other groin is available, it would be wise to avoid puncture in the groin with the bypass graft. An aortobifemoral bypass graft can be punctured, although there is the additional hazard of creating a graft infection. An infection involving a synthetic bypass graft can have devastating consequences. Therefore, the strictest of aseptic technique must be used when puncturing a previously placed bypass graft. The catheters should remain indwelling for as short a time as possible and catheter changes should be kept to an absolute minimum.

There is the occasional patient in whom an extra-anatomic bypass has been previously performed to revascularize the low extremity. It is important to understand the course of the bypass prior to attempting passage of guidewires or catheters.

If a dissection or intraluminal injury to an artery is recognized, the prudent use of anticoagulants or antiplatelet drugs will help to minimize the sequelae of the injury and allow healing of the luminal surface. A hematoma or sealed perforation would be an indication for withholding anticoagulants and antiplatelet medications at least initially. There is little role for pentoxifylline.

Careful initial evaluation of the arterial tree, avoidance of manipulation of diseased arteries, early recognition and treatment of arterial complications, and careful follow-up will reduce to a minimum the associated patient morbidity.

SUGGESTED READING

Crawford SE, Crawford JL. *Disease of the Aorta.* New York: Williams & Wilkins; 1984.

Doroghazi RM, Slater EE. *Aortic Dissection.* New York: McGraw-Hill; 1983.

Hershey FB, Barnes RW, Sumner DS. *Noninvasive Diagnosis of Vascular Disease.* Pasadena: Appleton Davis; 1984.

Jones EL, Craver JM, Michalik RA, et al. Combined carotid and coronary operations: when are they necessary. *J Thorac Cardiovasc Surg.* 1984; 87:7–16.

Kempczinski RF, Yao JS. *Practical Noninvasive Vascular Diagnosis.* 2nd ed. Chicago: Year Book Medical Publishers; 1987.

Miller DS, Beven EG, Gardner TJ, et al. Symposium: coexistent cardiac and peripheral vascular surgery. *J Vasc Surg* 1986; 3:681–694.

Nicolaides AN, Yao, JS. *Investigation of Vascular Disorders.* New York: Churchill Livingstone; 1981.

Sundt TM. *Occlusive Cerebrovascular Disease Diagnosis and Surgical Management.* Philadelphia: WB Saunders; 1987.

Preoperative Evaluation— Anesthesiologist's View

Thomas R. Eide, M.D.

8

The preoperative evaluation of the cardiac surgical patient by the anesthesiologist is an important step in the preparation of the patient for surgery. It begins with an often overlooked but extremely important aspect: the emotional and psychologic preparation of the patient. Most patients are apprehensive and scared of the surgical process. The patient is confronted with the acceptance of his own mortality, the loss of control of his body, possible permanent disability, and the thought of post-surgical pain. These are frightening unknowns to most patients. One of the primary purposes of the preoperative visit is to educate and provide a source of reassurance. This is accomplished by demonstrating a competent and caring image and discussing what the patient will experience on the day of surgery and in the intensive care unit during the postoperative period. A premedication of a narcotic together with a benzodiazepine can be given to decrease anxiety and provide sedation on the morning of surgery; however, there is no substitute for the personal interaction and reassurance the anesthesiologist can provide to the patient prior to the operation.

Another purpose of the preoperative evaluation is to gather information for assessing risk and formulating an anesthetic plan. The patient's history, physical examination, and laboratory data form the basis of the anesthetic plan.

An interview is conducted, directed toward the cardiac and respiratory systems. Important information obtained will include knowledge of the extent of the patient's cardiac disease, the past medical history, previous surgery including surgical and anesthetic complications, and current medications. Objective laboratory data are noted from the patient's chart (blood work, chest x-ray, electrocardiogram [ECG], pulmonary studies, and cardiac catheterization data) and informed consent for the anesthetic care to be provided is obtained. To obtain informed consent, the anesthetic plan along with possible complications, which are either common or severe, must be explained and discussed in language which the patient can understand.

Finally, a preoperative note is written in the patient's chart which briefly discusses the relevant medical and surgical histories, allergies, medications, and physical and laboratory findings. It is concluded with an assessment of physical status (ASA classification) and the invasive monitoring and type of anesthesia planned.

A safe, uneventful anesthetic and operative course is the desired goal.

PERIOPERATIVE RISK

Risk is the possible morbidity and mortality a patient is exposed to as a result of receiving an anesthetic and undergoing a surgical procedure. Studies which attempt to define and quantitate morbidity and mortality based on patient characteristics form the basis for understanding risk. These studies are extremely valuable in that they clarify which of the many conditions or disease states a patient has and are important predictors of outcome. Table 8-1 outlines the characteristics identified as contributing factors to an increased rate of complications in general surgical patients. These parameters have been studied in cardiac surgical patients and a somewhat different group of

---

Table 8-1   Conditions Associated with Increased Perioperative Risk for General Surgical Patients

Unstable angina
Severe hypertension
Congestive heart failure
Recent myocardial infarction (<6 mo)
Chronic obstructive pulmonary disease
Obesity

Table 8-2   Conditions Associated with Increased Intraoperative Risk in Cardiac Surgical Patients

Unstable angina
Left main coronary disease
Ventricular dysfunction (wall motion abnormalities)
Congestive heart failure
Increased left ventricular end-diastolic pressure (LVEDP)
Age over 60

characteristics has been found to effect perioperative morbidity and mortality (Table 8-2). Outcome in this group of patients is significantly determined by the amount of myocardial damage that has taken place prior to surgery and by the severity of underlying atherosclerotic and valvular disease. During the preoperative evaluation, the anesthesiologist will note these conditions and include them in the anesthetic plan.

SYSTEMS AT RISK

Complications associated with the administration of an anesthetic to a cardiac surgical patient together with the complications which occur during the intraoperative and postoperative periods tend to involve the cardiac, neurologic, pulmonary, and hematologic systems. The following discussions address the risk factors in these areas.

Cardiac risk factors

Poor ventricular function: Cardiac surgical patients can be divided into those with preserved ventricular function and those with impaired ventricular function. Numerous studies have pointed to the presence of poor preoperative ventricular function as causing a significant increase in perioperative complications.

When the anesthesiologist determines from the patient's history, physical signs, and symptoms or from objective laboratory data that a patient has poor ventricular function (Table 8-3), it is appreciated that this patient will have little tolerance to stresses encountered perioperatively.

The compromised myocardium may not tolerate an episode of perioperative ischemia from a difficult anesthetic induction. Furthermore, an incomplete revascularization, a

Table 8-3   Indications of Ventricular Dysfunction

History	Dyspnea at rest or with exertion
	Orthopnea
	Poor exercise tolerance
Physical examination	S_3
	Rales
	Wheezing
Laboratory evaluation	Decreased wall motion
	Increased LVEDP
	Reduced ejection fraction
	Left ventricular aneurysm
	Valvular heart disease

prolonged cardiopulmonary bypass time, or inadequate myocardial preservation (cardioplegia) may lead to myocardial damage. These will contribute to poor myocardial function when the patient is weaned from cardiopulmonary bypass and may result in the use of inotropic agents, an intra-aortic balloon pump (IABP), or a ventricular assist device and potentially increase complications intraoperatively and postoperatively. Hence, the presence of poor ventricular function is a major cardiac risk factor.

Perioperative myocardial ischemia: The patient about to undergo a coronary revascularization is particularly at risk to develop perioperative myocardial ischemia and as a result, may develop an intraoperative or postoperative myocardial infarction (MI). Slogoff and Keats have found that as many as 55% of patients scheduled for elective coronary revascularization develop perioperative ischemia and those who develop ischemia are at a significantly increased risk for postoperative MI.

The incidence of postoperative MI in groups of patients undergoing cardiac surgery has been reported to range from 1% to 5%. An MI in the surgical setting carries a higher rate of mortality than an MI in the general population and reduces postoperative ejection fraction and exercise tolerance.

Preoperative conditions associated with operative mortality were found (Coronary Artery Surgery Study) to be signs and symptoms related to myocardial dysfunction (decreased wall motion, clinical signs of congestive heart failure, increased ventricular filling pressures) and left main coronary disease.

These conditions are indicative of myocardial damage and extensive coronary atherosclerotic disease.

Minimizing the risk of perioperative ischemia and postoperative MI is crucial in this patient population. Many steps are taken by the anesthesiologist to accomplish this. They include providing an adequate premedication to decrease anxiety, making sure that all appropriate antianginal and antihypertensive medications are continued on the day of surgery, monitoring for the appearance of ischemia intraoperatively, and treating suspected ischemia early to avoid myocardial damage.

Valvular heart disease: Valvular heart disease may be the reason the patient is presenting for surgery or may be an incidental finding on physical examination or objective cardiac tests. The severity of the valvular lesion and its effects on the heart and pulmonary vasculature are seen in the cardiac catheterization report. The presence of critical stenosis with a small calculated valve area or the presence of a large regurgitant fraction are indicative of significant valvular dysfunction. A chronic valve abnormality may produce a hypertrophied or dilated heart and possibly pulmonary hypertension. When a valve is replaced, these chronic changes usually do not reverse themselves in the perioperative period. The ventricular dysfunction which is often present in this group of patients leaves little reserve for the stresses of a surgical procedure and places the patient at a higher risk for perioperative morbidity and mortality. Additionally, Slogoff and colleagues found an increased incidence of stroke thought secondary to the presence of air which enters the heart when it is opened to replace the valve.

Cardiopulmonary bypass: Cardioplegic arrest and the institution of cardiopulmonary bypass during the revascularization procedure is necessary for a motionless field to permit the surgical repair. Hypothermia and cardioplegia are necessary for myocardial preservation during this time.

The bypass period has associated complications which are both mechanical and physiologic. The mechanical complications are concerned mostly with pump lines and filters and the placement of the aortic and venous cannulas. A kinked or occluded venous cannula, an aortic dissection from an improperly placed aortic cannula, a malfunctioning pump head, and an improperly connected bypass circuit are possible complications of an extracorporeal circuit. Physiologic effects of bypass are evident in the intraoperative and postoperative periods. The major systems affected are cardiac, pulmonary, neurologic, and hematologic. A few examples are the following:

1. Potassium cardioplegia and hypothermia necessary for cardiac preservation during bypass may have residual cardiac depressive effects when weaning from cardiopulmonary bypass.
2. Associated electrolyte abnormalities such as hyperkalemia from the cardioplegia solution or subsequent hypokalemia secondary to the osmotic diuresis from mannitol may result in arrhythmias and conduction abnormalities.
3. Bleeding secondary to residual heparin, excess protamine, or platelet dysfunction may occur.
4. Neurologic dysfunction may arise from air or atheromatous plaque embolism or secondary to hypoperfusion during bypass.

Surgery in the setting of an acute myocardial infarction: A situation which occasionally arises is the patient presenting with an acute MI and continuing ischemia not responsive to emergency angioplasty, thrombolytic therapy, or IABP counterpulsation. Surgical revascularization may be considered. A major consequence of an acute MI is the appearance of severe myocardial dysfunction. This results in a dramatic increase in the use of inotropic agents, an increase in intraoperative ventricular arrythmias, and the use of the intra-aortic balloon.

According to Katz, coronary bypass in the setting of a recent MI (less than 30 days) is associated with a higher mortality rate from myocardial failure.

Neurologic risk factors

The cardiac surgical procedure is associated with an incidence of stroke of 1% to 1.5% when defined as a continuing neurologic dysfunction 1 year after the procedure. Factors implicated in this are the presence of carotid occlusive disease, perioperative hypotension, and embolism from atheromatous plaque or air. Indeed air introduced into the aorta or into the heart itself has been implicated as the primary factor in most focal deficits. As a standard part of the cardiac surgical procedure, the surgeon performs what are called air maneuvers to eliminate air from the heart, aorta, and coronary grafts.

There are, however, cerebral deficits that are subtle and not focal which can be detected by sensitive neuropsychiatric testing. These deficits in perception and behavior may be present in 16% of patients in the immediate postoperative period but usually subside within a year of the procedure.

Conditions associated with cerebral dysfunction in the postoperative period are thought to be related to poor cardiac status preoperatively, prior organic brain syndrome, increased time spent on cardiopulmonary bypass, intraoperative hypotension, and increased age.

It should also be noted that the cardiac surgical population has an increased incidence of vascular disease and of primary importance is the presence of significant carotid artery disease which has been reported to be approximately 6% in this group. An elective bypass procedure carries an incidence of postoperative stroke of approximately 1.0% in patients with no known carotid disease and increases in patients with asymptomatic carotid bruits, transient ischemic attacks, or stroke. It is, therefore, important, if a history of transient ischemic attacks is elicited or a carotid bruit found, that these patients undergo further studies to determine if significant carotid disease is present and if it should be corrected prior to cardiac surgery.

Pulmonary dysfunction

Preoperative pulmonary dysfunction will greatly affect the postoperative pulmonary status of the patient. The patient having a median sternotomy for a cardiac surgical procedure will develop a restrictive lung abnormality and a 75% reduction of vital capacity 12-18 hours after the operation. A normal vital capacity of 55-85 mL/kg may be reduced to the 15 mL/kg point where respiratory insufficiency would develop if the patient were breathing spontaneously. It is for this reason that patients are normally supported with mechanical ventilation during the postoperative period. A reduced functional residual capacity and an inability to mobilize bronchial secretions contribute to the possibility of producing atelectasis and pneumonia in the postoperative period.

Preoperative pulmonary conditions greatly contribute to this possibility. A preoperative history of smoking, sputum production, or obstructive or restrictive lung disease will greatly contribute to postoperative pulmonary dysfunction and it reasonably follows that pulmonary conditions should be identified and corrected prior to elective cardiac surgery. A preoperative respiratory history, pulmonary function testing such as a forced expiratory spirogram and possibly an arterial blood gas where impaired gas exchange is suspected will help to identify patients at risk for postoperative complications. A forced vital capacity (FVC) of less than 20 mL/kg, a forced expiratory volume at 1 sec (FEV_1)/FVC of less than 50%, as well as signs and symptoms of pneumonia, bronchitis, or atelectasis place a patient at high risk for pulmonary dysfunction postoperatively. Therapeutic interventions such as cessation of smoking and preoperative chest physical therapy for the mobilization and clearance of bronchial secretions and antibiotic therapy for any suspected underlying bronchial or pulmonary infection will usually result in an improvement of vital capacity and reduce the possibility of developing postoperative pulmonary dysfunction.

Hematologic dysfunction

Postoperative bleeding is of particular importance to the cardiac surgical patient because of the physiologic changes of cardiopulmonary bypass and the requirement for heparinization. According to Bick, bleeding in the postbypass patient can be due to lack of surgical hemostasis, the presence of a circulating anticoagulant (excess heparin or excess protamine), clotting factor deficiency secondary to dilution from the pump prime volume or consumption, or a platelet abnormality.

Complete anticoagulation with heparin is required for a patient to be placed on cardiopulmonary bypass since the bypass circuit does affect plasma proteins and activates the coagulation system. The heparin administered prior to and during bypass is reversed with protamine sulfate. If the heparin is incompletely reversed or if too much protamine is administered, excess bleeding may result (protamine is a mild anticoagulant).

When excess bleeding presents in the postoperative period with normal coagulation times (prothrombin time [PT] and partial thromboplastin time [PTT]), a platelet dysfunction must be suspected. Cardiopulmonary bypass is associated with a time-dependent depression of platelet function thought secondary to activation and degranulation from the bypass circuit material. Platelet infusion is indicated in this setting. Clotting factor deficiency is usually not the etiology of postsurgical blood loss (when disseminated intravascular coagulation is not present). Clotting factor levels do decrease during bypass; however, sufficient levels are usually present to yield adequate hemostasis. Routine infusions of fresh frozen plasma are not indicated for the uncomplicated cardiac surgical patient.

Recently, thrombolysis with streptokinase or tissue plasminogen activator has been introduced as a treatment modality for acute MI. A patient requiring surgical revascularization shortly after receiving a thrombolytic agent would present the possibility of active fibrinolysis. This condition is considered in these patients bleeding postoperatively. Treatment for this includes fresh frozen plasma, cryoprecipitate, and ϵ-aminocaproic acid.

Renal dysfunction

The preservation of existing renal function is a major concern for any surgical patient. The cardiac surgical patient presents the additional problems of renal changes during cardiopulmonary bypass and the maintenance of renal function during the postoperative period when these patients may have depressed myocardial performance and require inotropic support.

Although there are many possible etiologies of postoperative renal dysfunction after cardiac surgery, (i.e., embolic events, hypotension, allergic reactions, or toxins), the most common etiology is a dysfunction secondary to depressed cardiac output. Steps taken to minimize renal dysfunction in this group of patients include actively supporting cardiac function during the perioperative period. Preserving renal function by maintaining a specific mean arterial pressure while on bypass, inducing an osmotic diuresis with mannitol, as well as instituting pulsatile flow on bypass are controversial issues with literature both pro and con.

It should be recognized that patients with severe renal disease who are dialysis dependent are more difficult to manage intraoperatively and postoperatively due to the presence of electrolyte, acid–base, and coagulation abnormalities which are characteristic of the disease process and may require early postoperative dialysis.

LABORATORY DATA FOR RISK ASSESSMENT

Objective laboratory data are important in the preoperative evaluation. Cardiac catheterization data, in particular, are extremely helpful in defining the severity of cardiac disease present. The anesthesiologist will look at the catheterization data to understand the extent and severity of the coronary artery disease present (triple vessel, left main, etc.) and the presence of myocardial dysfunction by description of wall motion and ejection fraction. Changes in the pulmonary vasculature or valve abnormalities will also be noted. This type of information is important for the anesthesiologist to plan his anesthetic technique taking these factors into account. For example:

1. The presence of wall motion abnormalities indicating depressed myocardial function in the presence of severe left main coronary disease may necessitate the placement of an IABP prior to induction of anesthesia. The anesthesiologist will avoid pharmacologic agents with known myocardial depression and hemodynamic states that stress the myocardium such as increases in heart rate or systemic vascular resistance (SVR).
2. The presence of abnormal coagulation studies may indicate the need for specific blood products after bypass.
3. An arrhythmia or conduction disturbance on the ECG would alert the anesthesiologist to the probable use of an antiarrhythmic agent or the use of a pacemaker during the induction period as well as during the weaning process.

INTRAOPERATIVE MONITORING

Standards of intraoperative monitoring have been established to ensure patient safety. The cardiac surgical patient will undergo a major thoracic procedure and require intensive care postoperatively. Monitors of vital organ function are essential for the safe administration of an anesthetic and for the management of these patients perioperatively.

Intraoperative ischemia and cardiac dysfunction are primary concerns in this patient group and the array of monitoring in the cardiac operating room is directed toward minimizing these factors (Table 8-4).

The most sensitive indicator of myocardial ischemia is decreased wall motion. This can be monitored intraoperatively with transesophageal two-dimensional echocardiography which is currently being introduced into clinical practice. The placement of this device is via an esophageal catheter and will yield information regarding changes in wall motion and

Table 8-4   Intraoperative Monitoring

Monitor	Purpose
Arterial line	Continuous blood pressure and arterial blood gases
Pulmonary artery catheter	Ischemia detection, intravascular volume, cardiac output, core temperature
Bladder catheter	Renal function (urine output)
Pulse oximeter	Adequate ventilation and pulmonary function
ECG	Monitor rhythm
End-tidal CO_2	Adequate ventilation
Transesophageal two-dimensional echo-cardiography	Detects ischemia (wall motion abnormalities) Reveals intracardiac air Evaluates valvular function Detects bidirectional blood flow (shunt flows—atrial, ventricular septal defects)

ventricular dimensions. The next most sensitive means to detect myocardial ischemia is the change in cardiac filling pressures observed with the pulmonary artery catheter. An increase in LVEDP, as detected by an increase in pulmonary capillary wedge pressure, is a sign of ischemia. The pulmonary artery catheter can also perform a thermodilution cardiac output. Because changes in filling pressures frequently occur before ischemic ECG changes appear and before changes in systemic blood pressure take place, the anesthesiologist will follow cardiac filling pressures during the induction and maintenance of anesthesia, to detect ischemia and treat it early and appropriately.

THE DAY OF SURGERY AND THE CARDIAC ANESTHETIC

The preoperative evaluation by the anesthesiologist is performed the evening prior to surgery during which pertinent laboratory data are reviewed (Table 8-5), an anesthetic plan formulated, and informed consent obtained from the patient.

The day of surgery for an elective coronary revascularization patient will begin with the administration of a premedication prior to being transported to the operating room together with the cardiac medications the patient is receiving chronically (calcium channel blockers, nitrates, β-blockers, antihypertensives).

Upon the patient's arrival in the operating room, a

Table 8-5 Cardiac Surgical Preoperative Checklist

Complete blood count with platelet count
PT, PTT
Bleeding time
Electrolytes and SMA-12
Arterial blood gas ⎫ If history is suggestive
Pulmonary function tests ⎬ of pulmonary disease
Chest x-ray
ECG
Urinalysis
Cardiac catheterization results
Other cardiac tests
Thallium stress results
Echocardiography
Premedication orders for sedation
Review medications to be given on day of surgery

Table 8-6 Preanesthetic Hemodynamics

Problem	Possible Interventions
Low cardiac output	Reduce SVR with vasodilator
	IABP
	Inotropic agent
	Increase preload (volume)
Hypertension	β-Blocker
	Vasodilator
Tachycardia	β-Blocker
ECG changes (ischemic)	IV nitroglycerine
	Sublingual nifedipine
	β-Blocker
	IABP

large-bore peripheral intravenous line, a radial arterial catheter, and a pulmonary artery catheter via an internal jugular vein are inserted. With invasive monitoring in place, important information about the patient is obtained such as a thermodilution cardiac output, SVR, heart rate, and systemic blood pressure. It is at this point that critical decisions are made to reduce the risk of anesthetic induction. If abnormal parameters of low cardiac output, tachycardia, high SVR, or ST segment changes are present, they are corrected prior to the administration of the anesthetic to minimize the risk of ischemia during this period (Table 8-6).

Table 8-7 Myocardial Oxygen Balance	
Supply	**Demand**
Coronary blood flow	Afterload (blood pressure)
Blood hemoglobin content	Preload (LVEDP)
Hemoglobin O$_2$ saturation	Heart rate
Oxyhemoglobin dissociation curve	Contractility

A mask airway is initiated with 100% oxygen and a large dose narcotic anesthetic, combined with a nondepolarizing neuromuscular blocking agent, is administered. Shortly thereafter, the patient's trachea is intubated. Vital signs are continuously monitored and supplemental anesthetic agents are administered periodically.

The term "cardiac anesthetic" has become synonymous with the titration of anesthetic agents in the presence of invasive hemodynamic monitoring (arterial and pulmonary artery catheters) toward the goal of providing hemodynamic stability and optimizing the relationship of myocardial oxygen supply and demand (Table 8-7). For example:

1. Tachycardia produces a profound increase in myocardial oxygen consumption and is treated aggressively during anesthetic administration.
2. Arterial hemoglobin oxygen saturation is a major determinant of blood oxygen content and oxygen delivery to the myocardium. Changes in oxygen saturation seen on the pulse oximeter usually reflect problems with ventilation and are quickly treated.
3. Changes in afterload are followed and appropriately treated. If SVR (afterload) is abnormally low, coronary perfusion pressure and myocardial oxygen supply are reduced. If SVR is abnormally high, cardiac work and myocardial oxygen demand increases.

The widely accepted anesthetic for the cardiac patient is a high-dose synthetic narcotic such as fentanyl or sufantanil. Although postoperative mechanical ventilation is usually required, a high-dose narcotic technique provides superior hemodynamic stability as it does not intrinsically depress myocardial function nor does it release histamine which results in venous and arterial dilatation. Potent inhalational agents such as enflurane or halothane may be given either as supplemental agents or as the primary anesthetic agent to patients with preserved myocardial function. The potent inhalational agents decrease myocardial oxygen consumption and can be beneficial; however, they are also myocardial depressants and patients with little myocardial reserve may not tolerate them.

SUMMARY

The preoperative evaluation consists of preparing the patient emotionally, including obtaining informed consent; obtaining relevant medical information and assessing risk; formulating an anesthetic plan; premedicating the patient to reduce anxiety; and reviewing orders of chronic medications. It is the responsibility of the anesthesiologist to be involved in each of these areas. Addressing them will reduce the risks of morbidity and mortality in the adult cardiac surgical patient.

SUGGESTED READING

Bick RL. Hemostasis defects associated with cardiac surgery, prosthetic devices, and other extracorporeal circuits. *Semin Thromb Hemost* 1985; 3:249–280.

Katz NM, Kubanick TE, Ahmed SW, et al. Determinants of cardiac failure after coronary bypass surgery within 30 days of acute myocardial infarction. *Ann Thorac Surg.* 1986; 42:658–663.

Kennedy JW, Kaiser GC, Fisher LD, et al. Multivariate discriminate analysis of the clinical and angiographic predictors of operative mortality from the Collaborative Study in Coronary Artery Surgery (CASS). *J Thorac Cardiovasc Surg.* 1980; 80:876–887.

Slogoff S, Girgis KZ, Keats AS. Etiologic factors in neuropsychiatric complications associated with cardiopulmonary bypass. *Anesth Analg.* 1982; 61:903–911.

Slogoff S, Keats AS. Further observations on perioperative myocardial ischemia. *Anesthesiology.* 1986; 65:539–542.

Surgical Risk—Surgeon's View

Frank Seifert, M.D.
Thomas Bilfinger, M.D.

9

When surgeons evaluate patients for open heart procedures, they will customarily offer an estimate of the risk of death, the risk of complications, and the likelihood of cure or palliation. They may contrast this to the inherent risks of continued medical management, and they might project the long-term outlook for the patient if treated surgically. Overwhelmingly, what the patient remembers after such consultation is the stated risk of death, expressed as a simple proportion or percentage. This risk is approximated by the in-hospital or 30-day mortality rate. It is inclusive of serious morbidity, because most serious morbidity such as extensive stroke or myocardial infarction (MI) results in the patient's death before hospital discharge. However, in the cardiac patient it implies something more than the operative mortality. It is perceived as an answer to the patient's straightforward query, "Doctor, what are my chances ?" Although the in-hospital mortality expressed as a percentage carries a negative connotation, subtracted from 100, the chances of surviving the operation are readily obtained and equated with success. The implications of successful survival must be distinguished from the inverse of the in-hospital mortality, and we will refer to these implications as the surgical outlook.

In-hospital mortality is only a measure of hospital survival. It does not measure other end points, such as relief of cardiac symptoms, nor does it predict long-term results. A statistically accurate and complete statement of the surgical outlook for a given patient would require actuarial analysis based on a population matched for diagnosis, operation, and risk factors. Results are not expressed as a simple proportion, but as a time-dependent curve describing freedom from a particular event. For the cardiac surgical patient, important events are death and cardiac symptoms such as angina and congestive heart failure. Not one, but two or three curves may be required to describe a patient's situation. Comparison of these curves is mathematically possible but complex. Indeed, describing a single curve, giving it tangible value to the patient, can be challenging. Furthermore, the availability of actuarial data for the diverse subsets of cardiac surgical patients is limited. Actuarial analysis is a powerful research tool, but it is not an answer to the patient's query about his chances.

In-hospital mortality, on the other hand, is represented by a single number, has been estimated in thousands of different patient subgroups, and is readily compared by chi-square testing. The nature of cardiac disease and of current cardiac surgery is such that an in-hospital survivor of cardiac surgery is likely free of symptoms and will probably survive for a few years. Support for this assumption comes from actuarial analysis, which has repeatedly demonstrated that the probability of death is greatest in the perioperative period. An exception to this assumption is the patient with severe, irreversible myocardial dysfunction. Patients with extensive MI, severe valvular regurgitation, or cardiomyopathy may survive operation but are unlikely to realize functional improvement. They are also less likely to gain protection from sudden death. Taking note of this exception, the implicit extension of the meaning of in-hospital mortality provides a pragmatic tool, a simple estimate of the surgical outlook. This estimate of outlook may be used as the basis for making informed decisions regarding surgical intervention and as an instrument of quality assurance.

ESTIMATING RISK

The ideal circumstances by which a surgeon could render an estimate of in-hospital risk for a procedure would consist of a personal experience of thousands of similar cases. Few surgeons have such a large personal experience. Instead, most surgeons rely on published statistical data from single or multiple institutions and adjust this data based on their personal experience and the experience of their own institution. The problem with published data is that there is often an inherent bias, and few institutions are apt to publish "bad" results. Bias in results can be introduced because of variation in the quality of the hospitals, surgeons, or patients. With the exception of highly specialized forms of cardiac surgery such as transplantation or neonatal heart surgery, hospital and surgeon quality is fairly constant throughout the country. The last decade has demonstrated that most adult cardiac surgery can be performed successfully even at the community hospital level. What accounts for the majority of variability in reported results is the composition of the patient population. A hospital where 40% of the coronary patients go from coronary care unit to operating room will have different results for bypass surgery than a hospital where most of the coronary patients are referred from out of town. To compare the results of cardiac surgery in such a way that variation in the severity of illness is accounted for, risk factor analysis must be used.

Two recently published studies of risk factors influencing operative mortality during adult cardiac surgery are noteworthy in that reporting was obligatory and complete. Both involved a large number of patients over a short period of recent time. They were initiated as instruments of quality assurance to relate preoperative risk factors to hospital mortality. The report of the Bureau of Health Care Research of the New York State (NYS) Department of Health analyzed 16,337 cardiac surgical cases performed during the calendar year 1989 in the 28 hospitals licensed to perform such surgery in the state. The Veterans Administration (VA) Cardiac Surgery Consultants Committee reported on 10,480 cases performed over a 2-year period in 47 of the 50 VA centers authorized to perform cardiac surgery. The aggregate operative mortality rate in both studies was approximately 5%. Risk factors were analyzed in a univariate fashion to determine their influence on in-hospital mortality and in a multivariate fashion to establish the odds ratio and to construct a predictive model. Data from studies such as these is an excellent starting point for estimating the surgical risk of a given patient.

Pure coronary bypass surgery had a 3.7% mortality in NYS and a 4.8% mortality in the VA study, confirming an upward trend in mortality as compared to 10 years ago. This trend has been attributed to increasing age and severity of disease in the coronary population by many other recent studies. The higher VA mortality figure is probably the result of combining left ventricular aneurysm resection patients in the coronary subgroup; these patients were tabulated as "all others" in NYS, with a 14.1% mortality rate. Independent studies of left ventricular aneurysm resection with or without bypass report 10% to 15% mortalities with congestive heart failure as a negative risk factor and angina as a positive risk factor. Postinfarction ventricular septal defect, also tabulated as "other" in NYS and excluded in the VA study, has reported mortality rates between 20% and 40%; anterior MI is a positive risk factor and posterior MI a negative risk factor. Great vessel surgery is the last component of the NYS "other" category, and independent reports of operative mortality for this type of surgery vary depending on the site of surgery; ascending aortic replacement carries a 10% risk, whereas arch replacement may be as high as 30%.

Surgery for valvular heart disease was not subcategorized in the VA study and included valve plus coronary operations as well as great vessel operations, and had a 9.2% operative mortality rate. Mitral and aortic valve replacement alone had a 5.8% and 7.1% mortality, respectively, in NYS, and multivalve operations had an 11.2% mortality rate. If coronary bypass was added to either mitral or aortic valve replacement, 20.1% and 6.0% mortalities resulted. The inordinate rise in mortality for mitral plus coronary operations undoubtedly reflects the high risk of patients with ischemia–related mitral regurgitation. In independent studies of mitral plus coronary surgery where ischemic mitral disease was excluded, 8% to 10% mortality rates are generally reported.

Aside from the type of cardiac surgery performed, the VA and NYS studies reaffirmed the overwhelming preponderance of left ventricular ejection fraction (EF) and patient age as determinants of operative mortality. The respective risk for EFs greater than .50, between .40–.49, .30–.39, .20–.29, and less than .20 were 2.6%, 4.3%, 6.9%, 10.5%, and 24.7%. The odds ratio, the coefficient multiplied by a standard of comparison (in this case, the risk for a patient with an EF greater than .50) was 1.45, 1.90, 2.27, and 5.42 for the later four subdivisions. Age was related to mortality in a nonlinear fashion, and odds ratios could not be calculated (one has to define a baseline age for comparison). The respective mortalities for patients 59 years or less, 60–64, 65–69, 70–74, 75–79, and over 80 years were 3.0%, 4.2%, 4.8%, 6.9%, 8.1%, and 11.5%.

In addition to analyzing the continuous variables of age

and left ventricular EF, both studies screened and tested numerous discrete risk factors; a discrete risk factor is either present or absent, it does not take on a value. The strength of a discrete risk factor is best compared by the odds ratio derived from multivariate analysis, which corrects for the influence of other variables. In the following paragraphs, numbers stated in parenthesis are the univariate (uncorrected) mortalities of patients with and without the risk factor, and are presented to put the odds ratio in perspective. Both studies found priority of operation (i.e., emergency operation) and cardiac reoperation to be the most powerful qualitative predictors of in-hospital mortality. In the NYS study, emergencies were subcategorized as structural defects causing shock, catheterization laboratory accidents, and angioplasty accidents. Emergencies causing cardiogenic shock such as postinfarction ventricular septal defect, ruptured papillary muscle, and gunshot wound were 6.36 times more likely to result in in-hospital mortality (45.2% versus 4.5%). Catheterization laboratory accidents requiring emergency surgery were 2.10 times more likely to cause death (18.6% versus 5.0%). Interestingly, percutaneous transluminal coronary angioplasty (PTCA) accidents requiring emergency surgery did not experience a significant increase in in-hospital mortality (6.3% versus 5.1%). Cardiac reoperation was 2.92 times more likely to result in death (25.6% for third time, 17.4% for second time, 10.9% for first time, versus 4.4% for no reoperation).

Dialysis dependence, despite a few studies suggesting little increase in risk for cardiac surgery, had a highly significant odds ratio of 2.80 in the NYS study (22.8% versus 5.0%). Intractable congestive heart failure (NYHA class IV), recent MI (less than 7 days old), and unstable angina (preoperative intravenous nitroglycerin requirement) were also correlated with mortality, with odds ratios of 1.80, 1.60, and 1.58, respectively (20.2% versus 4.3%; 13.2% versus 4.7%; 9.6% versus 4.4%). An MI greater than 7 days old was not found to be a risk factor of significance (4.7% versus 4.6%). Both studies found preoperative intra-aortic balloon pump (IABP) placement to be significant, increasing the associated risk by 1.45 times (21.2% versus 4.7%). No attempt was made to separate prophylactic from required IABP placement.

Previously unreported, both studies demonstrated an increased risk in patients with chronic obstructive pulmonary disease (COPD), with an odds ratio of 1.49 (8.8% versus 4.8%). Forced expiratory volume in 1 sec (FEV_1) less than 75% of predicted values or an absolute FEV_1 less than 1.25 was used as an inclusion criterion. Significant left main coronary stenosis was also a significant predictor in both studies, but NYS used greater than 90% for inclusion, whereas the VA study used greater than 50%. For NYS, the odds ratio was 1.35 (7.6% versus 4.9%). Diabetes requiring medication, female sex, and a history of hypertension were significant in the NYS study, with odds ratios of 1.52, 1.54, and 1.25, but were not significant in the VA study. A history of cerebrovascular disease or of peripheral vascular disease was significant in the VA study, with odds ratios of 1.8 and 1.9, but not studied in the NYS study. Neither study was able to demonstrate a significant association of morbid obesity and in-hospital mortality.

In summary, the strongest predictors of in-hospital mortality for cardiac surgical procedures are the type of procedure, left ventricular EF, patient age, emergency priority, reoperation, dialysis dependance, class IV congestive heart failure, MI within 7 days of operation, and unstable angina. Of significance was preoperative IABP placement, left main coronary stenosis, COPD, and cerebral or peripheral vascular disease. Of possible significance is diabetes, female sex, and hypertension.

Unfortunately, one cannot simply add or multiply the univariate risk of in-hospital mortality or the odds ratio for all the factors that pertain to a given patient; the logistic equation must be solved to obtain the answer. NYS has distributed a small computer program that will solve the logistic equation based on the 1989 data for the risk factors given above. Calculated from the equation or estimated from the univariate statistics, a risk factor analysis is the best starting point in assigning a given patient a risk of in-hospital mortality. But one must adjust this figure based on the surgeon's and the hospital's experience and an understanding of nature of the data and statistical tools used. For example, a 53-year-old woman with prosthetic valve endocarditis needs a mitral valve re-replacement. Her EF is 65% and she has severe COPD. The NYS logistic model predicts an in-hospital mortality of 5%, suggesting that operation is quite reasonable; despite the strong negative predictors of re-operation and COPD, the patient's young age and high EF seem to negate these influences. However, the model cannot account for the fact that the patient has been on home oxygen for 1 year, that her pulmonary functions are 25% of predicted (COPD as a discrete risk is coded with pulmonary function values below 75% of predicted) and that any operation would render this patient respirator dependent for the rest of her life. The NYS model would also predict a 24% in-hospital mortality for a 65-year-old man with unstable angina, left ventricular aneurysm, and an EF of 18%. One would question the efficacy of operation based on this mortality figure. However, basal segment contractility is excellent, angina has a positive influence on results of left ventricular aneurysm resection, and the residual aneurysm volume skews calculation of EF. This man's in-hospital mortality rate is more likely between 5% and 10%, and operation is quite reasonable. Obviously, statistical data are important and should serve as a starting point, but they cannot supplant the judgment of the surgeon.

MAKING DECISIONS

When utilizing an estimate of surgical risk in clinical decision-making, one must be aware of the variability of making such estimations. Statistically, the variability of a proportion or probability is measured by confidence limits, which define an upper and lower boundary for the estimate and the likelihood that the estimate will fall between these boundaries. For example, the in-hospital mortality rate for aortic valve replacement in NYS was 7.1% (80 deaths in 1121 procedures); the 95% confidence limits are 5.6% and 8.6%, which implies that there is only a 5% chance that the risk of in-hospital mortality would fall outside these boundaries if the operations were to be repeated under the same conditions. The confidence limits narrow if the level of certainty is decreased; 70% confidence limits (implying a 30% chance that the probability will fall outside of the boundaries) for aortic valve replacement are 6.3% to 7.9%. The confidence limits widen if the sample size (the number of operations) decreases; if 8 deaths occurred in 112 operations, the probability is still 7.1%, but the 95% confidence limits are 2.3% and 11.9%. When a surgeon estimates the in-hospital mortality for an individual, the level of certainty of the estimate will depend on how closely the patient approximates a large well-defined study population. An uncomplicated coronary bypass patient with no risk factors will very likely be subject to a 3.4% to 4.0% risk (95% confidence limits for the

3.7% coronary artery bypass graft mortality of NYS). However, if the patient requires a complex operation and has two or three defined or undefined risk factors, he presents a unique situation, and although the surgeon tells the patient the risk is 15%, the confidence limits for such judgmental estimates might imply a risk as low as 7% or as high as 20%. In such situations, stating a range of risk is perhaps more prudent than ascribing a single number.

Having defined an estimate of the in-hospital mortality for a given operation on a specific patient, one must decide whether to offer the surgery to the patient. This requires a comparison of the results of surgery (the inverse of the in-hospital mortality) to the outlook with alternative forms of therapy. Alternative therapy consists of medical management but may include PTCA with coronary disease patients or percutaneous valvuloplasty in selected valvular heart disease patients. Results of alternative therapy should reflect intermediate term (months to years) mortality (or inversely, survival) in keeping with the concept of surgical outlook. Ideally, data from large randomized trials such as the Coronary Artery Surgery Study are utilized and provide levels of significance through chi-square testing to different treatment results. However, very few randomized trials involve cardiac surgery, and more often information from an independent medical study is compared. If confidence intervals are available, a significant difference is usually implied if the 70% confidence limits of the two treatments do not overlap (a 70% confidence limit correlates with one standard deviation for a proportion). A more pragmatic guideline supporting operation is to have the in-hospital surgical mortality equal to or less than one-half the expected medical mortality.

The question of when to withhold operation because of high expected risk of mortality is a difficult one. One cannot follow the above guidelines oblivious to the wishes of the patient and the patient's family, or to considerations of age or functionality. Few surgeons will operate if the expected mortality rate is in excess of 50%, even if the medical alternative predicts certain death. Yet some circumstances, particularly in a younger patient, justify such a bold undertaking. And 50% as the upper limit of operability may be too high for an older patient with limited functionality to begin with. These issues defy mathematical analysis and require an assessment of the individual merits of each specific situation. They demand of the physicians involved the highest degree of professionalism as well as a realistic outlook regarding the goals of medical intervention.

The availability of risk factor analysis data like that in the NYS study has provided a basis for making legitimate comparisons between surgeons or between institutions. A given operative record can be analyzed and weighted to reflect the severity of disease present. The predicted mortality rate based on a logistic model such as that of NYS for each operation is calculated and then averaged. The actual mortality rate divided by the averaged predicted mortality rate and multiplied by the aggregate mortality rate of the model yields the risk adjusted mortality rate. If the actual mortality rate is higher than the predicted rate, the adjusted rate is assigned a number higher than the actual rate and conversely. For example, if a hospital had performed 247 operations with 13 deaths, the actual mortality rate is 5.26%; however, the predicted mortality rate for these patients averages 7.76%, giving a risk-adjusted mortality rate of 3.44%. This would imply that this particular hospital performed somewhat better than the average performance of hospitals upon which the model was based. Risk-adjusted mortality rates allow a fairer basis for comparison than crude mortality rates because they minimize the bias of institutional or surgical selection of patients.

SUGGESTED READING

Grover FL, Hammermeister KE, Burchfiel C, et al. Initial report of the veterans administration preoperative risk assessment study for cardiac surgery. *Ann of Thorac Surg* 1990; 50:12–28.

Hannan EL, Kilburn H, O'Donnel JF, Lukacik G, Shields EP. Adult open heart surgery in New York state—an analysis of risk factors and hospital mortality rates. *JAMA* 1990; 264:2768–2774.

Parsonnet V, Dean D, Bernstein AD. A method of uniform stratification of risk for evaluating the results of surgery in acquired heart disease. *Circulation* 1989; 79(Suppl. I), I-3:I-12.

Myocardial Preservation Techniques

Alan R. Hartman, M.D.

10

The average patient requiring surgical myocardial revascularization currently is different than he or she was 10 years ago. The depth of illness has increased, and the indications for referral to a surgeon have become more strict. The Coronary Artery Surgery Study (CASS) results have typically focused referrals to patients with triple vessel and left main coronary artery disease, especially those with compromised left ventricular function. Likewise, with the introduction of powerful calcium channel blockers and β-blockers, only those patients in whom these antianginal medications fail are referred to surgery. Thus, patients selected have severe disease and impaired myocardial function, often further depressed by antianginal medications with negative inotropic effects.

Hence, the value of myocardial preservation techniques has become the cornerstone of successful cardiac surgery. Important consideration must be given to every element of the myocardial preservation process, for not doing so can frequently spell the difference between survival and death.

There are many elements of myocardial preservation, and it is certainly not limited to the type or technique of cardioplegia used. We will discuss a coronary bypass operation from beginning to end with emphasis on each contribution to the overall myocardial preservation process.

PREOPERATIVE PERIOD

The time from the cardiac catheterization with the definition of the coronary anatomy to the induction at anesthesia will be called the preoperative period. Frequently, the patient is on the medical service, either in the coronary care unit or telemetry unit, depending on the severity of angina or the extent of coronary disease. Obviously, the major objective is surgical intervention prior to irreversible myocardial damage, but during the time that lapses between the catheterization and surgery there is ample opportunity for significant myocardial ischemia and damage.

When studying unstable angina patients, our catheterization laboratory has a low threshold for institution of intra-aortic balloon pump (IABP) counterpulsation. This will frequently be done prior to the coronary angiography. The two important elements of IABP counterpulsation are the augmentation of coronary flow during diastole by the displacement of blood with the helium-filled balloon and the lowering of myocardial wall tension and, therefore, myocardial oxygen requirements with the afterload reduction achieved by balloon deflation. Increasing myocardial oxygen delivery while simultaneously decreasing the oxygen demand will almost uniformly quiet unstable angina patients. This has the added benefit of stabilizing the preoperative period and allows for safe transfer to the operating room. The anesthetic induction will usually be better tolerated and will make crash initiation of cardiopulmonary bypass less likely. Finally, the presence of the IABP usually allows for a safer prebypass period, which allows for harvesting of the internal mammary artery (IMA) and better planning of the operative procedure with examination of the epicardial anatomy.

The liberal use of intravenous nitroglycerin, heparin, and antianxiety medications is advocated. If very high doses of nitroglycerin are required, then strong consideration for IABP should be given. Recent studies have demonstrated the value of heparin in preinfarction patients, making certain that therapeutic prolongation of the partial thromboplastin time is achieved. We frequently do not stop the heparin at all and keep the infusion going even at time of anesthetic induction, especially in critical or subtotal coronary stenosis. The value of benzodiazepines cannot be overly stressed. These patients by nature are frequently very nervous, and waiting in bed on their back with anxious family members hovering over them before the operation frequently precipitates anginal events. These patients need to be medicated with sedatives of sufficient quantity that will make them sleepy. Most of the time, nurses may undermedicate these patients. I insist on repeated dosing until the patients are clearly very comfortable. Using benzodiazepines of different classes or combined with morphine may be more effective than one alone.

The guiding principle is to limit the frequency and severity of myocardial ischemia as much as possible prior to the surgery so as not to precipitate acute injury at time of operation or to be forced into an emergency situation because of bad planning during the preoperative period.

ANESTHETIC PERIOD

This topic is covered extensively by my anesthetic colleagues elsewhere in this book; however, several points relate to myocardial preservation. All the coronary procedures are performed while the patient is monitored with thermodilution pulmonary arterial catheters. Early signs of ischemia are treated with intravenous nitroglycerin, or if this fails or hemodynamic instability ensues, IABP is instituted. Frequent cardiac outputs are calculated using the thermodilution technique. Caution is advised regarding potential spurious results if the wrong calibration factor or if the injectate temperature is not cold. We like to correlate the cardiac output with mixed venous oxygen determinations sampled from the pulmonary arterial port. Generally, a Po_2 above 35 mm Hg is considered acceptable while below 28 mm Hg is a very ominous sign.

Frequent communication with the anesthesiologist is imperative, especially when engrossed in IMA mobilization or saphenous vein harvest. Sudden deterioration in hemodynamics or acute onset of myocardial ischemia must be communicated to the surgeon, so that a change in the conduct of the operation can be instituted immediately. I usually inquire as to the electrocardiogram (ECG) and hemodynamics of the patient at 15-minute intervals. Finally, it is extremely important for the surgeon to have full view of the monitors during the entire procedure.

Most anesthetists use high-dose narcotics for anesthesia. This appears to be extremely safe, is beneficial for cardiac hemodynamics and myocardial oxygen consumption, and allows for early extubation of stable patients.

INTRAOPERATIVE PERIOD

Coronary bypass conduits

It is generally known that the IMA is the choice bypass graft, followed by saphenous vein. Early results using gastroepiploic artery seem encouraging, but long-term follow-up is not available. Lesser saphenous vein is used if greater saphenous is not usable, and cephalic vein from the upper extremities is the least desirable for autologous conduits. We use bilateral IMAs as frequently as possible and can usually complete three or sometimes four bypasses with these choice conduits. What may not always be appreciated by the cardiologist and internist is that in the setting of active and severe myocardial ischemia, pursuing IMA revascularization can be potentially dangerous, resulting in perioperative infarction or even death. There are three reasons for this. First, the harvesting of the IMA generally takes longer than saphenous vein harvest. For patients who are hemodynamically very unstable, early institution of cardiopulmonary bypass may be the only factor that terminates myocardial ischemia, and this should be done as quickly as possible while another surgeon harvests the saphenous vein. Secondly, since the most ischemic myocardial zones are also the ones that have critical coronary artery stenoses, these vessels need to be bypassed first so as to deliver protective cardioplegia and allow repletion of adenosine triphosphate stores. The IMA does not allow for this. Because it arises from a systemic vessel, the subclavian artery, cardioplegia cannot be delivered through this conduit. It is for this reason, that the IMA graft is anastomosed last to the coronary artery vessel. For ischemic myocardium that is in the distribution of severely stenosed or totally obstructed vessels, no cardioplegia may be delivered at all, resulting in continued ischemia and myocardial infarction (MI). Therefore careful consideration must be given to IMA grafting in the setting of severe ongoing myocardial ischemia. Saphenous vein revascularization in this subset of patients will lead to superior short-term results and perioperative survival, despite its limited long-term patency rates. Continued work with retrograde cardioplegia may obviate these concerns, but for very ischemic patients, a strong argument can still be made for saphenous vein bypass.

Cardiopulmonary bypass

The pump–oxygenator is required to technically manipulate the heart so as to perform the distal coronary artery anastomoses.

However, the heart-lung machine is also an extremely valuable tool in myocardial preservation through its regulation of body temperature, control of perfusion rates and perfusion pressure, and the venting of intracavity cardiac chambers. Briefly, the heart-lung machine is a series of roller pumps, reservoir bags, oxygenator, and heating/cooling unit interposed between a venous drainage point (usually the right atrium) and the arterial return (usually the ascending aorta). Cannulae are used to cannulate the right atrium, vena cavae, and ascending aorta, respectively. Tubing is usually added to allow for suctioning of blood from the field that can be returned to the patient after passing through filters.

Technologic advances in the oxygenating membranes have permitted longer pump runs while limiting the damage to the blood elements.

Temperature: Interposed between the venous return and the arterial input is the oxygenator and the heating/cooling coils. The temperature of the perfusate and blood can be lowered during the cooling phase of cardiopulmonary bypass to moderate levels of 30°C or 32°C or profoundly to 12°C. Coupled with ambient room temperature cooling and surface body cooling with water blankets, the body temperatures can be easily manipulated. The protection this affords the ischemic myocardium is multifold. The most obvious effect of lower tissue temperature is lowering the metabolic rate and therefore the oxygen requirements. This protects ischemic myocardium when the blood flow is reduced because of native disease or surgically induced by cross-clamping the aorta. The lower the temperature the lower the metabolic rate, the better tolerance toward ischemic situations. Additional protection from cooling is provided by topical pericardial hypothermia usually in the form of cold saline that is 4°C. The colder the blood temperature of the patient and the tissues and cavities surrounding the heart, the less likely the myocardium will rewarm, making ischemia more tolerable.

Perfusion pressure-perfusion flow rate: The other benefit of low body temperature is the ability to significantly reduce the perfusion flow and pressure. This prevents blood that courses through noncoronary collaterals and the bronchial arterial system from flooding the operative site and filling the cardiac chambers. By avoiding this, it makes for more precise surgical technique and prevents the washout of the protective cardioplegia solution. Noncoronary artery collaterals and bronchial arterial circulation can be extremely well developed in patients with chronic ischemic myocardial disease. The ability to reduce the perfusion flow rate and pressure as the body temperature is lowered adds considerably to the myocardial preservation technique.

Venting: The blood return to the pump oxygenator is not only from the right atrium and vena cavae, but also from vents which are catheters placed in cardiac chambers that return intracavity blood back to the pump reservoir. Vents can be placed in a number of cardiac structures, depending on the procedure and the surgeon's preference or philosophy. The more common locations are the main pulmonary artery, the aortic root, and the left ventricle, either indirectly through the left atrium traversing the mitral valve or directly through the apex of the heart. The effect of venting the heart has three distinct benefits. By suctioning blood that continuously accumulates, it keeps the operative site free of blood and allows for precise placement of sutures. Secondly, it prevents warm intracavity blood from bathing the endocardium which would have the adverse effect of raising the endocardial temperature, making it less tolerant to ischemia. Finally, intracavity venting of blood prevents the distention of the ventricle which can occur with the cardiac return of a large volume of blood from noncoronary collaterals, bronchial circulation, administered cardioplegia, and blood escaping the right venous cannulae. Ventricular distention will cause high intracavity pressures resulting in endocardial necrosis.

Cardiopulmonary bypass alone has salutory effects on ischemic myocardium by limiting the work the heart does to perfuse the body. Early institution of cardiopulmonary bypass in acute ischemic events coupled with severe hemodynamic instability is not only lifesaving but may also salvage ischemic myocardium. The weaning from cardiopulmonary bypass also is critical with regard to limiting myocardial necrosis. Generally, the patient needs to be fully warmed to 37°C, and enough time should elapse to allow the heart to replenish its myocardial oxygen debt. An additional requirement for weaning from bypass is a stable rhythm, either native or temporarily paced.

Cardioplegia

Chemically-induced diastolic arrest is the basis of cardioplegia. It is during this relaxed nonworking myocardial state that energy expenditure is the least and oxygen requirements minimal, hence ischemia best tolerated. The cardioplegic solution is cold thereby achieving the added benefit of myocardial hypothermia.

Many different types of cardioplegic solutions have been developed. Multiple pharmacologic additives have been tested, as well as the substrate of the solution. The substrate used today is either crystalloid or dilute blood. Potassium chloride in a concentration of 20-30 mEq/L is usually used as the primary agent inducing cardiac arrest. Other agents such as procainamide, calcium channel blockers, and vasodilators have been incorporated and have shown varying success.

Initial rapid induction of diastolic arrest and myocardial hypothermia is accomplished by injecting the cardioplegic solution into the root of the aorta, which has been segregated from the systemic circulation by a cross-clamp. We generally infuse 1000–1500 mL over several minutes. The cardioplegic solution is generally 4-6°C and we try to achieve myocardial temperatures of less than 12°C. Depending on the coronary artery pathology, myocardial temperature gradients may be present. Early bypassing of the responsible coronary vessel in this myocardial region is performed, with reinfusion of the cardioplegic solution down the bypass graft. This generally will ensure complete myocardial protection.

The frequency of readministration of the cardioplegic solution is also critical to good myocardial protection. Reinfusion at 15–20-minute intervals is performed to maintain low myocardial temperature, to replenish the high intracoronary potassium levels needed to maintain diastolic relaxation, and finally to wash out any accumulated toxic metabolic products.

Generally, cardioplegic solution is injected into the root of the aorta, delivering the solution to the coronary ostia, provided that there is no aortic insufficiency. In patients who have concomitant aortic valve insufficiency, an aortotomy needs to be performed to allow direct cannulation of both coronary ostia for the delivery of cardioplegic solution. Careful monitoring of injection pressures is crucial to ensure that intimal damage to the coronary vessels will not occur.

An alternative to antegrade cardioplegia through the aortic root or coronary ostia is retrograde cardioplegia that is infused through the coronary sinus. The theoretical advantage of this technique is the ability to deliver cardioplegia to myocardium that is in the distribution of severe obstructive coronary lesions. It also is valuable when the IMA is used, so that cardioplegia can be given to this region of myocardium despite not being able to give it through the graft. The full spectrum of this technique is yet to be proven.

As previously mentioned, control over systemic flow from the pump-oxygenator is critical in preventing myocardial rewarming and cardioplegia washout from noncoronary collateral flow. When systemic hypothermia is used to below 30°C, then flow rates can be reduced by half, resulting in less return to the heart from the noncoronary collaterals and bronchial artery systems.

Although preservation techniques for cardiac surgery have advanced considerably, a carefully planned and efficiently executed operation is of prime importance. Myocardial damage progresses as the ischemia time is prolonged, and no preservation technique will compensate for this. Additionally, the avoidance of ventricular fibrillation during the procedure is generally protective. The high energy expenditure associated with ventricular fibrillation can significantly deplete myocardial energy reserves even in the cold empty heart. Finally, it is commonly acknowledged that subendocardial blood flow is diverted during ventricular fibrillation, which could lead to endocardial ischemia or necrosis.

SUGGESTED READING

Axelrod HI, Murphy MS, Galloway AC, et al. Percutaneous cardiopulmonary bypass limits myocardial injury from ischemic fibrillation and reperfusion. *Circulation*. 1988; 78: (suppl V): III 148–152.

Cheung EH, Arcidi JM, Jackson ER, et al. Intracavitary right heart cooling during coronary bypass surgery: A prospective randomized trial. *Circulation*. 1988; 78: (suppl V): III 173–179.

Kirklin JW, Barratt-Boyes BG. Cardiac Surgery. New York: John Wiley; 1986, 29–108.

Koshal A, Bearlards DS, Ross AD, et al. Urgent surgical

reperfusion in adult evolving myocardial infarction: A randomized controlled study. *Circulation.* 1988; 78: (suppl III): I-171–I-178.

Sabiston DC, Spencer FC. Surgery of the chest 5th ed. Philadelphia: Saunders; 1990; 1107–1125.

Aortocoronary Bypass

Alan R. Hartman, M.D.

11

The surgical procedure most commonly performed by most cardiac surgeons is coronary artery bypass grafting (CABG). Since first introduced, its successful outcome has been improved due to advances in myocardial preservation (see Chapter 10) and as a result of accumulated experience regarding choice of conduit, graft design, and other technical features. Although a standardized technique, the decision-making elements of aortocoronary bypass grafting are still complex and can influence morbidity and mortality rates of the operation. Similarly, graft patency can be influenced by subtle technical detail and by pharmacologic intervention. Once the patient is out of the operating room, continued vigilance for immediate and late postoperative problems is the priority of the cardiac surgeon, frequently in consultation with medical colleagues. Despite a complex procedure with numerous steps and potential for disaster, the vast majority of aortocornary bypass operations can be executed trouble-free with excellent outcomes.

CHOICE OF APPROACH AND TECHNIQUE
The internal mammary artery

All CABG procedures are approached through a midline sternotomy incision. As mentioned in Chapter 10, the hemodynamic stability of the patient at time of surgery may dictate the choice of bypass conduit. Excluding these unstable emergency situations, the internal mammary artery (IMA) is the prime bypass conduit. The IMAs ordinarily run parallel to the sternum and may be sacrificed as a blood supply to that location and used to serve as a source of blood to the myocardium. The IMA is a branch of the subclavian artery (the latter artery is the way it is approached angiographically). Due to its intimate relationship with the chest wall, mobilizing the artery is time consuming, adding 30 to 45 minutes to the operative procedure. All branches connecting to the chest wall must be carefully ligated to avoid bleeding. In the unstable patient where time is of the essence, saphenous vein may need to be used instead. Additionally, IMA utilization may be avoided in patients who are obese, diabetic, and elderly for fear of wound complications, although in our experience this has not been borne out. More compelling objections for not using the IMA are for patients who are hemodynamically unstable, with multisystem organ failure, and in chronic steroid use.

Patency rates for the IMA have been excellent with 10-year follow-up demonstrating 90% to 95% to be open. The reasons for this success have not been clearly delineated, but there are many hypotheses. The caliber of the IMA closely approximates that of the coronary vessels. Most of the time the IMA is used as a living pedicled flap, containing not only the artery, but also its venous drainage and lymphatic vessels, based on muscle and fascia. This is distinctly different from the explanted collagen tube that saphenous vein represents. However, early results relating to use of the IMA as a free graft seem to demonstrate early patency rates equivalent to the pedicled grafts. Study of the IMA has identified various factors which may contribute to superior patency rates. This artery is almost uniformly spared of atherosclerosis even when attached to the heart. Endothelial relaxing factor has recently been identified in these arteries, and this may prevent platelet deposition, an important etiology in graft closure.

Excluding the previously discussed circumstances, the IMA should be used whenever possible. Not only are the patency rates superior to vein, but long-term survival and event-free intervals have been increased when the IMA has been used to bypass at least one coronary artery. Many of the previous concerns over the use of the IMA have not been substantiated, such as age, infection in diabetics, or in chronic obstructive lung disease. Furthermore, the postoperative sternal pain does not appear to be significantly greater, either. Most patients will have anterior chest wall paresthesias related to the IMA harvest, but this disappears with time.

The trend has been toward the increased use of both IMAs. The left IMA is frequently reserved for the left anterior descending artery, diagonal, or an obtuse marginal. The right IMA can be used for the right coronary artery, left anterior descending artery, obtuse marginal, or the posterior descending artery. When using the right IMA to bypass an obtuse marginal, the graft is brought through the transverse sinus behind the aorta and pulmonary artery. When using the right IMA to bypass the posterior descending artery, extra length needs to be gained, and this is done by mobilizing the distal IMA as it becomes the superior epigastric artery in the rectus sheath. Additional length can be gained by splitting the mammary pedicle endothoracic fascia transversely in several locations.

At the present time, sequential anastomotic technique does not appear to improve patency rates over single graft to coronary anastomoses. However, the sequential anastomotic technique allows an increased number of coronaries to be bypassed with the IMA, which may be a distinct advantage.

Many of the patients coming for CABG surgery these days are those who have had previous saphenous vein grafts that have failed. Redo surgery has prompted the more liberal use of bilateral IMA grafting, as well as the search for other arterial conduits that share similarities with the IMA.

Using both left and right IMA and doing sequential anastomotic technique, between two and four coronary vessels can be bypassed with the IMAs alone. In our center we have not experienced any of the theoretical untoward effects of bilateral IMA usage, such as sternal devascularization or increased sternal wound infections.

Long-term patency rates of the IMAs have averaged 95% at 10–12 years. When problems develop with the IMA, it is usually as a result of an initial problem with the anastomotic site (possibly related to a misplaced suture) and usually is detected early when the patient complains of recurrent angina and ischemia is documented. Often this problem can be corrected with angioplasty. Neointimal hyperplasia at the site of anastomosis is a persistent problem and is probably best treated by the use of perioperative antiplatlet drugs (i.e., aspirin and dipyridamole).

Alternate Arterial Conduits

The *right gastroepiploic artery* is a terminal branch of the gastroduodenal artery from the common hepatic artery and runs toward the left on the greater curvature of the stomach. This vessel has recently been used with regular frequency for CABG. It appears to have many similarities to the IMA, although it is a little smaller in diameter. Short-term follow-up for less than 2 years has been excellent.

The *lateral costal artery* is a branch of the IMA which courses along the midaxillary aspect of the chest wall. Its incidence is reported to be 27% in cadaver series. We recently described the use of the lateral costal artery for bypass purposes, using it for direct myocardial revascularization as an alternative to saphenous vein. This anomalous vessel can be as large as the IMA and is harvested in the same fashion, as a pedicled graft.

The cardiovascular surgeon now has in his armamentarium a large number of arterial conduits to choose from, and soon we may see the day when veinless bypass surgery will be routine.

The saphenous vein graft

Location of vein: In cardiovascular surgery today, the greater saphenous vein as an aortocoronary bypass conduit is still being used very frequently, usually in conjunction with the IMA. The vein is harvested from the leg, ligating all branches, reversed in direction, and perfused with physiologic heparinized solution. The vein courses from anterior to the medial malleolus and runs the entire length of the leg draining into the femoral vein at the groin. Because of the presence of valves, reversing the vein is imperative to ensure reliable flow of blood. When examining the vein, one is ascertaining its patency, wall thickness, distensability, and overall diameter. All vein is not created equal, and there are definite priorities as to where to harvest. Preoperative examination of the saphenous vein by the operating surgeon is crucial and when at all possible the patient should be standing. Of course, excluding the presence of saphenous vein varicosities or previous vein stripping is mandatory. If the greater saphenous vein does not appear usable, or has been previously harvested, examination of the lesser saphenous vein on the back of the calf is critical.

If one were to grade vein as to its quality and long-term patency rates, greater saphenous vein (longest in body) would lead the list, followed by lesser saphenous vein, and a distant third would be arm vein or cephalic vein. Cephalic vein has had very disappointing short- and long-term results and should be used only in extenuating circumstances.

When using the greater saphenous vein, some debate remains as to whether the thigh or below-the-knee segment is of better quality. Generally, the thigh vein will be of larger diameter and thinner wall compared to the calf vein. If one is overly concerned about the disproportionate size of the vein compared to the coronary arteries, then staying below the knee is worthwhile. Additionally, in a young patient, where you may anticipate the need to redo CABG surgery in the future, using the below-the-knee segment will preserve the thigh vein for later use.

Harvesting the vein: The harvesting of the vein is a critical aspect of the coronary operation and should *not* be left to the least experienced member of the operating team. Exact attention needs to be given to the ligation of branches and careful distention of the vein to prevent endothelial necrosis. We prefer not to have the vein harvested too far in advance of its implantation, so as to prevent hypoxic injury to the endothelium. There has been debate as to whether the vein distention fluid should be blood versus crystalloid, but this is probably less important than the pressure of injection, which should not be greater than normal systemic blood pressure. The lengths of the vein segments are generally measured on cardiopulmonary bypass, but keep in mind that additional length is needed when the heart is full of blood.

Patency rates: Although 5-year patency rates for saphenous vein have been in the 60% to 70% range, in certain circumstances its usage is preferable and safer than IMA usage. One of those circumstances is the rare instance of a catastrophic event in the cardiac catheterization laboratory or a patient in extremis and cardiogenic shock, where cardiopulmonary bypass has to be instituted immediately and CABG performed quickly. It is at these times that the quickly harvested saphenous vein is superior to the more tedious and slower mobilization of the IMA. The additional advantage that needs to be reemphasized is the ability of the saphenous vein to deliver cardioplegia and blood to an ischemic area of myocardium immediately after the anastomosis is constructed. This is not possible with the IMA when it remains attached to the subclavian artery and continues drawing its blood from the systemic circulation. Retrograde cardioplegia may circumvent this problem, but is still being studied for its efficacy with regard to this problem.

When CABG is performed in conjunction with valve replacement, repair, or ventricular aneurysmectomy, saphenous vein is the choice conduit. The reasons again relate to adequate myocardial preservation and the ability to deliver cardioplegia to the myocardium distal to coronary stenoses, ensuring adequate cooling and diastolic arrest of the jeopardized myocardium. The coronary bypasses are always performed prior to the secondary procedure, again to ensure adequate myocardial preservation. Retrograde cardioplegia holds promise in circumventing this problem, potentially allowing for the use of the IMA in these complex operations.

Endarterectomy

Coronary bypass is frequently performed in patients with distal coronary artery disease, especially in diabetics. This often necessitates the addition of a localized endarterectomy at the site of anastomosis or more extensive endarterectomies of both the proximal and distal coronary vessels. Endarterectomy of an artery refers to the coring of the intima and associated atherosclerotic plaque. The length is variable and may be localized or extensive. What remains is a portion of the media and adventitia. The bypass graft is then anastomosed to the arteriotomy that was created for performing the endarterectomy. The role, safety, and efficacy of endarterectomy have been debated, and are still not entirely clear. Endarterectomy of the right coronary artery and its distal branches has been studied the most, and this appears to be reasonably effective. Some have argued that patency rates are lower and perioperative infarction rates higher in those endarterectomized coronaries. However, many of these vessels would not be bypassable unless endarterectomy was performed. Extensive endarterectomy of the left anterior descending and circumflex vessels has been championed by Dudley Johnson, with reportedly excellent results. Again, many of these patients would not be bypassable without the adjuvant use of endarterectomy.

Graft flow

Graft flow measurements in the operating room are done in several ways. For the IMA, we always measure free flow after the papaverine injection. Generally, flows of 180–300 mL/min are the norm. Flows less than 100 mL/min are redilated with papaverine. If the flow remains low, it is worthwhile to disconnect the IMA from the subclavian artery and use it as a free graft. In this regard, it is always imperative to measure the blood pressure in both arms to exclude a pressure gradient. Gradients greater than 30 mm Hg should arouse suspicion for subclavian artery stenosis which may very well effect flow in the IMA on that side.

Vein graft flow is generally measured after weaning from cardiopulmonary bypass. Flow velocity is measured using either an electromagnetic flow meter or a Doppler. Doppler technique tends to be more accurate and reproducible, although it is more expensive. Reasons for documenting graft flow are several. It is used to assess the adequacy of a graft and may be of predictive value of graft patency. If graft flow is lower than the surgeon anticipated, then searching for a technical problem at the time of surgery may be helpful. Finally, excluding technical problems, pharmacologic manipulation may have a salient effect on graft flow in terms of reversing spasm or dilating the distal coronary capillary bed.

Graft patency

Pharmacologic intervention: While the surgeon may have successfully revascularized the blocked coronary arteries, it is now up to the patient and the referring physician to assist in maintaining their patency. Cessation of smoking, proper diet, and monitored exercise are critically important. Additionally, protection against thrombosis and neointimal hyperplasia through the use of antiplatlet medications is imperative. Finally, modifications of the atherosclerotic process through cholesterol- and lipid-lowering drugs may be indicated. Chesebro demonstrated increased short-term patency rates of bypass grafts when dipyridamole was started preoperatively and aspirin was initiated in the recovery room immediately postoperatively. Aspirin and dipyridamole are then continued indefinitely after discharge. Close follow-up of serum cholesterol, triglycerides, and low density lipoprotein levels seems to be important with regard to ongoing atherosclerosis and its involvement of newly created bypass grafts. If these lipid levels stay elevated despite diet modifications, then strong consideration needs to be given to adjuvant drug therapy. Current recommendations for desirable lipid levels may not be strict enough for patients having undergone CABG.

POSTOPERATIVE CONSIDERATIONS AND COMPLICATIONS

Despite the increasing complexity of the patients referred for surgery, CABG is still considered a low mortality operation. Obviously, subgroups of patients stratify to high-risk groups and this includes octogenarians, ejection fractions less than 30%, and multisystem organ failure preoperatively.

New York State has looked at crude mortality rates and has attempted to standardize mortality according to risk stratifications. The present average mortality rate for the 30 hospital centers doing more than 16,000 open heart procedures is 5% with that for CABG alone being 3.7%. Morbidity rates are yet to be calculated but generally also vary directly with risk stratification. Most common morbidity events include minor pulmonary problems, atrial arrhythmias, and vein harvest site seromas, hematomas, and cellulitis. Less frequent but more serious problems include acute tubular necrosis, sternal infections, strokes, perioperative myocardial infarctions, and malignant ventricular arrhythmias.

The length of hospital stay is directly related to postoperative problems but generally is anywhere from 6 to 10 days; elderly patients will need 2 weeks while receiving physical therapy. Patients with postoperative complications stay in hospital and on the surgical service until the problem is resolved.

Intra- and postoperative complications

Inability to wean from cardiopulmonary bypass: Inotropic support in conjunction with intraortic balloon pump (IABP) counterpulsation is usually successful for weaning from pump. We generally use dobutamine and intravenous nitroglycerin as the first-line drugs. Epinephrine and Inocor are added in succession if indicated. Use of the IABP is considered anytime high-dose or multidose pharmacologic support is needed for weaning from bypass. If both these measures prove inadequate for support, then use of a left ventricular assist device is the next level of support. Any institution that does heart surgery has at its disposal a left ventricular assist device, by simply using a roller pump interposed between the left atrium and the femoral artery or aorta.

Arrhythmias: The most common postoperative arrhythmias are atrial arrhythmias, usually atrial premature beats, atrial flutter, atrial fibrillation, and paroxysmal atrial tachycardia. Several prophylactic maneuvers will limit these problems, including close observation of the serum potassium level, especially in the immediate postoperative period where postpump diuresis can be significant. Additionally, the early reinstitution of β-blockers in patients on these drugs preoperatively will prevent a rebound phenomenon. If atrial arrhythmias do occur despite the above measures, then rapid digitalization for rate control and the adjunct use of intravenous β-blockers or certain calcium channel blockers is used to achieve a reasonable ventricular rate. Finally if the arrhythmias persist we start intravenous procainamide, which is one of the highly effective drugs for atrial arrhythmias that can be given intravenously, important in the anesthetized patient.

Ventricular arrhythmias are generally treated with lidocaine or procainamide if coexisting atrial arrhythmias are present.

Postoperative bleeding: Reexploration for bleeding has remained remarkably infrequent despite the fact that more of our patients are on aspirin preoperatively or may have recently received thrombolytic therapy. Indications for reexploration may vary slightly from center to center but generally any bleeding that causes hemodynamic compromise or cardiac tamponade needs immediate exploration. Any sudden increase in hemorrhage in a patient who previously had insignificant bleeding is reason for immediate attention and early reexploration. Finally, any hourly output that persists at 200–300 mL/h for over 5-6 hours most probably deserves reexploration.

Infection: Most common infections include minor ones either related to the urinary tract or vein harvest site. More significant problems include pneumonias, bacteremias, and intra-abdominal processes. The most significant wound problems are sternal infections, which occur in 1% to 3% of cases, with elderly diabetic females thought to be at greatest risk. Once identified, these wound infections need immediate operative debridement and are usually closed primarily over antibiotic irrigation catheters. This type of treatment has a better than

90% success rate with failures treated with redebridement and rotation of myocutaneous flaps.

Pericarditis: This is a frequent finding and may or may not pose a significant problem. It seems that use of the IMA may contribute to an increased incidence of pleuropericarditis. Most frequent findings are friction rubs, pleuritic chest pain on inspiration, and the occurrence of pleural effusions consisting of transudates. Observation and expectant treatment is usually all that is necessary; however, some patients require nonsteroidal anti-inflammatory agents such as ibuprofen or indomethacin. Only a rare patient will require a pulse of steroids with a rapid taper of 10–14 days.

Renal failure: Acute tubular necrosis still occurs with regular frequency and seems to be more common in patients with preexisting renal dysfunction. Also patients with multiple arterial atherosclerosis tend to have occult renal artery stenosis making them susceptible to alterations in renal perfusion on the heart-lung machine. In general, acute tubular necrosis occurring as an isolated phenomenon in the face of an adequate cardiac output will be self-limited and of no long-term consequence. This is in contradistinction to renal failure occurring in association with low cardiac output and multisystem organ failure.

SUGGESTED READING

Adult Cardiac Surgery in New York State in 1989. An analysis of risk factors and hospital mortality rates. New York State Department of Health. (Unpublished data).

Foster ED, Kronc AT. Alternative conduit for aortocoronary bypass grafting. *Circulation.* 1989; 79(suppl I):I-34–I-39.

Foster V, Chesebro JH. Aortocoronary artery vein graft disease. Experimental and clinical approach for the understanding of the role of platelets and platelet inhibitors. *Circulation.* 1985; 72(suppl V):V-65–V-70.

Grandin CM, Campeau L, Thornton JC, Engle JC, Cross FS, Schreiber H. Coronary artery bypass grafting with saphenous vein. *Circulation.* 1986; 79(suppl I):I-24–I-29.

Green G. Use of internal thoracic artery for coronary artery grafting. *Circulation.* 1989; 79(suppl I):I-30–I-33.

Hartman AR, Mawulwade K, Dervan JC, Anagnostopoulos CE. Myocardial revascularization with the lateral costal artery. *Ann Thorac Surg.* 1990; 49:816–818.

Kirklin JW, Barratt-Boyes BG. Cardiac Surgery. New York: John Wiley & Sons; 1986.

Loop FD, Lytle BW, Cosgrove DM, et al. Influence on the internal mammary artery graft on 10 year survival and other cardiac events. *N Engl J Med.* 1986; 314:1–6.

Loop FD, Lytle BW, Cosgrove DSM, Golding LA, Taylor PC, Stewart RW. Five (aorta-coronary) internal mammary artery grafts. *J Thorac Cardiovasc Surg.* 1986; 92:227–831.

Lytle BW, Loop FD, Cosgrove DM, Easley K, Taylor PC. Long term (5 to 12 years) serial studies of internal mammary artery and saphenous vein coronary bypass grafts. *J Thorac Cardiovasc Surg.* 1985; 89:248–258.

Lytle BW, Loop FD, Thurer RL, Goves LK, Taylor PC, Cosgrove DM. Isolated left anterior descending coronary atherosclerosis. Long term comparison of internal mammary artery and venous autograph. *Circulation.* 1980; 61:869–874.

Parsonnet V, Dean D, Bernstein AD. A method of uniform stratification of risk for evaluating the results of surgery in acquired adult heart disease. *Circulation.* 1986; 79(suppl I):I-3–I-10.

Pym J, Brown PN, Chenrette EJP, Parker JO, West RO. Gastroepiploic coronary anastomoses—A viable alternative bypass graft. *J Thorac Cardiovasc Surg.* 1987; 94:256–299.

Sabiston DC, Spencer FC. Gibbons Surgery of the Chest. Philadelphia: WB Saunders; 1983.

Tector AJ, Schmahl TM. Techniques for multiple internal mammary artery grafts. *Ann Thorac Surg.* 1984; 38:281–286.

Valvular Heart Surgery

Frank Seifert M.D.

12

With a decline in the incidence of rheumatic fever and syphilis during the first half of this century, it was hoped that the incidence of valvular heart disease requiring surgical intervention would decrease. This has not been the case. There has been an increase in the frequency or at least in the recognition of degenerative valve disease. Bacterial endocarditis has persisted as a significant source of valve-related morbidity despite advances in antibiotic therapy. Intravenous drug abuse and the ready access to the vascular space afforded modern medical practice has worsened this morbidity. In selected areas of this country and in third world nations, the consequences of chronic rheumatic valvular disease are still seen. Lastly, a population of patients treated during the past three decades with valve replacement have proven that the ideal prosthetic heart valve has yet to be created, and these patients may require a second or even third surgical intervention as valve-related complications occur. It will remain important for physicians to be conversant with the surgical management of patients with valvular heart disease for a number of decades to come.

PATHOLOGY

Acquired valvular pathology is traditionally classified according to whether the process results in stenosis of the effective valve orifice or to whether regurgitation is present. This is somewhat artificial, as many pathologic processes result in some degree of both lesions. Clinically manifesting itself 10–40 years after an episode of rheumatic fever, chronic rheumatic valvulitis can produce both lesions and can afflict the mitral, aortic, and tricuspid valve in descending order of frequency. It is the only process which can produce leaflet fusion at the commissures, and therefore the only important cause of mitral and tricuspid stenosis. Fibrosis, thickening, and contracture of leaflets can lead to loss of coaptation and regurgitation. With mitral valve involvement, chordae tendineae can thicken, fuse, contract, or rupture. Calcification can amplify the severity of any of these lesions. Although the incidence of rheumatic fever has decreased dramatically, the consequences of chronic rheumatic valvulitis is still seen with some frequency. Only 50% of the patients presenting with significant rheumatic valvular disease have a positive history of rheumatic fever.

In contradistinction to rheumatic disease, valvular damage as a complication of infective endocarditis usually produces regurgitant lesions. Only in rare situations, as with hemophilus parainfluenza or fungus, can bulky vegetations simulate mitral stenosis. Leaflet perforation, disruption of leaflet insertion, mechanical interference with coaptation, or rupture of the papillary muscle apparatus can occur. The predilection of endocarditis is for the aortic, mitral, tricuspid, and pulmonary valve in descending order, though intravenous drug users have an inordinately high incidence of tricuspid valve involvement. In advanced cases, endocarditis can form subannular abscess cavities that further distort valvular competence and may even perforate the ventricle. Preexisting valvular abnormalities enhance the likelihood of endocarditis, and a dental procedure is all too frequently associated with the initiation of infection.

Calcific aortic stenosis, or Mönckeberg's aortosclerosis, is one of the most common forms of degenerative aortic valve disease. It characteristically presents in the sixth and seventh decades, and the cause is unknown. It is not related to atherosclerosis, as Mönckeberg thought. Unlike rheumatic aortic stenosis, where actual fusion of the commissures occurs, calcification and fibrosis of the leaflet and annulus restrict valve motion. The leaflets may be greater than 1 cm thick and calcification can extend into the annulus, the ventricular septum, or on the anterior leaflet of the mitral valve. Bicuspid aortic valves, occurring in 3% of the population, may undergo a degenerative process of thickening and calcification that also leads to aortic stenosis. The process is distinct from calcific aortic stenosis and appears to be secondary to hemodynamic stress. Less frequently, the same process in a bicuspid valve results in aortic regurgitation. Stretching of aortic leaflets secondary to annular dilatation is a more frequent cause of aortic regurgitation and is usually associated with hypertension.

Degenerative causes of mitral regurgitation include a wide spectrum of pathologic changes, inclusively referred to as myxomatous changes. Portions of a leaflet may thicken or become redundant. Chordae tendineae can elongate or rupture. Prolapse of a whole leaflet or a portion of a leaflet may result. Annular dilatation may be symmetrical or asymmetrical. When regurgitation is predominantly caused by anterior leaflet prolapse, it may represent the end stage of the mitral valve prolapse syndrome, also known as Barlow's syndrome, which can be identified in benign stages in over 1% of the population. Senile mitral annular calcification, by distorting the flexible geometry of the valve, can also result in significant mitral regurgitation.

Processes remote to the heart valves can lead to significant regurgitant pathology. Atherosclerotic coronary artery disease can cause significant mitral regurgitation. Ventricular dilatation can enlarge the mitral annulus. Papillary muscle and posterolateral wall ischemia or infarction can further exacerbate incompetence. Rupture of a papillary muscle or one of its heads is a particularly fulminant presentation of mitral regurgitation. Retrograde dissection of the ascending aorta can lead to disruption of commissural support and acute aortic regurgitation.

PHYSIOLOGY

As with valvular pathology, it is convenient to categorize the myocardial adaptation to such pathology as a result of either stenotic lesions or of regurgitant lesions. Cardiac chambers can dilate as a compensatory response to volume overload. This enhances contractility by changing the Starling relation of the myofibrils, and is seen as the most prominent feature of regurgitant pathology. Pressure overload allows for myocardial hypertrophy, increasing the numbers of sarcomeres per myofibril, and this is the predominant feature of stenotic valvular lesions. Unfortunately, neither mechanism protects the myocardium long term. If the pathologic stress is unabated, the dilated chamber fails as myofibrils become overstretched, and the hypertrophied chamber fails as a consequence of diminished cellular nutrition. This is, of course, an oversimplification. Some hypertrophy does occur in response to regurgitation, and some chamber dilatation develops in response to stenosis.

Aortic stenosis, insidious in onset and marked by left ventricular hypertrophy, first manifests itself as forward failure. Syncope, angina, and a general decrease in the patient's activities all are secondary to decreased cardiac output. As the ventricle thickens further, decompensation in the face of chronic pressure overload occurs, the end-diastolic pressure rises, and backward failure is manifest as pulmonary edema. If the patient does not succumb to myocardial infarction (MI) or arrhythmia precipitated by the disproportion between coronary flow and myocyte demand, marked elevation of left ventricular diastolic pressures occurs and dilatation is manifest. This stage has been termed the cardiomyopathy of overload and is the terminal decompensation of a hypertrophied myocardium. Depending on how long the patient survives at this stage, chronic pulmonary hypertension and right ventricular dilatation may develop. Backward failure may be exacerbated by atrioventricular (AV) value incompetence secondary to ventricular dilatation. Sudden death is all too often a consequence of this tenuous balance of compensatory mechanisms.

Mitral stenosis, in contrast, manifests backward failure from the outset, increasing left atrial size and transmitting increased pressure to the pulmonary capillary bed. Atrial fibrillation and the risk of systemic embolization occur early, but cardiac output is maintained. As the pressure in the left atrium and pulmonary capillaries increases, pulmonary edema ensues. Patients become susceptible to recurrent pulmonary infections and to hemoptysis, which can be life-threatening. Chronically, right ventricular overload and dilatation result in tricuspid regurgitation. Peripheral edema, ascites, and anasarca are the sequelae. Forward failure occurs late, as a consequence of right ventricular decompensation, which cannot supply adequate filling pressure to the otherwise normally functioning left ventricle. Ventricular arrhythmias and sudden death may occur.

Unlike the pressure overload of stenotic valvular lesions, regurgitant lesions of both the aortic and mitral valve impose a volume overload on the left ventricle. To compensate for forward failure caused by loss of the regurgitant volume, the left ventricle must increase its stroke volume. A moderate degree of myocyte hypertrophy suffices initially to supply this increased volume and the condition may be tolerated for many years with only mild symptoms of exercise intolerance. With decompensation, dilatation begins, end-diastolic pressure increases, and ejection fraction (EF) falls. Forward and backward failure develop concurrently and pulmonary edema is experienced. Chronicity leads to right ventricular overload and with decompensation to the signs of right ventricular failure seen with stenotic lesions. Aortic regurgitation has one important additional component not seen in mitral regurgitation. The incompetent aortic valve lowers aortic diastolic pressure, and coronary artery perfusion is predominately a function of this pressure. As with aortic stenosis, aortic regurgitation can cause angina and MI.

INDICATIONS FOR SURGICAL INTERVENTION

The general goals of surgical intervention for valvular heart disease are to arrest myocardial deterioration, to alter hemodynamics in such a way that myocardial recovery is maximized, and to augment the event-free survival of the patient. In most instances valve replacement will arrest further myocardial deterioration regardless of the stage of the disease. However, to gain functional improvement, replacement must be appropriately timed. Despite numerous invasive and noninvasive parameters to guide this decision, judgment must be exercised on an individual patient basis. Too early an intervention substitutes prosthetic valve or anticoagulant morbidity for the morbidity of the disease. As a general rule, most patients should be symptomatic, usually with mild congestive failure and grade II symptoms. Modern prosthetic valves, though far from perfect, have achieved a level of reliability that no longer justifies waiting for established failure and significant (i.e., grade III) functional deterioration. Marked decrease in EF is the only absolute contraindication to valve replacement because it is the strongest predictor of perioperative death. So-called fixed pulmonary hypertension with systemic pulmonary artery pressures is not a contraindication provided there is a reasonable expectation of improving left ventricular function; pulmonary hypertension does, however, imply increased operative risk, greater likelihood of postoperative morbidity and prolonged hospital stay.

Symptomatic aortic stenosis is an absolute indication for valve replacement, because life expectancy after the development of symptoms is severely limited. The life expectancy after the development of failure, angina, and syncope has repeatedly been demonstrated to be no greater than 2, 3, and 5 years, respectively. These patients generally have a valve area less than 1 cm^2 and a mean aortic gradient of greater than 50 mm Hg. Although some investigators have questioned the need for valve replacement in the asymptomatic patient who meets these hemodynamic criteria, the small but real incidence of sudden arrhythmic death mitigates this conservatism. The timing of valve replacement for chronic aortic regurgitation is more difficult because moderate regurgitation (2-3+) is tolerated well for years, and the transition to severe regurgitation, with an attendant increase in operative mortality and decrease in functional recovery, is often insidious. Symptomatic patients with failure or angina should undergo valve replacement. Asymptomatic patients should be followed at regular intervals (e.g., every 6 months) with echocardiography. An increase in left ventricular end–systolic diameter above 5.5 cm or a decrease in fractional shortening warrants catheterization, and decrease in EF or elevation of end–diastolic pressure mandates valve replacement. The role of measuring change in left ventricular EF with exercise as a determinant of the need for valve replacement probably requires further study before adoption as a standard. Severe depression of EF below 30% is the major contraindication to aortic valve replacement for both lesions. A few aortic stenosis patients with EF values in the 20s are still surgical candidates, particulary if improvement can be demonstrated after percutaneous valvuloplasty, thus ruling out cardiomyopathic dysfunction.

Symptomatic heart failure remains the primary indication for mitral valve replacement. A gradient greater than 8–10 mm Hg and a valve area of less than 1 cm^2 correlate with this level in mitral stenosis. Patients who do not meet these hemodynamic criteria at rest and still have significant symptoms will often demonstrate a significant gradient if exercised during the catheterization. Most patients will be in or have experienced atrial fibrillation. Characteristically, EF is preserved in predominant mitral stenosis, even in the presence of systemic pulmonary artery pressures. Mitral commissurotomy as an alternative to valve replacement is a consideration in the younger patient without evident calcification, and probably should be considered earlier in the course of the disease when symptoms are only grade II. Mitral regurgitation, like aortic regurgitation, is more difficult to assess with regard to the timing of surgery. Patients tolerate mild to moderate regurgitation for years, but unlike the aortic regurgitation patient, mitral regurgitation patients should have an initial increase in EF. Subsequent decline in this parameter below 50% with 3–4+ regurgitation should prompt repair or replacement, particularly if associated with an elevated left ventricular end-diastolic pressure. Decline in EF below 40% signifies a marked increase in surgical risk and limitation of functional recovery, and an EF below 30% is considered a contraindication to surgery. This lower limit of operability is a recognition of two factors. First, ventricular adaptation to chronic mitral regurgitation involves an afterload mismatch that is eliminated by restoration of competency. In response to the increased afterload, the compromised ventricle decreases its EF further. Secondly, traditional mitral valve replacement requires severance of the chordae tendineae, and the loss of ventriculochordal continuity will further decrease the EF by 10% to 15%. The evolution of techniques to preserve the chordae tendineae and the development of mitral reparative techniques have challenged this lower limit of operability.

PROSTHETIC HEART VALVES

Prior to operation, consideration of the type of prosthetic device to be used is mandatory. This is true even if a commissurotomy or repair is anticipated, for often such conservative plans must be aborted because of unexpected pathologic findings. Such consideration must take into account the data available on the various prosthetic choices, technical considerations, preferences of the cardiologist or internist who will follow the patient, and most importantly, the expectations and preferences of the patient. Over a dozen mechanical and two heterograft prosthesis types are currently available in this country. Mechanical valves are either caged-ball or caged-disc, tilting-disc, or bileaflet in design. Heterograft valves are fashioned by mounting a glutaraldehyde-treated pig aortic valve on a Dacron-covered metal stent. Cryopreserved aortic homografts are also used by some groups and should be treated as a type of prosthesis. Unfortunately, analysis of the available data of a given prosthesis is confounded by inconsistent definitions of valve failure or of valve complications, variations in statistical methods, and incomplete follow-up. Instead of trying to survey all the prosthesis options, we will concentrate on some generalizations and explore three well-studied options.

All mechanical valves require lifelong anticoagulation to prevent thromboembolism generated on the valve surface and to prevent valve thrombosis, regardless of the heart rhythm. Most mechanical valves require a prothrombin time (PT) of 2 to 2.5 times control to prevent these complications, though the newer bileaflet valves require a PT of only 1.5 to 2 times control. Linearized rates of thromboembolism in anticoagulated patients vary widely, from 3% to 6%/y. Valve thrombosis in the anticoagulated patient with a mechanical prosthesis is nearly always fatal, but the incidence for most models is less than 1%/y. Prolonged periods without anticoagulation (e.g., 2 months) in patients with mechanical valves carry a nearly 10% risk of death from thromboembolism or thrombosis. In addition to the aforementioned risks, the inherent risk of morbidity or mortality from anticoagulant-related hemorrhage must be added, and this rate is variously reported at 3% to 5%/y. Porcine heterografts, on the other hand, do not require anticoagulation in an absolute sense, as there is no risk of valve thrombosis. Anticoagulation during the first 2-3 months after implantation is strongly recommended, because of a tendency to thromboembolism during this period of endothelialization of the Dacron sewing ring. After this period, long-term anticoagulation should be provided for those patients who remain in atrial fibrillation, usually at a PT of 1.5 to 2 times control level. The incidence of thromboembolism and of anticoagulant hemorrhage in patients so managed is on the order of 1.5% and 1%/y. This relative independence from anticoagulation with a low rate of thromboembolism is the major advantage heterograft prosthesis has over mechanical prosthesis.

Most mechanical valves in use today have a theoretical life expectancy far in excess of the life expectancy of the patients in whom they are implanted. Intrinsic valve failure does occur secondary to wear, stress fractures, or freezing of moving components, and unfortunately it is usually catastrophic. It has been a powerful motivator of model revision, particularly in regard to disc type valves. Newer bileaflet valves have the inherent advantage that if intrinsic failure occurs, it likely involves only one leaflet, and the patient is more apt to survive the episode. Fortunately, the overall incidence of intrinsic failure in mechanical prosthesis is small. Intrinsic valve failure occurs with porcine valves, and the mechanism is fibrocalcific degeneration of the leaflets. This appears to be a time-dependent phenomenon, but affects 17% to 35% of the valves at 10 years and 60% of the valves at 15 years, necessitating reoperation. The process is gradual, and patients usually develop stenotic hemodynamics. Occasionally the fracture of a calcified leaflet presents with sudden onset of regurgitation. In either case, the patient usually survives this mode of failure. Degeneration of porcine valves is accelerated in patients younger than 30 years and in the presence of renal failure because of abnormal calcium metabolism and appears to be slower in patients over 60 years of age. It is clear from actuarial data that porcine valve prostheses wear out and that all recipients of porcine valves will need replacement, probably 10-15 years after the initial implantation. Mechanical valves have a distinct advantage over porcine valves in this regard.

Prosthetic valve endocarditis is a constant risk to the valve replacement patient, and prophylactic antibiotics are required for all dental and surgical procedures. No good evidence indicates that any prosthesis type, either mechanical or heterograft, is more resistent to endocarditis. The incidence of prosthetic valve endocarditis is approximately 1%/y. There are, however, significant differences between prosthesis types in the hemodynamic performance of smaller sized valves. Below 29 mm for mitral valves and 23 mm for aortic valves, heterografts and caged-ball valve prostheses have significant residual gradients. These prosthesis types should not be used in smaller sizes unless the patient has a small body surface area. The bileaflet prosthesis is most noteworthy in this regard, with essentially no gradient documented even in 19 mm aortic and 25 mm mitral sizes.

The Starr-Edwards Silastic caged-ball valve is the oldest and most studied prosthesis, and good data are available from a number of institutions regarding model 1260 (aortic) and 6120 (mitral) for periods up to 20 years postimplantation. Ten-year actuarial freedom from all valve morbidity and mortality is 40% to 50%, and this number decreases about 10% for 15 and 20 years postimplantation. The incidence of thromboembolism and anticoagulant-related hemorrhage is high and the valve is bulky with residual gradients in small sizes. This valve is seldom implanted now. The Hancock valve has one of the lowest incidences of thromboembolism and is the only valve type (i.e., heterografts) that does not mandate anticoagulation per se. Actuarial freedom from all valve morbidity and mortality at 10 years is 60% to 75%. For a decade this was the valve of choice at many institutions, but it is clear that fibrocalcific degeneration will temper its widespread implantation. Newer techniques of glutaraldehyde fixation are hoped to slow the degenerative process. The St. Jude bileaflet valve is the newest and rapidly the most popular valve available, despite limited follow-up. Although designed with hopes of not requiring anticoagulation, unacceptable complication rates have occurred in pilot studies with antiplatelet agents alone; a need for lower levels of anticoagulation (1.5 to 2 times control) is a distinct advantage over other types of mechanical prostheses. This valve appears to have the best hemodynamic performance of any valve made, and machine testing suggests a nearly infinite mechanical life expectancy. Only a single study has been published with 8-year actuarial freedom from all morbidity and mortality stated at 70% to 80%. It is clear that the perfect valve prosthesis does not exist and that currently the valvular heart disease patient must bear the inherent risks of morbidity and mortality that replacement entails.

PREOPERATIVE PREPARATION

The patient with well-compensated heart failure requires little preoperative preparation for valve surgery. Digoxin and diuretics are continued up to the time of surgery. Aspirin-containing medications are prohibited for 5–7 days before surgery because of their effect on platelet function. Patients on coumadin discontinue this drug 4 or 5 days before surgery, to allow PTs to return to normal. Frequently, anticoagulated patients are admitted a few days early and systemic heparinization is started to prevent thromboembolism. The heparin is then discontinued 3 or 4 hours prior to surgery. Pulmonary, hepatic, and renal functions are assessed, and where appropriate, carotid Doppler flow measured. The patient should be free of active infection or at least 3 or 4 days into treatment of minor infections. Sepsis requires completion of the prescribed antibiotic course to reduce the chance of prosthetic valve endocarditis.

Patients in florid heart failure seem to benefit greatly if they can undergo days or weeks of preparation before valve surgery. Bed rest, diuresis, afterload reduction, and control of atrial fibrillation all seem to have a positive influence on operative morbidity and mortality. Sometimes a period of support with catecholamines or even with intra-aortic balloon pump (IABP) counterpulsation (except in aortic regurgitation, where it is contraindicated) just prior to surgery is helpful. Aortic stenosis is the major exception to this rule of trying to maximize medical therapy before valve surgery, as diuresis and afterload reduction are hazardous undertakings with this lesion. One must also constantly assess the effectiveness of such medical preparation; some patients simply will not improve, and delay of surgery will have a negative influence.

AORTIC VALVE SURGERY

Surgical therapy for aortic valve disease is limited at this time to aortic valve replacement. In the past, both debridement for calcific aortic stenosis and repair for aortic regurgitation have been attempted, with little reproducible success. Recent attempts using an ultrasonic probe to perform aortic valve debridement have ended with an unacceptable rate of aortic regurgitation developing within 2-4 months of operation. Work continues on standardizing a technique for the repair of aortic regurgitation, but no new information is forthcoming.

The aortic valve is approached through a midline sternotomy utilizing cardiopulmonary bypass and systemic hypothermia. A clamp is placed across the aorta just in front of the innominate artery to interrupt coronary blood flow; an initial dose of cold blood or crystalloid cardioplegia is administered through the aorta proximal to the clamp. If aortic regurgitation is present, the heart is fibrillated first by pouring 4°C saline solution over the ventricles and the clamp is applied just as fibrillation starts; an initial dose of cardioplegia is administered directly into the coronary orifices using special cannulae. The pericardium is flooded with 4°C saline solution to provide additional topical cooling to the heart, and additional doses of cardioplegia are administered every 20 minutes into the coronary orifices during the ischemia period. This combination of systemic and topical hypothermia combined with intermittent intracoronary cardioplegia is critical to maintain myocardial temperature in the vicinity of 10-12°C. It is in this manner that myocardial preservation is maximized, and to a large extent, the low operative risk of aortic valve replacement is attributable to these developments.

Aortotomy is performed just above the valve annulus, and valve excision is accomplished leaving a 2- or 3-mm rim of tissue. In heavily calcified valves, extensive debridement is necessary so that the annulus is soft and flexible, allowing coaptation with the prosthesis. Care must be exercised, as too vigorous a debridement can perforate the heart, aorta, or the anterior leaflet of the mitral valve. Excessive manipulation of annular deposits at the junction of the right and noncoronary cusps can result in permanent heart block, as this region is contiguous with the AV node. Debridement generates numerous fragments of calcium that can fall into the coronary orifices or the ventricle, with disastrous consequences. Ventricular debris can be and is lavaged out after completion of debridement, but coronary debris can only be avoided by diligence.

The final selection of a prosthesis type may be modified by certain technical factors. If the annulus is very small relative to the patient's body surface area, a bileaflet prosthesis should be selected, for other prostheses will leave residual gradients. A Konno procedure (aortoventriculoplasty to enlarge the annulus) is rarely indicated in adults now that bileaflet valves are available. The prosthesis must be seated on the annulus below the coronary orifices. Highly scalloped annuli are seated more easily with the flexible stent of heterograft valves. As the aortotomy is closed, air must be worked out of the heart by a series of maneuvers designed to prevent embolization. Removal of the aortic clamp restores coronary perfusion and cardiac action. Most often the heart begins to beat spontaneously; if fibrillation is present, defibrillation is performed. If bradycardia or heart block are present, atrial or AV sequential pacing is started. While the heart is recovering from its ischemic insult, residual air is vented from the highest point in the ascending aorta, but since the right coronary orifice cannot be protected, right ventricular air embolism can and does occur. Usually, the right ventricle recovers with continued bypass support. The patient is weaned from cardiopulmonary bypass and the sternotomy closed.

The operative mortality rate for elective aortic valve replacement is generally reported at 3% to 5%. The strongest predictor of mortality in nearly every series was preoperative functional class. Additional predictors of operative mortality include EF, age, and whether the primary lesion was regurgitation (negative) or stenosis. Major complications after aortic valve replacement include cerebrovascular insult (from air, particulate debris, or aortic atheroma traumatized by the clamp), MI (from air, particulate debris, or poor preservation), bleeding, and permanent heart block. The respective incidences of these complications are 3%, 2%, 5% to 10%, and 4%. Unlike other open heart patients, postoperative bleeding in the aortic valve patient carries a negative influence on perioperative mortality, which is 10% in this subgroup. Overall, the rehabilitative power of aortic valve replacement is most impressive, with over 80% of the patients returned to class I or II status up to 8 years postoperatively. Most impressive is the fact that 70% of the improved patients started in functional class IV preoperatively.

Concomitant ascending aortic disease

Aortic valve replacement is sometimes combined with resection of the ascending aorta and Dacron tube graft replacement. This is indicated if there is a true aneurysm or if ectasia of the ascending aorta exists with a maximal diameter greater than 7 cm. The tube graft is inserted proximally at the aortic isthmus. When dilatation involves the sinuses of Valsalva and particularly in Marfan syndrome, a composite replacement of the aortic root is performed, using a tube graft which has an aortic valve prosthesis sewn into one end. This requires reimplantation of the coronary arteries, which is done to the side of the graft. Composite replacement is necessary in Marfan syndrome because leaving the sinuses of Valsalva has been shown to promote sinus aneurysms. Dissection of the ascending aorta with significant regurgitation is the one situation where aortic valve repair is likely to work successfully. The mechanism of regurgitation in dissection is loss of commissural support caused by separation of the layers of the aortic wall at the isthmus. Resuspension of the commissures with graft replacement above is all that is required in most circumstances. Because all of these procedures are more complex and time consuming than simple aortic valve replacement, they necessarily engender a higher operative mortality, generally in the range of 10% to 15%.

MITRAL VALVE SURGERY

Three surgical procedures are in general use to treat mitral valve disease: commissurotomy, valve repair that is inclusive of annuloplasty techniques, and valve replacement. All procedures are performed through a midline sternotomy. Although this is not the most direct approach to the mitral valve, because cardiopulmonary bypass with systemic hypothermia is required, it is the approach which maximizes the surgeon's control of the operation and therefore patient safety as well. Myocardial preservation is carried out in a manner similar to aortic valve replacement except that direct cannulation of the coronary ostia is not necessary, and cardioplegia is infused into the ascending aorta proximal to the clamp. Cardiotomy is based on an incision that starts on the anterior surface of the right superior pulmonary vein and extends inferiorly to the inferior vena cava. Exposure of the mitral valve from its atrial aspect is achieved, but this may be difficult, for the surgeon is working under the right atrium, right ventricle, and great vessels. In patients with particularly deep chests or small left atria, further exposure is achieved by splitting the atrial septum or by dividing the superior vena cava. To accurately perform commissurotomy or valve repair, visualization of the whole plane of the mitral annulus is required, and if exposure cannot be achieved, it is preferable to perform valve replacement. Valve replacement can be accomplished successfully with exposure limited to one-quarter of the annulus at a time. After the mitral valve procedure is completed, cardiotomy closure, resuscitation of the heart, weaning from bypass, and closure are performed. The management of trapped air to prevent embolism is similar to that with aortic valve replacement.

Open mitral commissurotomy has entirely supplanted the original closed procedure. Although the closed procedure does not utilize bypass, the imprecise nature of the commissurotomy (it is in reality a "blind" finger fracture) and the significant incidence of thromboembolism and death led to its abandonment. Commissurotomy is appropriate early in the course of rheumatic stenosis, before calcification and deformation of the subvalvular apparatus, and can delay replacement for 10-15 years. The precise splitting of the fused commissures with a blade may now be combined with some of the techniques of valve repair. Significant regurgitation is the major contraindication to this procedure and also the most important complication, which should prompt valve replacement before the patient leaves the operating room. Operative mortality for open commissurotomy is very nearly 0%. The role of percutaneous balloon valvotomy in relation to commissurotomy remains to be defined. A nonsurgical therapy for mitral stenosis is appealing, but the percutaneous procedure is analogous to closed commissurotomy, and one would predict similar limitations. The incidence of postvalvuloplasty atrial septal defect approaches 50%, with uncertain significance.

Mitral valve repair refers to a collection of procedures used to address either mixed or predominantly regurgitant lesions in a conservative manner. Leaflet debridement, commissurotomy, division of secondary chordae, and chordal fenestration are used singly or together to return competence to a valve with restrictive leaflet motion without creating stenosis. Annuloplasty, mural leaflet resection, chordal shortening, and chordal transposition are used in valves with excessive leaflet motion. Repair is a time-consuming process that depends on repetitive testing of valve competence with a bulb syringe as the procedure progresses. Although echocardiography is valuable pre- and postoperatively to identify candidates for repair and to assess the results of repair, it has little utility guiding the repair itself. Carpentier is credited with synthesizing all of these techniques into a logical and reproducible approach to mitral valve repair. In particular, the measured annuloplasty performed over a sized Dacron ring, with plications confined to the mural annulus only, is to his credit. Repair is advantageous because morbidity associated with prosthetic heart valves is delayed or eliminated, the risk of thromboembolism is very low (0.3% to 0.5%/y), and ventriculochordal continuity is preserved (see below), thus preserving EF. The reported mortality rate of mitral repair is 2% to 3% in elective series. Long-term actuarial data are limited; 5-year freedom from valve replacement is greater than 90%, and from thromboembolism, 95%. At 5 years, 95% of the patients are in functional class I or II. A closer analysis of the data suggests that long-term results are less favorable for patients with a rheumatic etiology. However, repair appears to be the procedure of choice for patients with degenerative and ischemic mitral regurgitation and is also probably definitive.

Mitral valve replacement traditionally required excision

of the leaflets and division of the chordae tendineae at their insertion into the papillary muscles. With bulkier prostheses such as the Starr-Edwards, the papillary muscles were excised as well. Debridement of the annulus is usually unnecessary or quite limited. With senile mitral annular calcification, it is safer to leave the posterior leaflet in situ and to seat the valve on the soft part of the mural leaflet. An adequate prosthesis size must be selected to avoid residual gradients, and care must be exercised in the placement of sutures to avoid the circumflex coronary artery and the membranous septum, which could result in MI or heart block. Mitral valve replacement is now accomplished with an elective mortality rate of 4% to 8%. The overwhelming cause of perioperative death is heart failure. Predictors of operative mortality include functional class, age, and ischemic etiology. Actuarial survival is not as good as with aortic valve replacement, with 60% and 45% survival at 10 and 15 years, respectively. Chronic congestive heart failure is the major cause of late mortality. Only 60% of the patients in functional class III or IV preoperatively achieve class I or II status postoperatively.

Evidence indicates that division of the chordae tendineae in traditional mitral valve replacement causes a 10% to 15% decrease in EF independent of the decrease in EF caused by relief of afterload mismatch. Preservation of only the mural leaflet and its chordae seems to be sufficient to prevent this loss, and many centers are conserving the mural leaflet and its attachments routinely. This is easily achieved with heterografts, where struts protect the prosthesis from intrusion by residual subvalvular material. It is more difficult with mechanical prostheses where a single chorda can foul the prosthesis mechanism, and manufacturers specifically warn against such preservation. Imbricating techniques have been developed to allow preservation of the mural leaflet with mechanical valves, and they have been used successfully. It would seem that an attempt at mural leaflet preservation is mandatory in every patient undergoing mitral valve replacement. Perhaps if widely applied, the operative mortality rate of mitral replacement would start to approach that of aortic valve replacement, and there might be less residual heart failure. A further benefit of chordal preservation is the absence of reported posterior ventricular rupture. This rare perioperative complication is most feared, presents catastrophically, and is almost uniformly fatal.

A majority of the reported cases of posterior ventricular rupture are associated with division of the chordal attachments. Other causes include the use of too large a prosthesis and excessive elevation of the heart after prosthesis implantation.

MULTIVALVE SURGERY

Many patients, particularly those with rheumatic valvular disease, present with significant lesions of both the aortic and mitral valve. In general, the hemodynamic indications for double valve replacement are somewhat less for a given valve than if the valve alone is the sole cause of symptomatology. For example, a patient with long-standing 4+ mitral regurgitation and with class III symptoms is found to have a 30-mm aortic valve gradient. The aortic gradient alone would not constitute an indication for replacement, but if mitral replacement alone were performed, the increased forward flow across the aortic valve would probably yield a gradient in excess of 50 mm, and symptoms of failure would persist. Appropriate treatment would be combined valve replacement. Double valve replacement is technically a combination of the two separate procedures. It is time consuming and approaches the upper limits of safe ischemia time relative to the current state of myocardial preservation. The mitral valve is always seated first to eliminate the possibility of aortic annular disruption caused by retraction to expose the mitral valve on the implanted aortic prosthesis. The operative mortality rate for combined valve replacement is 10% to 20% and is basically a reflection of the greater severity of heart failure in these patients.

Isolated tricuspid valve disease is extremely rare. Functional tricuspid insufficiency, on the other hand, frequently accompanies left-sided valvular dysfunction associated with severe backward failure. In many instances, the tricuspid insufficiency and right-sided failure will resolve with successful aortic, mitral, or double valve replacement. In some patients, however, improvement of left-sided function is marred by persisting right heart failure and tricuspid regurgitation. No good diagnostic modalities separate these two groups of patients preoperatively; instead, the tricuspid valve is assessed at the time of surgery. A finger is introduced into the right atrial appendage and the regurgitation graded. If significant, the right atrium is opened, usually after left-sided valve replacement and with the aortic cross–clamp removed, and a measured annuloplasty using a Carpentier ring is performed. Since the tricuspid valve is not excised, one can err on the side of treating those patients who might have resolved their regurgitation simply with resolution of left-sided heart failure. In patients with long-standing right-sided failure and tricuspid regurgitation, ascites, and hepatic changes, little improvement in right heart function can be expected, and a heterograft prosthesis is sewn into place. This provides a more secure and long-lasting solution than annuloplasty. Heterografts in the tricuspid position allow for the passage of Swan-Ganz and pacing catheters, and evidence suggests that they deteriorate at a slower rate in the right heart than in the left. Although still used by some surgeons, the DeVega annuloplasty and commissural plication techniques have produced less satisfying results.

CONCOMITANT CORONARY ARTERY DISEASE

Over a decade ago, enhanced survival of aortic stenosis patients with significant coronary artery disease was demonstrated when bypass surgery was performed at the time of aortic valve replacement, rather than performing simple valve replacement, which had been the preceding practice. This principle has been generalized to all valve patients, albeit without supporting survival data. Any patient at risk because of age for coronary artery disease should undergo preoperative coronary arteriography, and concomitant bypass grafting should be performed for significant (greater than 50%) obstructing lesions at the time of valve surgery. This is usually done prior to valve replacement, so that the bypass grafts can facilitate the delivery of cardioplegia. Although many studies suggest a 2% or 3% increase in operative risk if revascularization is performed simultaneously, the enhanced myocardial preservation during the surgery should be looked at as a positive factor.

A notable exception to this trivial increase in operative risk is the patient with ischemic mitral regurgitation. Traditionally, this group has experienced an operative mortality rate variously reported between 20% and 30%. It is a group that is heterogeneous, with some patients presenting in cardiogenic shock secondary to rupture of a whole papillary muscle, whereas other patients included in these series have simple inferior or lateral wall dysfunction and 3+ regurgitation that revascularization alone would have corrected. Mitral valve repair using annuloplasty alone or in combination with leaflet resection or reimplantation of the papillary muscle has had a dramatic impact on this group of patients, with reported operative mortality rates of 10%. Undoubtedly the success of this procedure for patients with ischemic mitral regurgitation lies in the fact that the continuity between the chordae tendineae and the ventricle is preserved, thus preserving left ventricular EF. Additionally, an annuloplasty probably carries little negative influence on the function of ventricles that would recover without valve surgery, so the need to finely discriminate between these two groups of patients becomes less important.

VALVE REOPERATIONS

Following previous commissurotomy, valve repair, or valve replacement, the hemodynamic indications for reoperation remain similar to the indications for a first intervention. This rule applies whether the valve in question is a native valve or a heterograft valve that has degenerated. In experienced hands, such an undertaking can be performed with the same risk of the initial native valve replacement. The key factor seems to be the state of left ventricular function. Early series on valve reoperation reported 10% to 30% operative mortality rates, but in a large part this was a reflection of the fact that the initial operation was performed in the 1960s and early 1970s, when the art of myocardial preservation had not matured, and patients suffered significant decreases in myocardial function as a consequence. Modern techniques of cardioplegia combined with topical and systemic hypothermia have obviated this negative influence. Unfortunately, reoperation for mechanical valve dysfunction still carries an extremely high mortality, first because of the tenuous nature of such dysfunction, and secondly because reoperation cannot be rushed. Resternotomy is a tedious process, sometimes progressing but a few millimeters at a time, and the pressure of emergency reoperation for mechanical valve dysfunction frequently leads to catastrophic results.

ENDOCARDITIS

Native valve endocarditis is thought of as primarily a medical disease, with valve replacement reserved for "complications" of endocarditis, specifically congestive heart failure, systemic embolization, and persisting sepsis. Unfortunately, 10% to 40% of these patients develop "complications" and require surgery. Furthermore, the major predictors of operative death for valve replacement with endocarditis are indeed the indications for operation. It has been amply demonstrated that successful valve replacement can be performed in the presence of active endocarditis, that there is little reason to attempt to complete a 4-week course of antibiotics to achieve "healed" status. This fact has allowed clinicians to focus on specific subgroups of patients with known high failure rates of medical therapy to allow for early surgical intervention. Morbid complications such as subannular and intramyocardial abscess formation, which require extensive surgical procedures in addition to valve replacement, are minimized with an enhancement of patient salvage. These specific subgroups include patients with infection from *Staphylococcus aureus,* gram-negative bacteria, and fungi with significant valvular regurgitation (particularly aortic regurgitation). The recurrence rate of infection in patients so operated on is less than 5%. Recently, mitral valve endocarditis has been successfully treated in the active phase using valve repair techniques, and this approach might be adopted more widely. Applying a similar analysis to patients with prosthetic valve endocarditis, only in patients infected with *Streptococcus viridans* is there any significant likelihood of medical cure; all other cases of prosthetic valve endocarditis will require valve re-replacement, preferably early in the course of antibiotic therapy.

POSTOPERATIVE CARE

The postoperative management of the valvular heart disease patient begins in the operating room. At the time the patient is weaned from cardiopulmonary bypass, indispensable information is gained about cardiac contractility and correlation is made with clinically measurable hemodynamic parameters. Catecholamine support is started if contractility is weak, usually using dobutamine or amrinone. Various states of ventricular preload can be tested with relative ease as the patient is weaned off cardiopulmonary bypass. Pacing is established if the heart rate is slow or heart block exists. Afterload-reducing agents are added as blood pressure allows, usually starting with nitroglycerin, and adding nitroprusside or hydralazine as needed. Agents agonistic to pulmonary vascular resistance, such as dopamine, levarterenol, or high-dose epinephrine are avoided.

Within the intensive care environment, the emphasis is on maintaining stability with maximal cardiac output during the first 12-24 hours, or longer if failure has been severe. Pharmacologic afterload reduction has its major role here, and systemic resistance is reduced to less than 1000 dyne cm/sec. This is crucial for all valve procedures. For compromised ventricles, it is a simple way of enhancing cardiac output. For patients with mitral valve replacement, it reduces wall stress and the incidence of posterior ventricular rupture. For the aortic valve patient, the risk of aortotomy bleeding is reduced. Improvement in ventricular function is heralded by spontaneous diuresis or a fall in left-sided filling pressures. Catecholamine support, if present, is weaned off slowly. Diuresis is encouraged with furosemide, and extubation is delayed until the patient at least reaches preoperative weight. One must remember that the valvular heart disease patient almost always has some element of failure preoperatively and that the aim of postoperative diuresis is a weight several kilograms less than that preoperatively.

Anticoagulation is started on all valve surgery patients on the third postoperative day. This is true of heterograft valves and commissurotomy and mitral repair patients as well. Although some groups simply start coumadin and wait for the PT to prolong, a small but disturbing experience with early postoperative stroke associated with rhythm changes has led many surgeons to simultaneously use systemic heparinization until the PT is adequately prolonged. New atrial fibrillation will occur postoperatively in nearly half of all valve patients, and digoxin is routinely used. Procainamide has been useful in the patient who alternates between atrial fibrillation or flutter and sinus rhythm and also in the patient who has significant ventricular ectopy.

PATIENT FOLLOW-UP

Patients who have had valve surgery require considerably more follow-up than the coronary bypass patient, and the follow-up should continue at some level indefinitely. Patient education regarding anticoagulant complications and endocarditis prophylaxis should occur with every visit. During the first 2 or 3 postoperative months, attention is directed to the treatment of residual heart failure with diuretics and afterload-reducing agents and to the monitoring of anticoagulation. After 2 months, anticoagulation can be stopped in patients with hetero-graft valves and in commissurotomy and mitral repair patients, provided they are in sinus rhythm. Mechanical valve recipients will require frequent PT determinations for a longer period until a stable dose is established. Thereafter, PT monitoring can be decreased to every 2–4 months. Digoxin is often continued for 6 months to a year, or longer if left atrial size remains large or heart failure persists. Afterload-reducing agents are often continued indefinitely in the patient with failure. Patients are encouraged to exercise commensurate with their ventricular function. Encouragement is often needed, particularly in mitral valve patients, who may require a full 6 months before maximal benefit from the operation is experienced.

Because the perfect cardiac valve prosthesis has yet to be developed, most patients, if they live long enough, will experience a complication from their heart valve prosthesis. A change in hemodynamic status requires prompt investigation, usually with echocardiography, and possibly with catheterization. New regurgitant murmurs require that endocarditis be ruled out. A loss or decrease in the sounds of a mechanical prosthesis is an emergency requiring admission and possibly emergency surgery. Heterograft valves older than 5 years should probably be followed on a yearly basis with echocardiographic determinations of valvular gradients. Despite the burden placed on the patient of prosthetic valve complication, heart valve surgery has prolonged the lives of thousands of patients. With proper timing of operation and emphasis on newer conservative techniques, a majority of the future patients should be able to carry out normal lives.

SUGGESTED READING

Assey ME, Spann JF. Indications for heart valve replacement. *Clin Cardiol*. 1990; 13:81–88.

Cobanoglu A, Jamieson E, Miller DC, et al. A tri-institutional comparison of tissue and mechanical valves using a patient-oriented definition of "treatment failure". *Ann Thorac Surg*. 1987; 43:245–253.

Rahimtoola SH. Perspective on valvular heart disease: an update. *J Am Coll Cardio.* 1989; 14:1–23.

Rahimtoola SH. Valvular heart disease: a perspective. *J Am Coll Cardio.* 1983; 1:199–215.

Sethi GK, Miller DC, Souchek J, et al. Clinical, hemodynamic, and angiographic predictors of operative mortality in patients undergoing single valve replacement. *J Thorac Cardio Surg.* 1987; 93:884–897.

Postoperative Management

Alan R. Hartman, M.D.
Stephen C. Vlay, M.D.

13

INTRA- AND POSTOPERATIVE MANAGEMENT

Weaning and separation from the pump and oxygenator

In preparation for the separation and discontinuation of the heart–lung machine, several criteria must be met. The patient's core and rectal temperature should be 37°C to avoid any of the problems associated with hypothermia, primarily arrhythmias and coagulopathy. Oxygenation and ventilation must be resumed via the respirator, with good expansion of both lungs at 100% fraction inspired oxygen (FiO_2). A cardiac rhythm that will support an optimal blood pressure and cardiac output should be verified, preferably a sinus rhythm at a reasonable rate. If absent, then atrioventricular (AV) pacing should be initiated.

Finally a last check of all the vascular anastomoses is worthwhile, for repair is more easily accomplished on full or partial bypass than off pump.

The process of weaning the pump oxygenator is the gradual decrease of flow through the venous cannula allowing the heart to fill with blood, with the simultaneous decrease of flow from the arterial cannula, allowing cardiac ejection to increase. The heart is allowed to fill with blood to achieve pulmonary diastolic pressures that allow optimal systolic ejection and acceptable mean arterial pressure. It is at this point that cardiopulmonary bypass is terminated. Cardiac output is calculated immediately via thermodilution technique to verify adequacy of perfusion.

Frequently, pharmacologic agents are necessary to augment

contractility, support blood pressure, or decrease afterload to optimize cardiac output. Intravenous nitroglycerin is used on practically all coronary artery bypass (CABG) patients. Many of these patients are on high-dose nitrates preoperatively, and nitroglycerin is used to prevent rebound vasospasm. Additionally, preload reduction with its favorable effect on hemodynamics is warranted. If blood pressure remains elevated despite the use of high-dose nitroglycerin, then intravenous nitroprusside is used. This drug is primarily an arteriolar dilator and lowers peripheral vascular resistance, augmenting cardiac output. Avoiding extreme hypertension contributes to the maintenance of hemostasis at the anastomotic sites. If contractility seems sluggish, then inotropic agents such as dobutamine or low-dose epinephrine are used. Renal dose (2–3 μg/kg) dopamine is reserved for those patients with preoperative reduction in creatinine clearance.

Antiarrhythmic agents are not used prophylactically, except in those patients with preoperative malignant ventricular arrhythmias and in patients with ventriculotomies for aneurysm resection. An occasional patient will be extremely hyperdynamic and will benefit from judicious use of intravenous β-blockers.

If ventricular function appears poor at time of weaning from bypass, early institution of intra-aortic balloon pump (IABP) counterpulsation is valuable. It will decrease ventricular dilation, minimize endocardial necrosis, possibly limiting the dose of inotropic agents necessary, and decrease the potential for arrhythmogenesis. If more than 10 μg/kg dobutamine is needed, or if another agent such as epinephrine or amrinone is necessary, then we seriously consider IABP support.

After cardiopulmonary bypass has been discontinued and hemodynamic and cardiac output are acceptable, reversal of heparin with protamine sulfate is performed. An occasional patient may have an adverse reaction to protamine, resulting in profound systemic hypotension associated with pulmonary artery hypertension and even bronchospasm. Some of these patients may have identifying risks that should alert the physician. Diabetic patients who are using NPH insulin (which contains protamine) may possibly be sensitized and may be at increased risk for protamine reactions. Similarly, patients exposed to protamine from previous open heart procedures or cardiac catheterizations may also be at increased risk. Patients with chronic pulmonary hypertension may be more likely to have exacerbation of their pulmonary hypertension during protamine administration. For these patients, some evidence suggests that slow administration of the protamine through a catheter in the left heart (i.e., left atrial catheter) may avoid these pulmonary effects.

Transthoracic pacing wires

Temporary epicardial pacing wires are used and left in place on all cardiac procedures. It is recommended that at least two leads be placed on the right atrium and right ventricle. This allows for a backup lead in case one fails to capture and always allows for AV pacing—very necessary when cardiac output or ventricular function is compromised and pacing is necessary. Atrial leads also allow for the diagnostic evaluation of supraventricular arrhythmias, helping to differentiate between sinus tachycardia, paroxysmal atrial tachycardia, atrial flutter, and atrial fibrillation. Additionally, atrial leads allow for rapid atrial pacing, a therapeutic modality for several supraventricular arrhythmias. It is generally advisable to leave the temporary epicardial leads in place until a day or two prior to discharge since they do not hinder ambulation or recovery.

Chest tubes—mediastinal tubes

All cardiac surgeons leave at least one or more drainage tubes. The type and number frequently depend on the surgery performed. Generally, a single mediastinal tube is always placed substernally to drain blood from the operative site and sternal bone edges. If bleeding is considered to be likely, a second mediastinal tube may be in place, frequently insinuated between the inferior wall of the heart and the diaphragm. If either mediastinal pleura was entered, as one routinely does for the internal mammary artery harvest, then a chest tube is left in that side. Again, this is primarily for drainage of blood or serous fluid.

Mediastinal tubes are generally removed before the chest tubes. They are typically left in place 16–36 hours depending on drainage. It is our practice to extubate and elevate the chest prior to removal to allow for complete drainage of any residual accumulation. The chest tubes can be removed thereafter if drainage is small or a day later if drainage persists. It is helpful to have the patient sitting in a chair at least once prior to removal of the pleural tubes to help drain any accumulations.

Antibiotics

Prophylactic antibiotic administration in cardiothoracic surgery is not dissimilar from other surgical disciplines. We generally administer a cephalosporin, such as cefazolin, prior to the surgical incision, repeat it when coming off cardiopulmonary bypass and again every 8 hours. It is stopped when the pulmonary artery catheter introducer sheath is removed, generally 36–48 hours after surgery.

INITIAL MANAGEMENT IN THE CARDIOVASCULAR ICU

Blood pressure, cardiac output, pulmonary arterial pressure, and central venous pressure are the cornerstones of monitoring for the postoperative cardiac patient. Additionally, mediastinal and chest tube output as well as urine output are watched extremely carefully. This type of second–by–second assessment demands at least one nurse per patient and sometimes two or more nurses depending on the acuity of the patient's condition. It also demands a physician present and available at all times, preferably the surgeon.

Key objectives are to maintain maximal cardiac output and perfusion to all organs without increasing myocardial oxygen demands.

Heart rate

In the absence of heart block requiring AV pacing, prevention of rapid rates is extremely important. In the milieu of catecholamine release, an awakening patient, and perhaps β-blocker or calcium channel blocker withdrawal, sinus tachycardia or tachyarrhythmias are not unusual. This frequently can significantly increase myocardial oxygen consumption. In patients who have been on high-dose β-blockers or calcium channel blockers preoperatively, reinstitution at a lower dose is started immediately, providing cardiac failure is not apparent. Atrial arrhythmias are treated aggressively with potassium supplementation, digoxin, and possibly an antiarrhythmic agent.

Blood pressure

Mean arterial blood pressure is generally kept at least at 60 mm Hg, but elevations greater than 75 or 80 are aggressively treated to minimize myocardial oxygen consumption and to avoid bleeding from the numerous vascular anastomoses and

281

cannulation sites. In fact, even transient severe elevations in blood pressure can have dangerous consequences in the immediate postoperative state. All hypertension is considered dangerous and is treated aggressively and urgently. Most postoperative patients will be on intravenous nitroglycerin. Intravenous nitroprusside is added if necessary and regulated to keep mean arterial blood pressure at 60–70 mm Hg. Frequently, in the awakening postoperative patient with significant circulatory catecholamine response, hypertension can be problematic and even high-dose nitroprusside is ineffective. In this situation, additional agents may be used including intravenous hydralazine, intravenous β-blockers, calcium channel blockers, or angiotensin–converting enzyme (ACE) inhibitors. Morphine sulfate and benzodiazepine-type drugs may be needed to control pain or anxiety that may provoke hypertension.

Cardiac output

An adequate cardiac output generally depends on body surface area and should be expressed as cardiac index (L/m^2). This number should be greater than 2 L/m^2 and can be corroborated by measuring the mixed venous gas (the saturation of the pulmonary artery blood). This saturation should be greater than 70% with a Pao$_2$ of at least 35. Anything lower than this requires serious assessment with regard to adequacy of oxygenation and adequacy of cardiac output.

Pulmonary artery pressure

The preoperative pressure will have some bearing on the postoperative valve. If chronic pulmonary hypertension is present, then direct left atrial pressure measurements will be more informative. In essence, one constructs Starling curves, determining at what pulmonary artery pressure the cardiac output is maximal.

Generally, the lower the pulmonary arterial pressures, the smaller the heart, the less myocardial wall tension exerted, and the lower the myocardial oxygen requirement. Therefore, the lowest pulmonary arterial pressure yielding an excellent cardiac output is desirable.

Central venous pressure

The main information obtained from central venous pressure measurements is used to help diagnose early cardiac tamponade or to alert one to the possibility of right ventricular failure. When the central venous pressure equals or exceeds the pulmonary diastolic pressure, then there is cause for concern.

Continued treatment plans in ICU

The choice of drugs for achieving and maintaining adequate cardiac output and perfusion pressure is similar to that already discussed at the time of weaning from bypass. The major difference is the addition of supplemental vasodilators, if the nitroprusside dose becomes extremely high or ineffective. As mentioned previously, early use of the IABP in a patient with high-dose or multidose inotropic agents is always a consideration.

As a patient's cardiac output improves in the postoperative period, any inotropic agents are weaned as tolerated, and early use of β-blockers or calcium channel blockers are instituted to prevent a hyperdynamic state that will contribute to increased myocardial oxygen demand or arrhythmias.

Tachyarrhythmias are treated with potassium supplementation, digoxin, and either β-blockers or calcium channel blockers. Overdrive rapid atrial pacing is effective in atrial flutter and paroxysmal atrial tachycardia. Any arrhythmia causing severe hypotension and compromise should be cardioverted immediately. Bradyarrhythmias are treated with AV pacing using the epicardial leads.

Serious ventricular arrhythmias are treated aggressively with potassium supplementation, overdrive pacing suppression, or antiarrhythmic drugs if persistent. Occasionally a malpositioned pulmonary artery catheter or mediastinal chest tube may be the culprit and can be repositioned or removed.

All patients are placed on stress ulcer prophylaxis. Generally antacids plus an H_2-blocker are administered or sucralfate without antacids is used. These are continued at least until the patient is on a regular diet several days postoperatively. In high-risk patients or those with a peptic ulcer history, prophylaxis will be continued throughout the hospitalization.

Aspirin and dipyridamole are administered according to the recommendations of Chesebro. Dipyridamole is started preoperatively the day before surgery. When the patient arrives in the postoperative unit, dipyridamole is reinstituted via the nasogastric tube. Aspirin in a dose of 325 mg is given as a rectal suppository, beginning at least 2 hours after surgery if bleeding is nonproblematic. Chesebro has demonstrated improved early patency rates of bypass grafts using this regimen.

PROGRESSIVE CARE IN THE CARDIAC SURGICAL ICU

Most patients are extubated by the morning after surgery. If they can lift their head off the bed and hold it and have a tidal volume of 10 mL/kg and a negative inspiratory force of greater than 20 cm H_2O, then extubation is safe. After extubation, the need for vasodilators is frequently reduced. Conversion of the intravenous nitroglycerin to a patch or paste form is accomplished over several hours. Inotropic agents are weaned as tolerated, providing cardiac output and pulmonary artery pressures remain acceptable.

If the IABP is in place, then the weaning and removal of this is accomplished prior to extubating the patient, primarily because of the inability to properly place the patient in an upright position allowing for adequate pulmonary toilet.

The process of converting the intravenous vasodilators or β-blockers to an oral form depends entirely on the functioning of the gastrointestinal tract. In the absence of bowel sounds, the intravenous preparations are used. When bowel sounds are adequate and there is no nausea or gastric dilation, and the patient can swallow pills, then oral antihypertensive agents are begun to aid weaning the nitroprusside. The types and dosages of oral antihypertensives will vary, but generally ACE inhibitors are the first-line drugs followed by prazosin if additional control is needed. Alternatives include the use of diltiazem or nifedipine, depending on the individual hemodynamics of the patient. Avoidance of prolonged use and excessive doses of nitroprusside (which will frequently cause cyanide poisoning manifested by confusion and acidosis) is particularly important.

β-blockers are generally continued in an oral form to prevent tachycardia and tachyarrhythmias. The dose is determined by the resting heart rate and the response to mild exertion. If recurrent atrial fibrillation requires an antiarrhythmic agent, then long-acting procainamide may be used along with digoxin. For malignant ventricular arrhythmias, consultation with a cardiologist well versed in electrophysiologic studies is obtained.

Early mobilization and ambulation are keys to an expeditious recovery. As soon as the pulmonary artery catheter and intravenous nitroprusside or nitroglycerin are removed, patients are placed in a chair. Frequently this is accomplished the day following surgery except in the critically ill. For these patients, the goals and steps are the same, but will often take a longer time to accomplish.

Soon patients will be ready to start ambulation and gradually resume their activities of daily living. As they progress they will be assisted by postoperative teaching and will increase their physical activity. After the postoperative course is completed, the patient will return to the care of the cardiologist and referring internist or family physician.

BRIEF SYNOPSIS OF COMMONLY USED CARDIOVASCULAR DRUGS

This section provides a brief overview of drugs commonly used in the care of cardiovascular patients. The purpose is to provide the reader with some familiarity but by no means is it intended to be an inclusive description of the metabolism, precautions, contraindications, adverse effects, or dosing regimens. For these the reader is advised to consult a pharmacology textbook or the *Physician's Desk Reference.*

Prescribing medications involves both science and art. One must be aware of the pharmacologic properties and the indications for the drugs. The "art" of medicine is to know how to use the science of pharmacology to adjust the therapy appropriately. Used improperly, a potentially useful drug may be discarded with the incorrect designation—"patient failed to respond." Furthermore, physicians cannot become facile with the use of a drug unless they follow the patient over a period of time. No matter what drug is prescribed, monitoring for short-term and long-term side effects is necessary.

Nitroglycerin and nitrate preparations

Nitrates are direct-acting vasodilators acting primarily on the venous circulation. Relief of angina with sublingual nitroglycerin occurs via an increase in the venous capacitance and reduction in the venous blood return to the heart, causing a reduction in the intracardiac pressure.

Nitrates dilate large epicardial coronary arteries and collateral vessels. It should be remembered, however, in the diseased coronary artery, ischemia is the most potent stimulus to dilatation.

Table 13-1   Nitroglycerin and Nitrate Preparations

Nitroglycerin

Sublingual	Tablets 0.3–0.6 mg
	Spray 0.4–0.8 mg/inhalation
Oral	2.5–6.5 mg orally bid-tid
Transmucosal	1 mg tid
Topical	Ointment ½–2 inches q4–6h
	Patch 5–10 mg daily
Intravenous	5 μg/min with titration as required

Long-acting nitrates

Isosorbide dinitrate	
Sublingual	5–10 mg q3h
Oral	5–30 mg q6h
Erythrityl tetranitrate	
Oral/sublingual	5–15 mg q6h
Pentaerythritol tetranitrate	
Oral	10–20 mg q6h

Nitrates are useful for the acute or chronic management of myocardial ischemia and congestive heart failure. Oral nitrates may require higher doses to achieve effect, as compared to sublingual or topical forms, due to first-pass hepatic metabolism (Table 13-1).

Attenuation may occur with all continuous nitrates. The response of the vasculature to nitrates diminishes but is not related to drug level. Today when nitrates are prescribed, a nitrate-free interval is programmed into the regimen. Since most episodes of myocardial infarction (MI), sudden cardiac death, and also some cerebrovascular accidents, occur between the hours of 6 AM and noon, it is important to have maximal protection during the early morning and waking hours.

β-Blockers

β-Adrenergic blocking drugs have a variety of actions. They have a negative chronotropic effect (slow heart rate), a negative dromotropic effect (slow conduction at AV node), and a negative inotropic effect (decreased contractility). In addition, they have a direct antiarrhythmic effect and increase ventricular fibrillation threshold (the latter may not be seen in those with partial agonist activity).

Several key pharamacologic properties distinguish the

Table 13-2 β-Blockers

Intravenous*	
Propranolol	1-mg incremental doses
Metoprolol†	1–5-mg incremental doses
Esmolol†	Loading 500 μg/kg/min then 50 μg/kg/min × 4 min then titrate
Labetalol	0.25 mg/kg (usually 20 mg)
Atenolol†	5-mg incremental doses
Oral	
Short-half life	
Acebutolol‡ (3–4 h)	200 mg bid
Metoprolol† (3–4 h)	50–100 mg bid
Labetalol (3–4 h)	100 mg bid
Pindolol‡ (3–4 h)	5 mg bid
Propranolol (3–4 h)	10–40 mg q6h
Intermediate half-life	
Timolol (4–5 h)	10 mg bid
Carteolol‡ (6 h)	2.5–10 mg od
Atenolol† (6–9 h)	50 mg daily
Penbutolol‡ (5 h)	20 mg daily
Sotalol (8–10 h)**	80 mg q12h
Long half-life	
Nadolol (14–24 h)	20–80 mg daily
Betaxolol† (14–22 h)	10–40 mg daily

*Adjust dosage as per physiologic requirement.
†Cardioselective
‡Intrinsic sympathomimetic activity
**Not yet FDA approved

various β-blockers including half-life, the ability to be cardio-selective (more effect on the β_1-receptor of the heart), to be water or lipid soluble, and to have intrinsic sympathomimetic (partial agonist) activity.

Therapeutic uses include angina, hypertension, MI, atrial and ventricular arrhythmias, migraine, hypertrophic cardiomyopathy, or pheochromocytoma, although not every β-blocker is approved for each indication. Table 13-2 lists the available preparations.

Calcium antagonists

These drugs act by inhibiting the entry of calcium into cardiac and vascular smooth muscle through voltage-dependent cal-

Table 13-3	Calcium Antagonists

Nifedipine (Vasodilator, no effect on conduction, no net negative inotropic effect)

Nifedipine 10–30 mg po q6–8h

Long-acting nifedipine (gastrointestinal transport system) 30–90 mg po od

Nicardipine (Vasodilator, no effect on conduction, no net negative inotropic effect)

Nicardipine 20–40 mg po tid

Verapamil (Vasodilator, negative dromotrope, negative inotrope)

Verapamil intravenous (for PSVT) 5–10 mg (0.075–0.150 mg/kg body weight) IV given over at least 2 min

Verapamil oral 80–120 mg po q8h

Long-acting verapamil 240 mg daily

Diltiazem (*Mild* vasodilator, negative dromotrope, negative inotrope)

Diltiazem 30–120 mg po q8h

Long-acting diltiazem 60–120 mg bid

Bepridil (Antianginal agent with type 1 antiarrhythmic activity but little antihypertensive properties)

Bepridil 200 mg od

Isradipine (Vasodilator, no effect on conduction, no net negative inotropic effect)

Isradipine 2.5–5 mg bid

Comments

Nifedipine, Verapamil, and Diltiazem have been available for several years. Nicardipine was released last year. Bepridil and Isradipine have just been released as this text is in press so that it is too early to comment on their place in therapy.

---

cium channels. The drugs have three major properties. First, they are vasodilators of both the coronary and systemic resistance vessels. Most currently available agents have this property, and this explains their utility for angina and hypertension. In addition, calcium channel blockers are the drugs of choice for coronary spasm.

The second property is a negative dromotropic effect on calcium-dependent pacemaker cells, particularly the AV node. Only diltiazem and verapamil have this activity; the dihydropyridine types (nifedipine, nicardipine) do not. Intravenous verapamil was the drug of choice for terminating paroxysmal supraventricular tachycardia (PSVT) due to AV nodal reentry but now has been superceded by adenosine.

The third property is a negative inotropic effect, being most profound with verapamil and diltiazem. The dihydropyridine drugs have no net negative inotropic effect (except perhaps in the end-stage heart or in isolated muscle preparations) due to their potent vasodilator activity.

The available drugs are listed in Table 13-3.

Vasopressors

Vasopressors are drugs that elevate blood pressure and support the circulation. Occasionally they are used in combination with vasodilators to optimize the hemodynamics of a patient in heart failure or after open heart surgery. One must be cautious in the use of vasopressors, because excessive stimulation potentially exacerbates the imbalance between myocardial supply and demand, thereby causing ischemia. In settings of acute decompensation, the necessity for three individual vasopressors used simultaneously usually indicates an extremely unfavorable prognosis.

Epinephrine: Epinephrine (Table 13-4), a stimulator of both the α- and β-adrenergic receptors, is a standard drug during cardiopulmonary resuscitation (CPR). In fact, CPR probably represents the most commonly used indication for epinephrine. Epinephrine improves cardiac contractility, increases the perfusion pressure, stimulates cardiac activity, and may facilitate defibrillation by coarsening fine ventricular fibrillation. During CPR, it is essential to administer epinephrine every 5 minutes until the circulation is restored, with a dose of 0.5–1.0 mg (5–10 mL of a 1:10,000 solution). Usually it is administered intravenously but can also be given endotracheally if no venous access is available.

Epinephrine is not necessarily considered the drug of first choice by the cardiologist for the patient with hypotension, because of the potential detrimental effects of intense cardiac β-receptor stimulation. Nevertheless, some cardiac surgeons or anesthesiologists may have a lower threshold for considering epinephrine infusions particularly in the peri- or postoperative period, because they consider it more physiologic under those circumstances.

When epinephrine infusion is used, 1.0 mg epinephrine is mixed in 250 mL of D_5W and the tritration started at 1 μg/mL. The infusion is continued as long as necessary with tapering as soon as possible.

Norepinephrine: Norepinephrine (Table 13-5) is a potent vaso-constrictor. Pharmacologically it stimulates both α- and

---

TABLE 13-4   Epinephrine

Type Endogenous cathecholamine
   α- and β-adrenergic receptor stimulator

Actions
1. Relaxes bronchial smooth muscle (β_2)
2. Constricts bronchial arterioles (α)
3. Positive chronotropic effect (β_1)
4. Positive inotropic effect (β_1)
5. Peripheral vasoconstriction (α)
6. Dilates arterioles of skeletal muscle (β_1)
7. Reduces renal blood flow

Indications
1. Bronchospasm
2. Anaphylaxis
3. Prolong action of infiltration anesthetics
4. Restore rhythm in cardiac arrest

Dose
1. Supplied as 1 mg in mL (1:1000)
2. For anaphylaxis or bronchospasm 0.2-1.0 mg SQ
3. For cardiac arrest 0.5 mg in 10 mL normal saline IV or intracardiac

Major contraindications
1. Narrow angle glaucoma
2. Shock
3. General anesthesia with halogenated hydrocarbons or
   cyclopropane and in individuals with organic brain damage
4. In cardiac dilatation and coronary insufficiency

Special precautions
1. Incompatible with 5% saline

Adverse reactions
1. Profound vasoconstriction
2. Arrhythmias

Comments
   The authors are aware that epinephrine is occasionally administered as a positive inotropic agent by constant infusion in some patients after cardiac surgery though this indication may not be approved.

β-receptors. Norepinephrine is commonly used to support the circulation when the patient is hypotensive for a variety of reasons, and is particularly effective if the peripheral vascular resistance is low. Several dangers exist because of its potent vasoconstrictive effects. If extravasated into the tissues, it may result in local ischemic necrosis and sloughing. Internally, it may compromise renal and mesenteric circulation.

Table 13-5   Norepinephrine (Levarterenol)

Type Powerful endogenous catecholamine
      α- and β-adrenergic receptor stimulator

Actions
    Increases systemic blood pressure and coronary artery blood flow

Indications
    1. Restoration of blood pressure
    2. Adjunct to treatment of cardiac arrest and profound hypotension

Dose
    1. Add 4 mL norepinephrine to 1000 mL D_5W (4 $\mu g/mL$)
    2. Adjust dose as necessary from 2–4 $\mu g/min$

Contraindications
    1. Hypovolemia
    2. Mesenteric or peripheral vascular thrombosis
    3. Cyclopropane plus halothane anesthesia due to risk of inducing ventricular tachycardia/fibrillation

Special precautions
    1. Infuse into a large vein to avoid risk of necrosis due to profound vasoconstriction
    2. Check for extravasation

Adverse reactions
    1. Occasional reflex bradycardia
    2. Severe hypertension
    3. Increased peripheral resistance and decreased cardiac output

Comments
    One of the drugs of choice when the patient requires immediate restoration of blood pressure

The administration of norepinephrine preferentially occurs via a central vein. Norepinephrine is placed into solution with 8 mg in 500 mL D_5W or normal saline (16 $\mu g/mL$ solution) and the dose is titrated as necessary. Due to the effects on the renal and mesenteric circulation, drugs such as dopamine may be preferable unless high doses of dopamine are also necessary.

Isoproterenol: Isoproterenol (Table 13-6) is a synthetic sympathomimetic amine similar in structure to epinephrine, but its effects are almost exclusively limited to β-adrenergic receptors. Its actions center on the heart as well as the smooth muscle of the bronchi, alimentary tract, and skeletal muscle vasculature. The effect on the heart includes an increase in contractility and heart rate. Systemic and pulmonary vascular

291

Table 13-6   Isoproterenol

Type Synthetic sympathomimetic amine
(Almost exclusively) β-receptor stimulant

Actions

1. Stimulates heart, relaxes smooth muscle of bronchi, skeletal muscle, and alimentary tract
2. Positive inotrope and positive chronotrope
3. Increases venous return by decreasing venous compliance
4. Decreases systemic and pulmonary vascular resistance
5. Increases coronary and renal blood flows

Indications

1. Heart block and Adams-Stokes attack before definitive therapy (e.g., pacing)
2. Cardiac arrest (until pacemaker or cardioverter available)
3. Bronchospasm during anesthesia

Dose

1. 0.1–1.0 μg/kg/min
2. Dilute 10 mL (2 mg) in 500 mL D_5W
3. If bolus desired 1 mL (0.2 mg) in 10 mL normal saline or D_5W

Contraindications

1. Sinus tachycardia
2. Ventricular arrhythmias
3. Angina
4. Digitalis–induced arrhythmias

Special precautions

1. Start at low dose
2. Be certain patient is not hypovolemic
3. Do not administer with anesthetics such as halothane to avoid sensitivity of myocardium to sympathomimetic amine

Adverse reactions

1. Arrhythmias
2. Angina

Comments

May also be utilized in treatment of torsade de pointes

---

resistances decrease. Coronary and renal blood flows increase. Systolic blood pressure may increase, whereas diastolic blood pressure may decrease. Venous return to the heart increases as venous compliance decreases.

In a patient with pulmonary hypertension and increased afterload requiring chronotropic and inotropic support, isoproterenol may have a role, but one must be alert for angina or arrhythmias that may result.

Table 13-7   Dopamine

Type Endogenous catecholamine precursor of norepinephrine
Direct β_1-adrenergic receptor stimulator

Actions

Low dose

1. Positive inotropic agent
2. Renal and mesenteric vasodilatation
3. Effect on dopaminergic receptors

High dose

1. Positive inotropic effect
2. Renal vasoconstriction
3. Increased peripheral resistance
4. Decreased mesenteric blood flow
5. Effect on dopaminergic receptors

Indications

1. Decreased cardiac output in patients with heart failure
2. Hypotension, shock

Dose

1. Dilute
   200 mg in 250 mL = 800 μg/mL
   200 mg in 500 mL = 400 μg/mL
2. Start at 1–5 μg/kg/min. The dose will be determined by the blood pressure, the response, and the potential for adverse effects.

Contraindications Known hypersensitivity

Special precautions

1. Extravasation may cause tissue necrosis
2. Prolonged high-dose dopamine may compromise perfusion to extremities
3. Correction of hypovolemia important before prolonged dopamine therapy
4. Monoamine oxidase inhibitors prolong effects; use dopamine with caution and in low dose
5. Concomitant IV phenytoin may cause hypotension and bradycardia

Adverse reactions

1. Tachycardia
2. Ectopy
3. Angina
4. Dose related increases in heart rate, blood pressure

Comments

1. Facilitates AV conduction
2. In higher doses, α-adrenergic effects predominate
3. Monitoring pulmonary artery pressure in patients with congestive heart failure may facilitate management
4. Best infused through long IV catheter in large vein

Dopamine: Dopamine (Table 13-7) is an endogenous catecholamine precursor of norepinephrine. As a positive inotrope, it increases cardiac output. It does not decrease afterload and may cause some pulmonary artery vasoconstriction. The systolic blood pressure increases, but it has little effect on diastolic blood pressure. In low dose, renal and mesenteric blood flows increase. Urine output usually increases. At a high dose, renal and mesenteric blood flows decrease.

Dopamine remains a very useful drug in the armamentarium and is frequently used to support the circulation in patients after cardiac surgery or in those who are in congestive heart failure. The dose must be monitored carefully due to the divergence of effects on certain vascular beds at low dose and high dose.

Table 13-8   Dobutamine

Type Synthetic sympathomimetic agent
Selective β_1-agonist, (also mild β_2- and α_1-adrenergic agonist effects

Actions
1. Cardiac stimulation (positive inotropic effect)
2. Decreases peripheral vascular resistance

Indications
Increase cardiac output in patients with heart failure

Dose
1. Dilute
   250 mg in 250 mL = 1000 μg/mL
   250 mg in 500 mL = 500 μg/mL
   250 mg in 1000 mL = 250 μg/mL
2. Start at 2.5 μg/kg/min. Usual dose 2.5–10 μg/mL.

Special precautions
Incompatible with bicarbonate injections or alkaline solutions

Major adverse reactions
1. Tachycardia
2. Ectopy
3. Dose-related increases in heart rate, blood pressure

Comments
1. Does not release endogenous norepinephrine
2. Facilitates AV conduction
3. Does not affect dopaminergic receptors
4. May cause less tachycardia, decrease in diastolic blood pressure, and peripheral resistance than dopamine

---

Dobutamine: Dobutamine (Table 13-8) is a synthetic sympathomimetic amine that does not cause the release of endogenous norepinephrine (as compared to dopamine). It stimulates the cardiac β-receptors but the increases in heart rate and blood pressure are minimal. Dobutamine increases myocardial contractility but has limited effect on afterload and no effect on renal vasodilatation. There may be less potential for arrhythmia than with other agents.

Dobutamine is useful in the short-term management of patients in congestive heart failure and after cardiac surgery.

Amrinone: Amrinone (Table 13-9) is a positive inotropic agent whose activity is different from that of either digitalis or catecholamines. It operates through the inhibition of myocardial cyclic adenosine monophosphate (cAMP) activity. In addi-

---

TABLE 13-9   Amrinone

Type Inhibitor of cyclic adenosine monophosphate (cAMP) phosphodiesterase

Actions
1. Positive inotrope with vasodilator activity (not a β-adrenergic agonist) (does not inhibit sodium-potassium adenosine triphosphate activity)
2. Should increase cardiac output

Indications
Short-term management of congestive heart failure

Dose
1. Initiation of therapy with 0.75 mg/kg over 2–3 min
2. Maintenance infusion 5–10 μg/kg/min
3. Dilute in normal or half-normal saline

Contraindications
Patients with known sensitivity to amrinone or bisulfites

Special precautions
Do not dilute with dextrose (glucose) infusions prior to injection

Adverse reactions
1. Arrhythmias
2. Thrombocytopenia
3. Gastrointestinal

Comments
1. Slight enhancement of AV conduction
2. Continued use of amrinone beyond 24 h depends on its efficacy and the absence of adverse effects

---

tion to being an inotrope, it directly relaxes vascular smooth muscle, resulting in reduction of both afterload and preload.

Amrinone is not the first drug to use in the patient with hypotension or congestive heart failure. Often it is added as an additional agent after the patient is already receiving vasodilators, diuretics, digitalis, or other positive inotropes. The patient must be monitored for the occurrence of thrombocytopenia or arrhythmia.

Phenylephrine: Phenylephrine (Table 13-10) is a sympathomimetic amine occasionally used as an adjunct to anesthesia or to treat shock after volume has been replaced. At one time its vasoconstrictive properties were used to cause a vagally mediated reflex bradycardia and terminate PSVT, but now there are more optimal choices, such as the use of IV Adenosine.

Due to the concerns about coronary vasoconstriction, it is not a favorite choice of the cardiologist or cardiac surgeon.

Vasodilators

Vasodilators are useful for dilating the arterial or venous vascular beds, depending on the agent selected. Often they may be combined with a vasopressor to achieve optimal hemodynamics in a patient with congestive heart failure or in the postoperative period after cardiac surgery.

Nitroglycerin: The availability of the intravenous preparation of nitroglycerin (Table 13-11) changed the management of patients with myocardial ischemia, MI, and congestive heart failure. It is particularly invaluable after cardiac surgery and other vascular procedures.

At lower doses, venous effects predominate, but arterial effects start as the dose increases. The mechanism of action is relaxation of vascular smooth muscle. Venous pooling reduces venous return to the heart and reduces the left ventricular end-diastolic pressure. These effects are described as a reduction in *preload*. Reductions in the arterial blood pressure and the systemic vascular resistance reflect a decrease in the *afterload*.

The dose of nitroglycerin must be carefully titrated to achieve the desired therapeutic effects.

Nitroprusside: Nitroprusside (Table 13-12) is a potent vasodilator with immediate effects on reducing afterload, most likely

TABLE 13-10   Phenylephrine

Type Sympathomimetic amine

Predominant effect on alpha receptors

Effect on β_1-adrenergic receptors of heart only at high doses.

Does not stimulate β_2-receptors of the bronchi or peripheral blood vessels.

Actions

1. Constricts resistance vessels and increases total peripheral resistance, systolic and diastolic blood pressure (α)
2. Lesser effect on capacitance vessels
3. Some reduction in blood flow to vital organs, skeletal muscle, and skin
4. Some constriction of coronary and pulmonary blood vessels
5. Some reduction in renal blood flow due to constriction of renal blood vessels
6. Vagally mediated reflex bradycardia
7. Vasoconstriction lasts longer than that achieved by epinephrine or ephedrine
8. Although similar in vasoconstrictive properties to norepinephrine, it has little inotropic or chronotropic activity

Indications

1. Treatment of shock after adequate volume replacement. Probably should not be used in acute myocardial infarction
2. Certain uses as an adjunct to anesthesia. Refer to appropriate bibliography

Dose

Only the intravenous infusion rate will be mentioned with an initial rate of 0.1–0.18 mg/min and lower rates after stabilization 0.04–0.06 mg/min

Major contraindications

1. Severe hypertension
2. Acute myocardial infarction
3. Serious ventricular arrhythmias

Special precautions

1. Use with caution in the elderly, those who are hyperthyroid, or who have severe arteriosclerosis, coronary artery disease, heart block or bradycardia
2. Potentiated by MAO inhibitor

Adverse reactions

Headache, reflex bradycardia, arrhythmias, excitability

Comments

1. The reflex bradycardia may be blocked by atropine
2. In some patients who require continuous intravenous bretylium and develop hypotension, phenylephrine infusion may maintain the blood pressure

Table 13-11   Nitroglycerin

Type Vasodilator

Actions
1. Relaxes vascular smooth muscle
2. Dilates arterial, venous, and postcapillary beds
3. Reduces systolic, diastolic, and mean arterial blood pressure

Indications
1. Control of blood pressure in perioperative hypertension
2. Congestive heart failure associated with acute MI
3. Treatment of angina pectoris
4. Production of controlled hypotension

Dose
1. 50 mg in 500 mL D_5W or normal saline
2. Start at 5 μg/min and titrate upward as necessary

Contraindications
1. Hypovolemia or hypotension
2. Increased intracranial pressure
3. Constrictive pericarditis
4. Inadequate cerebral circulation

Special precautions
Use with caution in severe hepatic or renal disease

Adverse reactions
1. Headache
2. Severe hypotension

Comments
Monitoring intracardiac pressures allows optimal titration

related to arteriolar vasodilatation. The peripheral vascular resistance decreases. It also acts on the venous circulation to reduce preload. It is frequently used for improving hemodynamics in patients with congestive heart failure, although if the patient has acute MI, intravenous nitroglycerin may be the drug of choice.

Nitroprusside is often used alone or in combination with a vasopressor to optimize the hemodynamics of a patient after cardiac surgery. Careful attention to intracardiac pressures results in optimal benefit.

Hydralazine: Hydralazine is a dilator of arteriolar resistance vessels and has little effect on venous capacitance. It increases circulation in coronary, cerebral, renal, and splanchnic vascular beds. The drug may be administered by oral or parenteral means.

Table 13-12 Nitroprusside

Type Immediate-acting, IV hypotensive agent and Vasodilator

Actions
1. Immediate reduction of blood pressure in patients with hypertensive crises
2. For producing controlled hypotension

Dose
1. Dissolve 50 mg nitroprusside in 2–3 mL D_5W and dilute to 250–1000 mL D_5W
2. Average dose 0.5–10.0 $\mu g/kg/min$. Titrate as needed.

Contraindications
Known inadequate cerebral circulation

Special precautions
1. Deteriorates in light
2. Results in cyanide production

Adverse reactions
1. Profound hypotension
2. Tachycardia, bradycardia
3. Increased intracranial pressure

Comments
Rapidly metabolized to cyanide and thiocyanate through a reaction with hemoglobin

---

The oral dose starts with 10 mg every 6 hours. The parenteral dose is 20 mg intravenously or intramuscularly, but this must be carefully adjusted according to the patient's blood pressure and clinical condition.

Angiotensin-converting enzyme inhibitors

These drugs block the conversion of angiotensin I to angiotensin II and thus interfere with the eventual production of aldosterone. They are particularly useful in the patient with high renin hypertension in which high renin levels lead to high levels of angiotensin II (constrictor of vascular smooth muscle) and aldosterone (promotion of salt and water retention). These drugs also may prolong the life of bradykinin (a naturally occurring vasodilator) which is inactivated by ACE.

In addition to hypertension, they are useful for patients with congestive heart failure. By reducing afterload, they make it easier for the failing heart to maintain the circulation. Often the ACE inhibitor is combined with a diuretic. Some investigators

Table 13-13   Angiotensin-Converting Enzyme Inhibitors

Captopril
  For hypertension 12.5–25 mg po q8h
  For congestive heart failure 6.25 mg po q8h and titrate upward
Enalapril
  For hypertension or congestive heart failure
  If patient on diuretic, start at 2.5 mg po od and titrate upward
  If not, 5.0 mg po od and titrate upward
Lisinopril
  Approved for hypertension
  Start at 10 mg po od
Ramipril*
  Approved for hypertension
  Initial dose 2.5 mg then 2.5–20 mg od or bid as needed
Benazepril*
  Approved for hypertension
  Initial dose 10 mg, maintenance dose 20–40 mg od
Fosinopril*
  Approved for hypertension
  Initial dose 10 mg, maintenance dose 20–40 mg od

*Newly released

Table 13-14   Drugs Affecting Coagulation

Antiplatelet drugs
Aspirin	324 mg daily or higher dose
Dipyridamole	25–75 mg tid-qid
Sulfinpyrazone	(infrequently used)

Anticoagulants
  Heparin
  Warfarin
Thrombolytic agents
  Streptokinase
  Alteplase (tissue plasminogen activator)
  Urokinase
  Anistreplase (anisoylated plasminogen–streptokinase activator
    complex)

are evaluating the possibility that captopril administered after MI will reduce infarct expansion and reduce left ventricular size. In the Consensus study, enalapril prolonged survival in patients with heart failure. Lisinopril is the lysine analogue of enalapril.

Other ACE inhibitors are soon expected to be on the market. The currently available drugs are listed in Table 13-13. *Caution:* The dose of ACE inhibitors for congestive heart failure patients is usually lower than that used in hypertensive patients.

Cough is a common side effect. The development of proteinuria or leukopenia indicates the need for discontinuation.

Drugs affecting coagulation

Antiplatelet drugs: These preparations have been used as vasodilators to treat patients with ischemia. Aspirin has shown some benefit in patients with acute MI. Both aspirin and dipyridamole have been used in varying doses to reduce the risk of graft closure following CABG surgery and to reduce the risk of restenosis after angioplasty. The commonly used drugs are listed in Table 13-14.

Anticoagulants: Anticoagulants have been used in a variety of cardiovascular conditions using heparin intravenously for acute situations and warfarin when chronic anticoagulation is needed. When using these agents, the partial thromboplastin time, prothrombin time, platelet count, and hemoglobin/hematocrit level must be monitored.

Thrombolytic agents: These drugs have been used primarily for acute MI and to a lesser extent in patients with massive pulmonary embolism. The available agents are listed in Table 13-14. Great care must be utilized with these agents because the risk of systemic bleeding is present.

Table 13-15   Diuretics

Thiazide and similar agents
Hydrochlorthiazide
Chlorthalidone
Indapamide (also reduces peripheral resistance)
Metolazone (acts as cortical diluting sement; inhibits proximal tubular reabsorption of sodium)
Loop diuretics
Furosemide
Bumetanide
Ethacrynic acid (current use infrequent)
Diuretics that conserve potassium
Spironolactone (antagonist of aldosterone)
Triamterene (directly blocks sodium-potassium exchange in distal tubule)
Amiloride (similar mechanism to triamterene)

Some of these diuretics are used in combination to minimize the danger of hypokalemia.

Table 13-16   Other Drugs for Hypertension

A variety of drugs are available for the treatment of hypertension, some of which have already been mentioned. To be complete, we have listed other agents which act through mediation of sympathetic activity.

Methyldopa Acts as medulla to decrease sympathetic outflow

Centrally acting α_2-agonists

Clonidine

Guanabenz

Guanfacine

Peripherally acting α_2-Antagonist

Prazosin

Terazosin

Doxazosin

Sympathetic nervous system depressants

Guanethidine

Reserpine

Guanadrel

Other Direct Vasodilators

Minoxidil

Table 13-17   Antiarrhythmic Drugs (Currently available)

Type 1

1A Procainamide, quinidine, disopyramide, imipramine (tricyclic antidepressant), moricizine

1B Lidocaine, phenytoin, tocainide, mexiletine

1C Propafenone, encainide, flecainide

Type 2

β-Blockers

Type 3

Amiodarone, bretylium

Type 4

Calcium blockers (diltiazem, verapamil)

Other classes

Atropine

Adenosine

Digitalis

Diuretics

Diuretics are used in the management of hypertension, congestive heart failure, and other fluid overload states. Diuretics are no longer the drugs of first choice for the hypertensive patient but certainly may be useful in some cases either alone or in combination. Diuretics and digitalis are particularly useful in congestive heart failure.

The major concern with the use of diuretics involves the development of hypokalemia, hypomagnesemia, and hyperuricemia. A minimal effect may also be seen on serum lipids.

The available agents are listed in Table 13-15. Because the dose may vary considerably with the situation and the individual patient, average doses are not listed.

Antiarrhythmic drugs

The editor recognizes the danger of the inappropriate use of antiarrhythmic drugs (Table 13-17) and recommends consulting specific texts on the subject rather than presenting details here.

SUGGESTED READING

Ewy GA, Bresslen R. Current cardiovascular drug therapy. New York: Raven Books; 1984.

Gilman AG, Goodman LS, Roll TN, Murad F. Goodman and Gilman's the pharmacologic basis of therapeutics. 7th ed. New York: MacMillan Publishing Co; 1985.

Kirklin JW, Barratt-Boyes BG. Cardiac surgery. New York: John Wiley; 1986; 139–176.

Moreno-Cabral CE, Mitchell RS, Miller DC. Manual of postoperative management in adult cardiac surgery. Baltimore: Williams & Wilkins; 1988.

Opie LH, Chatterjee K, Gersh BJ, et al. Drugs for the heart. 2nd ed. Orlando: Grune & Stratton Inc; 1987.

Physician's desk reference. Oradell, NJ: Medical Economics Company; 1990.

Purdy RE, Boucek RJ. Handbook of cardiac drugs. Boston: Little, Brown; 1988.

Sabiston DC, Spencer FC. Surgery of the chest. 5th ed. Philadelphia: Saunders; 1990; 202–251.

Vlay SC. Manual of cardiac arrhythmias: A practical guide to clinical management. Boston: Little, Brown; 1988.

New Directions

Thomas Bilfinger, M.D.
Constantine Anagnostopoulos, M.D.

14

COST CONTAINMENT

Since 1953, when John Gibbon successfully closed an atrial septal defect using extracorporeal circulation, the short history of cardiac surgery has witnessed extraordinary developments. Cardiac surgery is largely responsible for the introduction of "high tech" into the operating room and there is no doubt that this technological development has not been just an academic exercise designed to satisfy some curious minds, given that a vast segment of the population has greatly benefited from it. As we enter the last decade of this century, it is also clear that limited monies are available for health care. A cost conscious society has begun to scrutinize cardiac surgery.

The government at all levels is exerting more and more control over the health care system. It is not easy to predict what form this control will take. In cardiac surgery the implantation of pacemakers, and now, the performance of coronary artery bypass grafting (CABG) are placed under strict Medicare/Medicaid guidelines. Third-party payers tend to follow these guidelines as well. In the near future a revised diagnosis-related group (DRG) schedule will go into effect with a drastic cut in the payment for such common procedures as CABG and valve replacements. For DRG 107 (CABG without cardiac catheterization) Medicare allots 11 days at a lump sum of $25,509; while in non-Medicare patients the State of New York allots 11 days and $17,000 including professional services. Already, cardiac surgery is one of the more closely supervised disciplines in terms of quality control, and this scrutiny will increase in the future. In certain states it is now mandatory to submit all cardiac cases and their outcomes to a state-wide quality assurance program. The inclusion of preoperative risk factors in these programs make these data more accurate. It may only be a matter of time until this policy of mandatory review will be introduced on a federal level. It has already been established that disciplines such as cardiac surgery, requiring intensive care, fare worse under the DRG system. Small institutions without cardiac surgical facilities tend to benefit if they transfer the patient after initial stabilization, while tertiary care facilities tend to lose. Such policies will soon lead to new rules and regulations for granting privileges prior to opening a new cardiac program. As alternatives so far unacceptable to the American public are models like Sweden or Great Britain, with waiting lists up to 2 years for elective CABG.

We are, therefore, in dire need of studies examining the cost effectiveness of cardiac surgery in terms of social reintegration. How many people return to work? How many people lose their jobs or become temporarily or permanently disabled? From the scarce available data we can conclude that, although medically fit, patients from a lower socioeconomic level tend to apply for disability. These are just some of the questions that are awaiting answers.

How to best apply cardiac surgery to an increasingly elderly population remains to be defined. Currently the risk is clearly related to left ventricular performance. In general terms it is therefore safer to perform an aortic valve replacement in a 90-year-old than to perform a CABG in an octogenarian. Age is a risk factor although impressive results in octogenarians have been reported. However, the question of the cost of intervention related to life prolongation is beyond the scope of cardiac surgery and requires ethical as well as philosophical answers.

In terms of education, we will need better informed and better trained surgeons. The American Board of Thoracic Surgeons is seriously considering extending the minimum requirement for board certification from 2 to 3 years in the near future. Recertification every 10 years is already mandatory. On the innovative side, increased cost control is leading to standardization of care which will continue. The future cardiac surgical intensive care unit will be marked by computer-guided monitoring equipment. Software is being developed that will allow automated integration of monitoring equipment with pharmacologic interventions. This development will be intensified by the acute shortage of nursing for which there is no forseeable end in the near future.

MYOCARDIAL AND NEUROLOGIC PROTECTION

A quiet and relatively bloodless field is a prerequisite for the optimal performance of cardiac surgery. At present, over 90% of CABG operations in this country involve cross-clamping of the ascending aorta continuously while the distal coronary anastomoses are constructed. Although alternative techniques are available, such as CABG surgery without cardiopulmonary bypass, with intermittent cross-clamping, or with the heart in fibrillation, and local control of coronary artery blood flow, they are not widely used. In more complex cardiac surgical procedures, the principles of myocardial protection are similar, but technical features and prolonged cross-clamp times make these procedures more hazardous. Despite its advantages, continuous cross-clamping of the ascending aorta during cardiac surgery is associated with some myocardial ischemia, and in a few cases, severe myocardial damage may result unless specific measures are taken to protect the myocardium during interruption of coronary blood flow. Over the past 5 years, diverse cardioplegic solutions have been proposed. The main variations in these solutions relate to ionic composition (sodium, potassium, chloride, calcium, and magnesium), osmolality (glucose and mannitol), onconicity (albumin and hydroxyethylstarch), membrane stabilizing agents (steroids and procaine), buffering capacity (tromethamine, bicarbonate, and histidine), oxygen level, hematocrit, and temperature. More recently, β-blockers, calcium channel blockers, and vasodilators (papaverine hydrochloride and nitroglycerin) have also been added to various cardioplegic "cocktails." No clinical trials have been large enough yet to allow a final judgment of a superior solution. As do most institutions in the United States, at Stony Brook we use blood cardioplegia for our adult patients. Part of the problem is that our means of assessing the effect on the myocardium of our protective agents are crude in the clinical setting and often the results are only available with a time delay. In the laboratory new methods such as bioelectrical tissue resistance have been shown to correlate well with myocardial water content and subcellular ultrastructure as sensitive indicators of early myocardial ischemia. If such methods can be introduced into clinical practice, we may finally have a tool to better assess how successful current myocardial protection is. The mainstay will remain with hypothermia. The optimum temperature of the myocardium in different disease states will be better defined; currently, the optimum is thought to be 10°–20°C. Methods to obtain this temperature will be refined. The role of blood versus crystalloid cardioplegia will be resolved as the role of blood as free oxygen radical scavanger is determined. Exactly how helpful retrograde coronary sinus administration of cardioplegic solutions is will be determined in the near future. So far, we have been treating all hearts similarly, as we have tried to achieve myocardial preservation with hypothermia and a cardioplegic solution. But there is no reason to believe that all hearts are similar. Myocardium in a heart with a congenital malformation is not necessarily the same as myocardium in adult ischemic heart disease or a hypertrophied myocardium with aortic stenosis. Already trends are becoming established, indicating that myocardial preservation may have to be adjusted to the underlying pathology. The future cardiac surgeon will have several cardioplegic solutions at his disposal as well as other techniques to maximize myocardial protection.

One major aspect that needs to be addressed in the future is the preservation of neurologic along with myocardial function. The most urgent and obvious need is for better protection of the spinal cord during aortic surgery. So far, no convincing superiority of any currently used method is apparent. Simple cross-clamping has the same incidence of paraplegia as the use of extracorporeal circulation or a heparin-bonded shunt. From experiments using somatosensory-evoked response techniques (a form of an electroencephalogram after peripheral nerve stimulation), we know that proximal spinal fluid hypertension appears to have a role in the etiology of paraplegia. Lowering the pressure could significantly prolong the tolerated ischemia time. Very little is known about the neurologic alterations caused by cardiopulmonary bypass and their long-term effects. Stimuli to our senses lead to increased myocardial performance with feedback loops to the brain. How temporary interruption of this loop is affected and if it influences the long-term results remain to be determined.

CORONARY ARTERIAL DISEASE

The past 15 years have witnessed great changes in the treatment of ischemic heart disease. The present decade should continue to show equally promising new approaches to diagnosis, management, and interventional therapy. Comparison of medical and surgical treatments for coronary artery disease is confounded by the progressively improving longevity provided by nonsurgical therapy alone, by the large crossover rates from medical to surgical treatment whenever randomization has been attempted, and by the nonstandardization of medical therapy. However, the conclusion that CABG significantly improves longevity for patients having advanced coronary disease or reduced ventricular function is gradually gaining credence. The national mortality rate for CABG is approximately 5%. Recent reports show an increase in mortality due to the fact that older patients with more multisystem disease and patients with more "unfavorable" anatomy are revascularized. The risk is closely related to left ventricular function. Ejection fractions below 25% are generally considered a prohibitive risk and only a few centers accept such patients. "Unfavorable anatomy" consists of very distal disease, where the result of revascularization is not predictable anymore. Very few patients get turned down for operation based on anatomic reasons alone. Whether a combined procedure of CABG with intraoperative angioplasty improves the results of this group of patients is a subject of ongoing studies. Prior to judging an institution based on its results, it is necessary to look at the risk factors present in the patient population of a given institution. It is no secret that university hospitals tend to attract higher risk patients than private institutions.

That some 10% to 15% of saphenous vein grafts obstruct early is distressing. The percentage increases to around 50% after the first decade. This natural history will lead to an increased number of reoperations. So far, the use of the internal mammary artery (IMA) mainly to the left anterior descending artery has shown good results in terms of intermediate and long-term patency. It is foreseeable that this method will lead to an increased use of this conduit with more complex applications such as sequential, bilateral, or free grafts. The use of bilateral grafts on a routine basis is hampered by several factors: the slightly, but well-documented, increased incidence in sternal wound infections, the limited reach of the right IMA for revascularization of the right system if one wishes to abstain from crossing the midline, and the short follow-up of free IMA grafts.

Currently, much attention is focused on the relative merits of angioplasty versus surgery. The roles of each modality will become better defined. In brief, angioplasty carries a 1% inhospital mortality rate with a restenosis rate of 12% to 48%, usually within the first 6 months. CABG carries a higher mortality rate with a considerably longer recovery period. The future of angioplasty lies in the improvement of the long-term results. Currently a general rule is that after three failed angioplasty procedures the patient should be referred for surgery. New technologies such as laser catheters have not yet clearly improved those results.

A major frontier of further progress is the emergency treatment of acute evolving myocardial infarction (MI). The role of surgery under these circumstances will become better defined. At present, it carries a substantially higher risk than elective surgery. This is mainly due to the fact that it still takes too much time to establish the diagnosis. It has recently been shown that if revascularization can be achieved within 2 hours after the onset of MI, the mortality can be kept low and the long-term results surpass those of elective revascularization after an established MI. Hence, if diagnosed late, the rule was established to wait 7-10 days after a transmural infarction prior to surgery. Emergency operations for failed angioplasties also carry a substantially higher risk with mortalities reported between 10% and 16%. The patient should therefore be informed that emergency CABG after failed angioplasty cannot be equated to an elective procedure. There is little doubt that the patients in the group with evolving MIs will be sicker, older, and much more fragile than in the past, and in turn will require more sophisticated perioperative care. Among other things, intra- and postoperative assessment of myocardial performance will become more precise with noninvasive or semi-invasive methods such as the esophageal Doppler monitoring and echocardiography. Open endarterectomy has given impressive results in studies by Johnson and Cooley; in other hands, the procedure has not led to significantly improved results. This technique appears to be highly operator dependent. Efforts to solve the problem of creating a graft without graft-worthy veins will continue. A promising solution without proven long-term results is the cryopreservation of homograft veins. After a few well-publicized cases in which the gastroepiploic artery was used, the technique has just recently been well described. It is too early to make a final judgment about the long-term patency of this artery. As a general rule, the use of artificial graft material has been disappointing. Transmyocardial tunnels have been reported.

VALVULAR HEART SURGERY

The 1970s brought a long succession of various types and models of prosthetic valves, each waxing and waning in popularity since their introduction. The currently popular valves are either tissue or mechanical valves. Tissue valves are less thrombogenic, but also less durable. A Veterans Administration cooperative study has found no difference up to 7 years between the two valve types. Although the ideal valve has not yet been found, it appears that patients with significant valvular pathology benefit greatly from surgery. New and exciting is the emergence of improved homograft valves, which show great promise, especially in the aortic position. In the mitral position the long-term results of valve repair over replacement have yet to be determined, but the outlook is promising even for the infected valve. Galloway and colleagues recently reviewed the experience with mitral valve repair and found that the incidence of valve replacement in repaired valves ranged from 3% to 16% at 5 years. Mortality and complications are very similar to valve replacement. The homograft with the present preservation techniques lends itself only poorly for replacement of a mitral valve. Methods using a fresh heterograft with vascular pedicle could overcome the current problems. We are still looking for a growing valve prosthesis for the infant with congenital valve anomalies. Rectus sheath is one readily available tissue source with properties that appear to allow growth. It is also imperative to clarify the indications for balloon valvuloplasty. The only group with consistently good results so far is the infant and pediatric group. It is conceivable that balloon valvuloplasty has a limited role at the other extreme of the age bracket, although preliminary results show only a short-term benefit.

CONGENITAL HEART SURGERY

In every other area of concern to cardiac surgery, major efforts directed at the prevention of disease are underway. Chromosomal genes for congenital heart disease are not known as they are for certain hereditary disease. Chromosomal manipulation cannot, therefore, be considered for future parents. The etiology of these diseases is generally thought to be "multifactorial" which implies that the cause is unknown and that multiple genes as well as environmental factors are involved. Two-dimensional echocardiography and gated magnetic resonance imaging in utero have made possible the assessment of cardiac anatomy in the fetus after 18 weeks of gestation. With these methods all four chambers of the heart and the position of the great vessels can be defined. Prenatal diagnosis of congenital anomalies has become a reality. Research groups are currently working on surgical correction in utero as well as transplacental catheter systems to correct certain anomalies. Meanwhile, new ethical values are becoming accepted by society.

In the near future the refinement of current concepts will progress through the efforts of cardiac surgeons, especially as these concepts apply to the difficult group of patients with only one functional ventricle. The concept of a passive conduit bypassing the right heart (Fontan physiology) can be extended to the ventricular side of the heart and, in conjunction with homograft techniques, passive conduits may become available. The recent reports of encouraging results with the arterial switch procedure for transposition of the great arteries await confirmation and refinement of the indications. New techniques such as extracorporeal membrane oxygenation will aid in gaining time pre- and postoperatively, and will, it is hoped, lead to improved results. A new category of patients will be the adolescent or young adult who has undergone surgery to correct a congenital cardiac malformation and eventually will need reevaluation because of the extended survival with many of today's procedures. Whether transplantation is the answer, and at what stage it should be implemented, remains to be defined. The current limitations hinge on our ignorance of the effects of immunosuppression in infants. Encouraging preliminary results are now being reported from Los Angeles in the field of pediatric cardiac transplantation.

ELECTROPHYSIOLOGIC SURGERY

By now, surgery for arrhythmias can no longer be regarded as experimental. The centers with experience in this field report high success rates. Even for centers without experience in arrhythmia surgery, the automatic internal cardioverter defibrillator (AICD) is now available. Several companies are developing improved smaller models with longer-lasting batteries. The new models will feature pacer capabilities. Percutaneous insertion of the electrodes and defibrillator coils will become possible. The cost of the device will substantially decrease. Currently just the hardware costs around $15,000. The AICD, together with pharmacologic agents, will restrict the need for more complex procedures such as subendocardial resection or laser ablation except as they become non-surgical.

CARDIAC REPLACEMENT

Here the progress can be discussed in terms of two main developments: the cardiac prosthesis and the cardiac transplant. The use of the cardiac prosthesis is hampered by the difficulties in material research. Blood surface interaction is still incompletely understood and all materials used to date, are considered thrombogenic. The Food and Drug Administration has toughened the already very complicated approval process which makes it almost impossible even for a well-endowed commercial sponsor to come up with a completely new project. Another important aspect is the development of a small independent energy source. Earlier plans aimed at using nuclear energy sources had to be abandoned more recently because of public pressures. The shift has therefore been toward exclusive use of electrical energy, recently applied clinically.

Cardiac assist devices can be used as bridges to transplantation and as such have had a fairly successful history. The most widely used, because of its simplicity and because of its low cost, is the Biomedicus pump, which is a modified roller pump with a simple circuit to bypass either the right or the left heart. As a final step in failing hearts, waiting until the heart recovers, the history of the assist device is less glorious. It fares best as a right ventricular bypass system. After a left ventricular bypass system, only 25% to 30% of patients leave the hospital alive and as a biventricular system, the failure rate is approximating 100%.

The clinical cardiac transplant effort was reinstituted on a much broader basis after the discovery of cyclosporine. Although the results have improved, it now is apparent that the patients are not exempt from their original disease. Atherosclerosis in the graft appears to be accelerated. In combined heart-lung transplants the rejection of the lung appears to be the rate-limiting factor. Future efforts to improve cardiac transplantation as therapy must include the implementation of new immunosuppression immunotolerant protocols, the development of methods to prevent graft atherosclerosis, and the creation of procurement systems that markedly increase the number of donor hearts available, including long-distance procurement. On a national scale additional facts have hampered the transplant effort. First, the availability of donor hearts is extremely limited. Donor sharing is a reality and often several institutions share the different organs of one person. Second, the public sector is not able and willing to pay for a cardiac transplant, contrary to a kidney transplant, so that only patients with private insurance are eligible for this modality.

FUTURE ETHICAL ISSUES

The ethical issues that surround the great developments in cardiac surgery are inescapable. The surgeon is not merely a technician, but a member of the health care team who must assume certain moral responsibilities for the well-being of patients. For instance, as we confront greater numbers of patients with HIV, we must decide the cost effectiveness and indications for cardiac surgery. Should this group of patients be mixed with other patients or should specially designated centers be created which are able to manage the manifold problems associated with HIV? Currently a big legal dispute is taking place over whether a physician is obligated to perform surgical procedures on HIV positive patients. With the improved awareness and testing of blood donors, the transmission of AIDS by blood components has become very rare. How are staff to be protected during cardiac surgery? Besides guidelines developed by the American College of Surgeons, every hospital should set up its own regulations.

The increasing number of intravenous drug users leads to more cases of endocarditis. How are we going to deal with the "repeat offender" who has an infected prosthesis? At what

313

stage is valve rereplacement no longer justifiable? Current data from around the nation suggest that the mortality rate for repeat offenders continuing their drug habit is above 60%.

Other complex ethical issues loom before us. Is there an maximum age after which we should no longer offer patients cardiac surgery? The American society, in contrast to every other society in this world, is very "operation happy." Will cost containment force us to deny certain patients the treatment they need? As we are exploring new health care systems, we will have to decide if we are willing to accept long waiting lists as in countries with national health care systems, or if health maintenance organizations should become mandatory and able to cover such relatively expensive procedures. Will lack of resources close the doors of hope for many? The obligations between the public and private sectors have to be redefined. Many questions that are not purely technical or even physiologic await answers. Cardiac surgeons must become actively involved now in the effort to resolve these moral and ethical issues.

SUGGESTED READING

Binet JP. New frontiers and new barriers. *J Thorac Cardiovasc Surg.* 1987; 94:647–655.

Crippen DW, Bonetti MM, Hoyt JW, Martin BR. Cost and survival rates of critical care regionalization for medicare patients. *Crit Care Med.* 1989; 17:601–606.

Garson A. The science and practice of pediatric cardiology in the next decade. *Am Heart J.* 1987; 114:462–468.

McGoon DC. Cardiac surgery in perspective. *Chest.* 1986; 89:737–742.

Pierce WS, Pae WE, Myers JL, Waldhausen JA. Cardiac surgery: a glimpse into the future. *J Am Coll Cardio.* 1989; 14:265–275.

Richenbacker WE, Myers JL, Waldhausen JW. Current status of cardiac surgery—a 40 year review. *J Am Coll Cardio.* 1989; 14:535–544.

Stapenhorst K. Thoracic and cardiovascular surgery—a rational and essential unity for scientific and practical clinical progress. *J Thorac Cardiovas Surg.* 1987; 35:267–269.

Index